1984

YEAR BOOK OF

**PLASTIC AND
RECONSTRUCTIVE
SURGERY®**

The YEAR BOOK of

Plastic and Reconstructive Surgery® 1984

Editor
FREDERICK J. McCOY, M.D.

Associate Editors
RAYMOND O. BRAUER, M.D.
B. W. HAYNES, JR., M.D.
ROBERT J. HOEHN, M.D.
STEPHEN H. MILLER, M.D.
LINTON A. WHITAKER, M.D.

YEAR BOOK MEDICAL PUBLISHERS, INC.
CHICAGO

The editor for this book was Jane Toomey, and the production manager was H. E. Nielsen.

THE 1984 YEAR BOOKS

The YEAR BOOK series provides in condensed form the essence of the best of the recent international medical literature. The material is selected by distinguished editors who critically review more than 500,000 journal articles each year.

Anesthesia: *Drs. Kirby, Miller, Ostheimer, Saidman, and Stoelting.*

Cancer: *Drs. Clark, Cumley, and Hickey.*

Cardiology: *Drs. Harvey, Kirkendall, Kirklin, Nadas, Resnekov, and Sonnenblick.*

Critical Care Medicine: *Drs. Rogers, Booth, Dean, Gioia, McPherson, Michael, and Traystman.*

Dentistry: *Drs. Cohen, Hendler, Johnson, Jordan, Moyers, Robinson, and Silverman.*

Dermatology: *Drs. Sober and Fitzpatrick.*

Diagnostic Radiology: *Drs. Bragg, Keats, Kieffer, Kirkpatrick, Koehler, Sorenson, and White.*

Digestive Diseases: *Drs. Greenberger and Moody.*

Drug Therapy: *Drs. Hollister and Lasagna.*

Emergency Medicine: *Dr. Wagner.*

Endocrinology: *Drs. Schwartz and Ryan.*

Family Practice: *Dr. Rakel.*

Medicine: *Drs. Rogers, Des Prez, Cline, Braunwald, Greenberger, Bondy, Epstein, and Malawista.*

Neurology and Neurosurgery: *Drs. De Jong, Sugar, and Currier.*

Nuclear Medicine: *Drs. Hoffer, Gottschalk, and Zaret.*

Obstetrics and Gynecology: *Drs. Pitkin and Zlatnik.*

Ophthalmology: *Dr. Ernest.*

Orthopedics: *Dr. Coventry.*

Otolaryngology: *Drs. Paparella and Bailey.*

Pathology and Clinical Pathology: *Dr. Brinkhous.*

Pediatrics: *Drs. Oski and Stockman.*

Plastic and Reconstructive Surgery: *Drs. McCoy, Brauer, Haynes, Hoehn, Miller, and Whitaker.*

Psychiatry and Applied Mental Health: *Drs. Freedman, Lourie, Meltzer, Nemiah, Talbott, and Weiner.*

Sports Medicine: *Drs. Krakauer, Shephard and Torg, Col. Anderson, and Mr. George.*

Surgery: *Drs. Schwartz, Najarian, Peacock, Shires, Silen, and Spencer.*

Urology: *Drs. Gillenwater and Howards.*

Table of Contents

The material covered in this volume represents literature reviewed up to July 1983.

Journals Represented

Acta Chirurgica Scandinavica
Acta Neurochirurgica
Acta Ophthalmologica
Acta Orthopaedica Scandinavica
Aesthetic Plastic Surgery
American Journal of Obstetrics and Gynecology
American Journal of Roentgenology
American Journal of Surgery
American Surgeon
Anesthesiology
Annales de Chirurgie Plastique
Annals of Emergency Medicine
Annals of Internal Medicine
Annals of Neurology
Annals of Plastic Surgery
Annals of the Royal College of Surgeons of England
Annals of Surgery
Annals of Thoracic Surgery
Archives of Internal Medicine
Archives of Otolaryngology
Archives of Surgery
British Journal of Plastic Surgery
British Journal of Surgery
Burns
Canadian Journal of Psychiatry
Cancer
Cleft Palate Journal
Diseases of the Colon and Rectum
European Surgical Research
Foot and Ankle
Head and Neck Surgery
International Orthopaedics
Johns Hopkins Medical Journal
Journal of the American Academy of Child Psychiatry
Journal of the American Medical Association
Journal of Applied Physiology: Respiratory, Environmental and Exercise
     Physiology
Journal of Bone and Joint Surgery (American vol.)
Journal of Dermatologic Surgery and Oncology
Journal of Hand Surgery
Journal of Head and Hand Pathology
Journal of Laryngology and Otology
Journal of Maxillofacial Surgery

Journal of Neurosurgery
Journal of Oral and Maxillofacial Surgery
Journal of Parenteral and Enteral Nutrition
Journal of Pediatric Ophthalmology and Strabismus
Journal of Pediatric Surgery
Journal of Surgical Research
Journal of Thoracic and Cardiovascular Surgery
Journal of Trauma
Journal of Urology
Lancet
Laryngoscope
Neurosurgery
New England Journal of Medicine
New York State Journal of Medicine
Ophthalmologica
Ophthalmology
Oral Surgery, Oral Medicine, Oral Pathology
Plastic and Reconstructive Surgery
Postgraduate Medical Journal
La Presse Médicale
Revue de Stomatologie et de Chirurgie Maxillo-faciale
Scandinavian Journal of Plastic and Reconstructive Surgery
Schweizerische Medizinische Wochenschrift
South African Medical Journal
Surgery
Surgery, Gynecology and Obstetrics
Transplantation
Western Journal of Medicine

1. Congenital Anomalies

Cleft Lip and Palate

1–1 **Six-Year Follow-Up Study of 155 Children With Cleft Lip and Palate.** Halfdan Schjelderup and G. E. Johnson (Bergen, Norway) reviewed the speech results obtained in patients with complete labiopalatal clefts (group II) and those with varying degrees of posterior median clefts of the palate (group III). Most group I patients had a cleft lip.

Group II cases are managed by orthodontic treatment in early infancy and closure of the soft palate at about age 2 years. Group III children are operated on at the same time. The Tennison method of lip repair has been used, with great care given to suturing the muscle layers in the best possible relationship to one another. The soft palate is closed by a "pushback" technique. In group II cases two flaps are raised, leaving the scar tissue in the midline, but in group III cases the entire mucoperiosteum of the hard palate is used as a single flap.

Clinical assessments were supplemented by x-ray and videotape assessment. The extent of bone formation in the alveolar cleft was estimated radiographically in 61 children with group II clefts.

Thirteen of 15 girls with class II defects had no nasality on clinical assessment and perfect closure on x-ray–video study. Thirty-one of the 46 boys had no nasality; 11 others had slight nasality; most had perfect closure. Two boys had severe nasality. Speech was perfect at follow-up in 21 of 29 girls with class III defects, and x-ray–video study showed perfect occlusion in all of them. Four others had slight nasality, and 1 had severe nasality. Retarded patients were not evaluable. Seventeen of 20 boys with class III defects had no nasal escape and perfect closure on x-ray–video assessment. One boy had slight and 1 had severe nasality. Overall, the speech results were slightly better in group III than in group II cases. Patients with slight nasal escape can benefit markedly from speech therapy. Bone formation in the alveolar cleft was found in 43 of the 58 evaluable group II patients. In 2 other cases the x-ray findings were equivocal. In 38 cases with bone formation in the cleft, a tooth had migrated into the new bone.

Five of the 45 children in group I had clefts that extended as far backward as the incisive foramen. In 4 of the 5, bone had formed in the cleft and a tooth had migrated into it.

▶ [Authors report the results of surgery and speech.—R.O.B.] ◀

(1–1) Br. J. Plast. Surg. 36:154–161, April 1983.

1–2 **The Tennison Lip Repair Revisited.** Excellent results have been obtained with the Tennison procedure for single clefts. Raymond O. Brauer and Thomas D. Cronin (Houston) have modified the procedure for use in repairing incomplete single clefts and extremely wide complete clefts. Infants aged 2 to 3 months are operated on, unless the vertical height on the normal side is 8 mm or less. The repair plan is based on the vertical height of the lip on the normal side. The repaired side is made 1 mm shorter than the noncleft side. A 1-mm offset of the incision is used just above the vermilion line. If the lip on the lateral side is too long, requiring vertical shortening, a full-thickness excision is made just below the ala during initial repair. In some wide clefts with the lip adherent to the maxilla, partial release of the lip is necessary before the repair is planned. Special attention is given to preserving the mucosa beneath the triangular flap. The nasal floor incisions should extend back into the nose as far as possible. If there is a soft tissue deficiency at the base of the columella, it may be possible to develop a small flap of skin and muscle.

The outcome in 1 case is shown in Figure 1–1. The Tennison oper-

Fig 1–1.—Operative plan in infant, aged 2 months, with complete cleft *(top)*. Same patient at age 15 years *(bottom)*. (Courtesy of Brauer, R. O., and Cronin, T. D.: Plast Reconstr. Surg. 71:633–642, May 1983.)

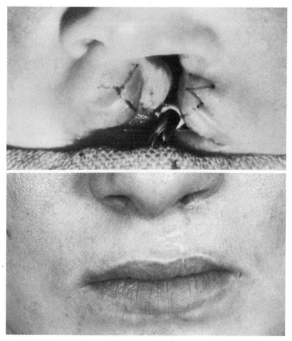

ation can be used to repair all clefts, from the most incomplete to the extremely wide complete cleft. A lip adhesion is unnecessary as a preliminary maneuver. Operation is performed with tracheal anesthesia and oral intubation to assess the deformity carefully. Patients aged 3 to 25 years have had the operation. The only lip revision has been correction of a whistle deformity in the vermilion, primarily on the normal side. Successful results have been obtained in blacks, Orientals, and Latins. Operation is no longer performed on the nasal deformity at initial repair, since lasting results are not obtained, and scars are left for later procedures.

▶ [The authors have presented one of the few long-term studies depicting a single lip repair, the longest being 25 years. This is something that has been needed for a long time.—R.O.B.] ◀

1–3 **Randomized Comparison of Triangular and Rotation-Advancement Unilateral Cleft Lip Repairs.** Barbel Holtmann and R. Chris Wray (Washington Univ.) undertook a prospective comparison of triangular and rotation-advancement repairs of unilateral cleft lip in 35 patients with complete or incomplete clefts. Sixteen triangular and 19 rotation-advancement repairs were performed between 1975 and 1978. Ten patients who had triangular repair and 6 who had rotation-advancement repair had complete clefts. Eight and 10 patients, respectively, had associated clefts of the secondary palate. Triangular muscle flaps were used in 31 patients. The two surgical groups were demographically and clinically comparable.

Postoperative complications were similar in the two groups. The preoperative nasal deformity was more marked in the triangular repair group, and the degree of improvement in nasal deformity was greater in these patients. Major secondary operations for nasal deformity were recommended for 10 triangular repair patients and 5 in the rotation-advancement repair group. Lip scar hypertrophy occurred in 9 patients who had rotation-advancement repair and in 2 who had triangular repair. In other respects the results of the two procedures were comparable.

No major differences in the early results of triangular and rotation-advancement repairs of unilateral cleft lip were found in this study. The single significant difference is probably the greater production of hypertrophic scars in patients who had rotation-advancement repair. Further follow-up is needed to assess the ultimate outcome of the nasal deformity. Both surgeons felt that the rotation-advancement repair permitted better "fine tuning" than the triangular flap technique, and that the philtral ridge was better simulated in the former procedure.

▶ [It is difficult to see why the downward rotational maneuver should result in the greater production of hypertrophic scars. The triangular flap is clearly indicated in the very wide clefts.—R.O.B.] ◀

(1–3) Plast. Reconstr. Surg. 71:172–178, February 1983.

1–4 **Cheiloplasty Employing Modified R. Millard and V. Veau Techniques.** Ch. F. Cazabatt (Concepción, Chile) observes that children with a large labiopalatine cleft often have difficult surgical, orthopedic, and esthetic problems. Forty-five such children seen between 1976 and 1982 were managed by a team consisting of a maxillofacial surgeon, an orthopedist, and a dentist. Use of elements of the Millard and Veau approaches led to improved immediate and later results, compared with methods involving closure of the cleft in several stages.

1–5 **Importance of the Musculus Nasalis and Use of the Cleft Margin Flap in Repair of Complete Unilateral Cleft Lip.** Sadao Tajima (Keio Univ.) believes that the nasal deformity cannot be managed independently of the cleft lip, and that both should be reconstructed in a dynamic manner. The skin marking of the lip itself is as in the rotation-advancement method, with a small triangular flap. On the noncleft side the rotation cut from the mucocutaneous junction up to the middle of the columella base is just medial to the estimated philtral ridge, and the cleft margin is hinged down over to the cleft side for oral lining of the nasal floor. On the cleft side the flap is designed so that as little tissue of the "sterile triangle" as possible is included. It is usually adequate to enlarge the triangular flap up to 2 mm. The cleft margin tissue and mucosa of the labial sulcus are made into a bilobed flap pedicled on the alar base. The intranasal incision passes just inside the piriform margin to free the lateral cartilage. The nose is corrected after dissection and closure of the lip repair. After subcutaneous undermining of the lower two thirds of the nose through a reverse U incision, the nasal fascia, rather than the cartilages themselves, is sutured.

Use of a bilobed cleft margin flap on the cleft side has proved to be effective in substituting for the lining defect of the piriform margin after elevation of the alae and lateral cartilages in cleft lip repairs. Subcutaneous undermining of the nose, without exposure of the cartilages, is the preferred approach. The nose subsequently grows without apparent disturbance, although the long-term outcome remains to be established.

▶ [The authors point out that it is a mistake to use the thin, depressed tissue at the tip of the B flap in the so-called "sterile triangle" area. I have seen several patients in whom this has been done in order to lengthen the B flap. This produces an unsightly depression which is pigmented with a few hairs and almost impossible to excise. The authors use a bilobed flap to cover the raw area created by the release of the alar base, a desirable procedure. It is difficult for me to agree with their dissection of the medial crura as this rarely results in a permanent correction. It does create scar for the later surgery.—R.O.B.] ◀

1–6 **Tibial Periosteal Graft in Repair of Cleft Lip and Palate.** A. Azzolini, C. Riberti (Parma), D. Rosselli, and L. Standoli (Rome), af-

(1–4) Rev. Stomatol. Chir. Maxillofac. 84:109–115, 1983.
(1–5) J. Maxillofac. Surg. 11:64–70, April 1983.
(1–6) Ann. Plast. Surg. 9:105–112, August 1982.

ter becoming dissatisfied with Skoog's maxillary flap procedure for repair of cleft lip and palate, began using the Stricker and Chancholle method of periosteoplasty. With this approach, they have repaired 68 unilateral clefts and 36 complete bilateral clefts.

TECHNIQUE.—A perfectly hermetic nasal layer is essential to insure that the graft will take. Preoperative orthopedic treatment may be necessary to provide a sufficiently wide cleft. The lateral graft edges are inserted in a groove prepared along the borders of the fissure and are then cured with transfixing stitches. The forward extremity of the tibial graft is tipped up along the hypoplastic border of the piriform aperture so that bone production can correct the hollow under the alar base of the nose.

Experience during a 6-year period indicates that the tibial periosteal graft procedure stimulates facial growth and permits harmonious dentomaxillary development. Bone production has been satisfactory in more than 80% of cases. The bone cleft is obliterated by newly formed bone. The teeth can migrate through the bone to assume their anatomical position in the arch. Imperfect preparation of the nasal layer and rhinopharyngeal infection can prevent the graft from taking. No difficulty in tibial bone growth was noted. The leg-skin scar was generally negligible, and no osteomyelitis occurred.

This technique reconstitutes and stabilizes the maxillary arch and provides good support to the floor of the nostril and the alar base of the nose. The entire alveolar and palatal bone cleft is closed in a single stage. The tibial periosteal graft is easier to handle than Skoog's flap. The oral layer is reconstructed, while the palatal mucoperiosteum is left free of scars.

▶ [This is an excellent source of bone but the iliac crest can be used with equally good results.—R.O.B.] ◀

1–7 **Early Results of Secondary Bone Grafts in 106 Alveolar Clefts.** H. David Hall and Jeffrey C. Posnick (Vanderbilt Univ.) report the early results of secondary bone grafting in 83 consecutive patients with 106 alveolar clefts who underwent unilateral or bilateral cleft lip-palate operations. Iliac bone grafting was combined with closure of the oronasal fistula if present. The timing of operation was based on development of about half the cuspid root adjacent to the cleft. Maxillary advancement was deferred until development was complete; such an operation was done in only 2 of the 83 patients. Patients with segmental collapse had preliminary orthodontic therapy. Cleft repair and procurement of bone were carried out at the same time. The incisions used in cleft repair are shown in Figure 1–2. The labial flap was replaced after bone was packed into the cleft.

Mean age at operation was about 12 years. Wound healing was good in nearly all cases. Only two cleft sites failed completely. The bone grafts were rapidly reorganized and were indistinguishable from alveolar bone within 4 months. Two patients had loss of the graft and

(1–7) J. Oral Maxillofac. Surg. 41:289–294, May 1983.

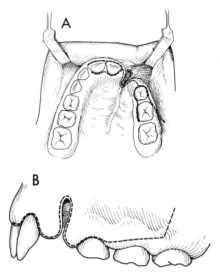

Fig 1–2.—Gingival and mucosal incisions on palatal (**A**) and labial (**B**) surfaces. (Courtesy of Hall, H. D., and Posnick, J. C.: J. Oral Maxillofac. Surg. 41:289–294, May 1983.)

recurrence of the oronasal fistula. About one fourth of the other patients had superficial dehiscence of the wound at the crest of the ridge. Morbidity was infrequent. Mean hospitalization was about 4 days both for patients with unilateral and those with bilateral involvement. Hip wounds were much less painful in the younger patients. All patients were able to return to their usual activities after about 8 to 10 days.

Secondary bone grafting of alveolar clefts was 98% successful in this series and was associated with infrequent morbidity. Preadolescent patients have had no significant complications, and operation would seem to be best done at a younger age. The authors suggest that bone grafting be done at age 12 years or earlier. Complications also can be reduced by moving the malposed central incisor into a more normal position by preoperative orthodontic treatment.

▶ [Not all patients require bone grafting of the cleft. For those who do, no established age has yet been suggested. The authors have made a contribution in this direction by demonstrating good results when the grafting is done at 12 years of age. The key to any grafting procedure is to be sure that the maxillary segments are not in any lingual crossbite and are properly related to the mandible.

The following article is a report on early bone grafting at 4 to 5 months using split rib grafts. Their results vary significantly from those previously reported in the literature. The patients showed good occlusion without any adverse effect on facial growth—R.O.B.] ◀

1–8 **Case for Early Bone Grafting in Cleft Lip and Cleft Palate.** The efficacy of early maxillary orthopedic procedures and primary osteoplasty in newborn infants with complete clefts is unclear, but the severity of orthodontic problems in patients with total clefts treated

(1–8) Plast. Reconstr. Surg. 70:297–309, September 1982.

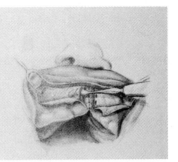

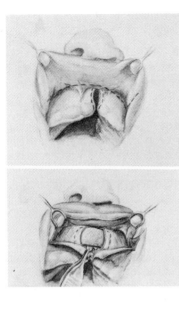

Fig 1–3.—*Above left,* incisions for insertion of alveolar bone graft in buccal sulcus and along margins of cleft. *Above,* flaps at margins of cleft turned back to form posterior wall of repair. Subperiosteal pocket dissected over premaxilla and lesser maxillary segment. *Left,* split-rib strut inserted across gap and bone chips for reinforcement inserted behind strut. (Courtesy of Rosenstein, S. W., et al.: Plast. Reconstr. Surg. 70:297–309, September 1982.)

conventionally is a cause of concern. Sheldon W. Rosenstein, Clarence W. Monroe, Desmond A. Kernahan, Bailey N. Jacobson, B. Herold Griffith, and Bruce S. Bauer (Children's Meml. Hosp., Chicago) have performed primary osteoplasty after insertion of an appliance within a few days of birth and repair of the lip at about age 6 weeks. Grafting is performed when good arch alignment is obtained, generally at age 4 to 5 months. Split-rib material is placed in the buccal sulcus and along the cleft margins as shown in Figure 1–3. No vomerine flaps are used, and the prevomerine suture is avoided. Palatal repair is done at about age 1 year; both the hard and the soft palates are closed at one sitting. Most patients have required only one prosthesis.

Data on 16 patients with a mean age of nearly 14 years were reviewed. All had complete unilateral clefts of the lip, alveolus, and palate. The SNA and SNB measurements were considerably below standard, as they were in a comparable sample of patients who did not have primary bone grafting. Anterior face height was not markedly abnormal in either sample. The ratio of maxillary to mandibular body length was considerably less than standard. The NAP, a hard tissue assessment of facial convexity, was minimally smaller in the grafted than in the ungrafted sample. The vertical ratios of upper face height to lower face height were similar in the two patient samples. The maxillary to mandibular ratios (expressed as percentage) were about the same. Seven study patients have completed orthodontic therapy and are in retention. Teeth have erupted in, around, and through previously cleft areas in a functional manner.

Primary osteoplasty has resulted in better maxillary segment alignment and better occlusion than if it had not been done in cleft cases, without adversely affecting facial growth. This approach should not be condemned because of individual failures.

1–9 **Rule of Thumb Criteria For Tongue-Lip Adhesion in Pierre Robin Anomalad.** Traditional operative criteria in Pierre Robin syndrome include an inability to breathe easily while resting or sleeping, periods of cyanosis secondary to respiratory obstruction, pneumonia, and failure to gain weight. These indications require considerable judgment in deciding when to abandon nonoperative care. Robert W. Parsons and David J. Smith reviewed 38 consecutive cases of infants admitted with Pierre Robin anomalad, all but 2 in 1968–1978; 30 in the past 5 years. All had micrognathia, glossoptosis, respiratory obstruction, and cleft palate. Three patients had hypertrophic pyloric stenosis, and 2 had pulmonary hypertension. No patient died.

Nineteen patients were referred with respiratory distress, and 19 primarily for feeding problems and failure to thrive. Six patients required surgery. Four had tongue-lip adhesions, 2 by the modified Routledge procedure, and 2 had tracheostomies performed for questionable indications. Seven other patients were admitted after 3 days of life and were discharged by the 14th day after showing a progressive gain in strength and an ability to control the tongue. These patients usually did not require gavage feedings, and were eating normally when discharged. No apnea or compromise in feeding was observed after a week in the hospital. Six other patients who were not operated on required long hospitalizations and had protracted morbidity. Four infants in all had endotracheal intubation. Two of them were seen with a tube in place and were extubated within 24 hours without difficulty. The other 2 infants had the tube replaced by a tongue lip adhesion, performed with an ensured airway.

Patients with Pierre Robin syndrome who gain weight and strength progressively and can control the tongue do not seem to require surgery. Surgery is indicated if a progressive gain in weight and ability to control the tongue in 7 days are not evident, or in any infant who requires endotracheal intubation for longer than 3 days. Using these indications, none of the infants in this review who did well in the long-term would have had surgery unnecessarily, and only one patient who probably would have benefited from surgery would not have been operated on.

1–10 **Reconstruction of the Nasal Orifice and Nasal Vestibule in Proboscis Lateralis** is described by G. Cotin, M. Bodard, B. Bouchenak, and N. Garabedian (Paris). Opening up of the inferior extremity of the lateronasal mucocutaneous cylinder into a funnel in a case

(1–9) Plast. Reconstr. Surg. 70:210–212, August 1982.
(1–10) Ann. Chir. Plast. 27:144–146, 1982.

of proboscis lateralis permitted it to be correctly inserted, and facilitated reconstruction of the nasal orifice.

A lozenge-shaped skin flap was traced on the atrophied surface, and its inferior pedicle was used to repair the nasal vestibule. Creation of a bony orifice provided ready communication between the single nasal fossa and the exterior. The cylinder was opened, a triangle of excess skin was resected, and the mucosa was retained and sutured to the edges of the incision. Subsequent retraction was prevented by cutting the endonasal mucosa, which was approached through the bony orifice, into two flaps, and turning these flaps outwards to provide a nasal vestibule with no raw areas.

Sectioning of the superior pedicle, opening out of the cylinder, and harmonization of the whole are planned as a second stage in conjunction with management of the associated facial malformations.

1–11 **Reliability of the Nasopharyngeal Fiberscope (NPF) for Assessing Velopharyngeal Function.** Endoscopy is an attractive approach to assessing the velopharyngeal mechanism. It is a generally noninvasive technique; information in the transverse plane can be obtained and extended observation is possible. Both speech and nonspeech activities can be observed, and the findings can be recorded photographically. Kaoru Ibuki, Michael P. Karnell, and Hughlett L. Morris (Univ. of Iowa) obtained simultaneous side-view nasopharyngeal fiberscopic and lateral cinefluoroscopic recordings from two normal subjects in order to determine the stability of NPF placement and the reliability and validity of the findings. The subjects, a man aged 50 years and a woman aged 24, were examined while performing inspiration and soft blowing and pronouncing six sustained phonemes.

The NPF was highly stable during the performance of several velopharyngeal activities. The tip of the NPF maintained relatively constant relationships within the vertebral complex. For most measures close agreement was obtained between two sets of measurements made by different investigators. Good agreement also was obtained between data obtained on different occasions. Measurements of fiberscopic velar motion along the pseudomidline and at the greatest velar displacement correlated closely with corresponding cinefluoroscopic measures of velar movement, distance between the tip of the NPF and soft palate, and velar displacement parallel to the long axis of the fiberscope. Measurements of left lateral wall movement were found not to be reliable.

The NPF is quite stable during various velopharyngeal activities. Measurements can be made from the still photos to evaluate several aspects of velopharyngeal function. Further studies are needed to determine the reliability of the NPF in examining cleft palate patients.

(1–11) Cleft Palate J. 20:97–104, April 1983.

It also will be important to study further whether the NPF provides reliable data on lateral wall movement.

▶ [The authors present a method which lacks the added dimension provided by the study done by David, et al. in the following abstract.—L.A.W.] ◀

1–12 **Nasendoscopy: Significant Refinements of a Direct-Viewing Technique of the Velopharyngeal Sphincter.** Objective assessment of the results of surgery on the velopharyngeal sphincter requires direct viewing of the sphincter during unhindered, continuous speech. D. J. David, J. White, R. Sprod, and A. Bagnall (North Adelaide, Australia) describe the use of a refined split-screen video technique involving color nasendoscopic imaging, lateral videofluoroscopy, and synchronous speech recording with the patient awake and in a supine position. A special signal processor is used to position the color nasendoscopic image. The findings are recorded on videotape. Speech is recorded with a tie-clip microphone. The procedure requires a nasendoscopist, usually a craniofacial surgeon, and also a second medical officer to apply topical anesthesia, a speech pathologist, a television operator, a radiographer, and a nurse.

This technique permits three-dimensional assessment of sphincter function with direct viewing. A wide range of patients can be examined in this way. Greater control of the patient in the supine position and of the nasendoscope results in a less traumatic procedure and a higher rate of successful examinations. Patients with cleft deformities, craniosynostosis syndromes, and facial microsomia syndromes have been examined, and the effects of midface advancement on sphincter function were ascertained. The procedure can be used to predict which patients will benefit from pharyngoplasty, and a permanent record of velopharyngeal function is obtained.

▶ [The authors present a refined method of simultaneous visualization through the nasopharyngoscope in color and with lateral fluorography. This represents a state of the art method for evaluating the velopharyngeal mechanism.—L.A.W.] ◀

1–13 **Sleep Apnea in Mandibular Hypoplasia.** Sleep apnea is a particular concern in patients with abnormalities that make them prone to airway obstruction. Charles L. Puckett, James Pickens, and John F. Reinisch (Univ. of Missouri, Columbia) report a case of first and second branchial arch syndrome and severe obstructive sleep apnea.

Boy, 5½, who had obstructive sleep apnea, had been born with the first and second branchial arch syndrome, Klippel-Fiel syndrome, and cleft of the lip and palate. The lip was repaired at age 3 months, and the palate at age 2 years. Macrostomia and the external ear deformities were repaired about a year later. Subsequently, a progressive pathologic condition of sleep developed, and an EEG was diagnostic of sleep apnea syndrome, with evidence of early cor pulmonale. The patient slept 16–18 hours a day, typically in a sitting position at night. The problem appeared to arise from glossoptosis involving the base of the tongue and the superior glottis. The base of the tongue

(1–12) Plast. Reconstr. Surg. 70:423–430, October 1982.
(1–13) Ibid., pp. 213–216, August 1982.

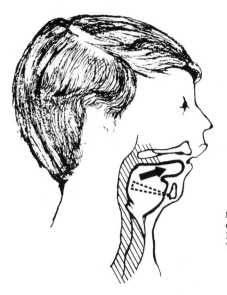

Fig 1–4.—Diagram showing position of fasciae latae sling *(broken line)* suspending base of tongue forward to mandible. (Courtesy of Puckett, C. L., et al.: Plast. Reconstr. Surg. 70:213–216, August 1982.)

was suspended anteriorly to the mandible using a strip of fascia lata (Fig 1–4). Obstructive symptoms abated postoperatively, and the patient was well 15 months after the operation. Currently, the patient rarely sleeps more than 10 hours a day, and appears to have normal physical and mental capabilities. Future surgery will be necessary to correct the micrognathia.

The earliest symptoms of this syndrome are snoring and daytime hypersomnolence. There also may be personality changes, altered consciousness during sleep such as deep levels of sleep with difficult arousal, and such findings as enuresis, hyperactivity, and somnambulism. In-hospital sleep monitoring and estimates of arterial gas can provide a definitive diagnosis. In the present case, the late development of obstructive symptoms was attributable to mandibular growth failing to keep pace with other orofacial growth, which created a relative, progressive micrognathia or retrognathia and predisposed to glossoptosis of the base of the tongue. The operation was designed to allow time to defer definitive mandibular reconstruction until growth is achieved.

▶ [Sleep apnea is a manifestation of hypoxia that may have profound importance to the patient. If sufficiently severe, it is life-threatening. More often it is subtle and requires adequate recognition and treatment, as the authors point out.—L.A.W.] ◀

1–14   **Incorporation of the W-Plasty in Repair of Macrostomia** is described by B. S. Bauer, G. H. Wilkes, and D. A. Kernahan (Children's Meml. Hosp., Chicago). Macrostomia, or transverse facial cleft, is an uncommon deformity for which a limited number of operations have been described. Macrostomia results from the failure of the mesoderm

(1–14)   Plast. Reconstr. Surg. 70:752–756, December 1982.

to completely penetrate the region of the bifurcation of the maxillary and mandibular processes. The extent of clefting can range from minimal lateral displacement of the commissure to complete division of the face. In most cases, the cleft ends medial to the anterior border of the masseter muscle. The cleft runs horizontally or obliquely upward. The goal of surgery is both functional and esthetic construction of the commissure. Repair should be done as early as possible to prevent feeding problems due to an incompetent oral sphincter. Other anomalies can be corrected later.

The site of the new commissure is best determined by inspection of the muscle and vermilion at the abnormal commissure. A small triangular flap is outlined on both lips with the base at the junction of the normal and abnormal vermilion. The incision is planned to excise abnormal tissue at the cleft margin and permit closure by a W-plasty (Fig 1–5). After excision of redundant vermilion and the skin extension into the cleft, the ends of the orbicularis oris and buccinator are dissected free, the buccal mucosa is trimmed and closed in a straight-line fashion up to the area of the commissure, and the muscle repair is performed up to the area of the new commissure. Skin closure is done using 6-0 nylon sutures, interdigitating the W-plasty flaps. The triangular mucosal flaps are trimmed as needed and turned into

Fig 1–5.—Repair of macrostomia: *(top, left)* marking of midline and site of new commissures; *(top, center)* excision of skin planned with triangular flaps at commissure and repair of skin by W-plasty; *(top, right)* straight line repair of buccal mucosa; *(bottom, left)* repair before closure of skin after repair of underlying muscle defect; *(bottom, right)* completion of repair of skin by W-plasty and commissure by inset of triangular flaps. (Courtesy of Bauer, B. S., et al.: Plast. Reconstr. Surg. 70:752–756, December 1982.)

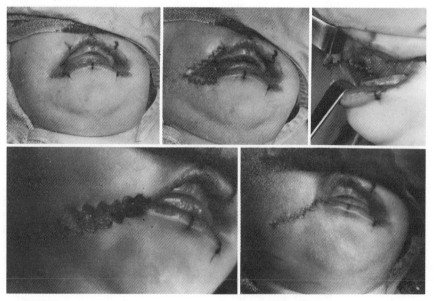

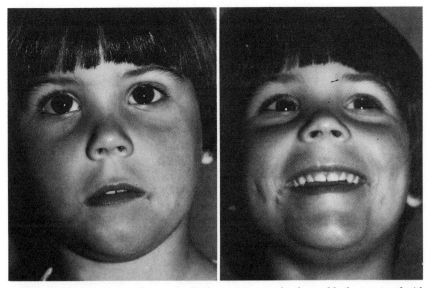

Fig 1–6.—Patient 4 years after repair. Good symmetry may be observed both at rest and with animation. No evidence of lateral creep of commissure is evident. (Courtesy of Bauer, B. S., et al.: Plast. Reconstr. Surg. 70:752–756, December 1982.)

place, with the lower flap placed more externally. The outcome in one case is shown in Figure 1–6.

This technique involves a thin mucosal repair at the commissure that closely approximates the appearance of a normal commissure, and staggered mucosal and skin scar lines to prevent lateral displacement of the commissure from contracture. The oral and buccal musculature is anatomically reconstructed.

▶ [I have never been impressed with this procedure because of the inherent danger of an overriding scar. In this instance one must question whether we are sending a boy to do a man's job, and whether a large Z-plasty would be better to use. The results presented here are excellent.—R.O.B.] ◀

1–15 **Fissural Cysts of the Maxilla and Mandible** are described by Elie Frederic Harouche (New York Univ.). Fissural cysts arise along the lines of fusion of the embryonic processes of the face, at points of junction of the developing head and neck structures. They are true epithelium-lined cysts. Nonodontogenic cysts are not rare, but they are asymptomatic and generally go unnoticed. The diagnosis is made when they are large and disfiguring, or infected and painful. The cysts are found on lines of fusion of the lateral nasal, globular, and maxillary processes. Both enclaving, or incomplete resorption of epithelial tissue, and delayed development of the growth center may explain the development of these cysts. They occur both in the midline

(1–15)   Ann. Plast. Surg. 10:224–230, March 1983.

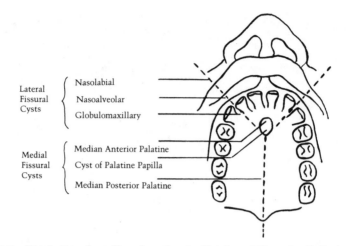

Lateral Fissural Cysts {
Nasolabial
Nasoalveolar
Globulomaxillary
}

Medial Fissural Cysts {
Median Anterior Palatine
Cyst of Palatine Papilla
Median Posterior Palatine
}

Fig 1–7.—Distribution of maxillary fissural cysts. (Courtesy of Harouche, E. F.: Ann. Plast. Surg. 10:224–230, March 1983.)

and laterally, at the junction of various facial processes (Fig 1–7). Growth of cysts later in life probably is induced by mechanical or infectious factors.

The lateral maxillary fissural cysts include nasolabial cysts, which are considered uncommon, and arise at the junction of the globular part of the medial nasal process and the maxillary process. Patients in the fourth to sixth decade of life generally are seen for a facial deformity or dental problem. There may be bony erosion of the nasal floor. These cysts are prone to infection. Globulomaxillary cysts are bony cysts of the maxilla developing at the junction of the globular part of the medial nasal process and the maxillary process, usually between the lateral incisor and canine. Medial lesions include the na-sopalatine cysts, the most common fissural cysts. These include both incisive canal cysts and those of the papilla palatina. Median palatine cysts probably are formed from epithelial remnants in the median palatine fissure of the maxilla. They usually are asymptomatic and present in later life, typically during dental examination. Mandibular fissural cysts are very rare. They arise in the mandibular symphysis, and are asymptomatic unless infected. A distinction from odontogenic jaw cysts is important.

Fissural cysts of the jaws are managed by eliminating infection, if present, followed by surgical excision or marsupialization combined with thorough curettage when appropriate. Aspiration is avoided. Excision is not warranted in asymptomatic dentulous patients with median anterior maxillary cysts, because malignant transformation has not been reported. Surgery is warranted in edentulous patients who require a prosthetic appliance. The prognosis after appropriate management is excellent.

HAND

1–16 **Management of Pouce Floutant.** The pouce floutant, or function-less underdeveloped thumb, may be associated with a hypoplastic radius. When small, it may be removed shortly after birth, but when large it may be lengthened and motored to provide a functional thumb. Ronald M. Match (Glen Cove, N.Y.) describes the management of 7 children with pouce floutant.

Patient, 1 year, had congenital bilateral hypoplastic thumbs (Fig 1–8) and cleft palate and lip. A first-stage lengthening of the larger pouce floutant on the right was carried out by interposing the proximal phalanx of the left fifth toe between the remnant of the first metacarpal and the proximal phalanx. A second-stage lengthening, done 11 months later, involved placement of the proximal phalanx of the right fifth toe into an osteotomy of the first metacarpal. At age 5, after cleft palate surgery, a third stage was done using the proximal phalanx of the left fourth toe. A year later the thumb was motored by an opponensplasty tendon transfer of the abductor digiti quinti. A residual anomalous abductor pollicis longus helped extend the thumb. Because of the smaller size of the left pouce floutant and a scissoring pattern of the left index and long fingers, pollicization of the left index finger was carried out. The skin flap from the fileted pouce floutant was used as an extra flap during the index pollicization.

Three of the seven hands had very small floating thumbs that were removed shortly after birth. Index pollicization later was done in these hands, and all had good function at follow-up, although a small neuroma remained in each case. Toe bones were used as grafts to interosteotomy sites in the four thumbs that were lengthened, or between the hypoplastic bones. Tendons later were transferred to provide adequate motion to the lengthened thumb. The abductor digiti quinti or a flexor sublimis tendon was used as a thumb abductor. Extension can be produced by an extensor indicis proprius transfer, although this was not necessary in the present patients. All children were very pleased with the functional and cosmetic results. Coordinated actions of the lengthened thumb and index finger were possible in all cases, although some children still used the index and long fingers to pick up small objects.

▶ [The result is good but one wonders if equally good function could have been achieved using alternative sources of bone graft, without sacrificing normal toes.— F.J.M.] ◀

GENITAL AND TRUNK

1–17 **Simplified Approach to Repair of Pediatric Pectus Deformities.** Conrad W. Wesselhoeft, Jr., and Frank G. DeLuca (Brown Univ.) in a 14-year period used a simplified approach to repair pectus deformities in children; the method involves insertion of a metal strut

(1–16) NY. State J. Med. 82:1749–1752, November 1982.
(1–17) Ann. Thoracic Surg. 34:640–646, December 1982.

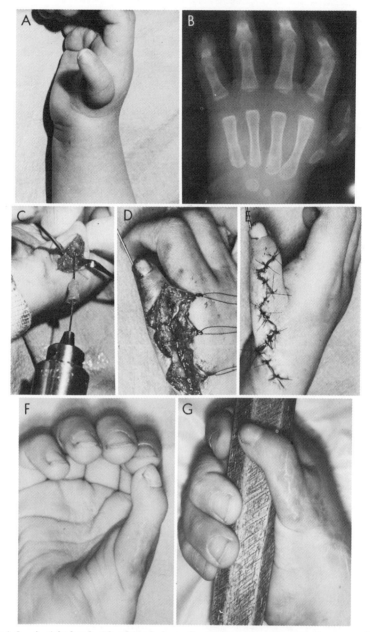

Fig 1–8.—A, right hand with relatively large, functionless pounce floutant. **B,** preoperative x-ray demonstrating hypoplastic thumb. **C,** first-stage lengthening performed by interposing the proximal phalanx of the left fifth toe between the thumb metacarpal and proximal phalanx. **D,** appearance of right thumb at third-stage lengthening; **E,** following third-stage lengthening; **F,** following abductor digiti quinti opponensplasty, opposition is possible. **G,** ability to grasp large objects is improved. (Courtesy of March, R. M.: NY State J. Med. 82:1749–1752, November 1982. Reprinted by permission of the NY State J. Med.; copyright by the Medical Society of New York.)

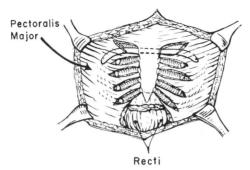

Pectoralis Major

Recti

Fig 1–9.—Strut seen in position beneath pectoral muscles. One end is placed far laterally, allowing later removal of the strut. (Courtesy of Wesselhoeft, C. W., Jr., and DeLuca, F. G.: Ann. Thorac. Surg. 34:640–646, December 1982.)

for internal fixation. Subperichondrial cartilage resection is carried out through small incisions made in the pectoral muscles, without sternal osteotomy; a malleable metal strut is passed transsternally and placed laterally beneath the pectoral muscles, with one end left easily palpable beneath the skin (Fig 1–9). The strut is removed in 4–6 months, often under local anesthesia. This procedure was carried out in 123 children; 38 of them under age 2. All operations were done chiefly for cosmetic reasons.

There were no deaths, and morbidity was minimal. In 5 children intraoperative pneumothorax developed, but only needle aspiration was required. One had postoperative atelectasis that cleared within a few days. Incisional keloid formation was fairly prominent in 5 children. Forty-eight children had the struts removed under local outpatient anesthesia. Most were left in place for 6 months. Seventy-five patients were followed for more than 5 years postoperatively; excellent cosmetic results were achieved in 70 with restoration of normal anterior chest contour, flattening of the abdomen, and a well-healed scar. Four patients had fair to good results. One patient had recurrence that warranted reoperation.

Use of this simplified technique of repairing pectus deformity in children has shortened operating time and reduced the need for extensive postoperative pulmonary physiotherapy. Excellent cosmetic results are usually obtained, and the patients' self-image improves substantially. Only 1 of the 75 children followed for 5 years or longer experienced significant recurrence. No deep infection or osteomyelitis complicated the procedure.

1–18 **One-Stage Repair of Hypospadias: Preputial Island Flap Technique.** L. Standoli (Rome) has evaluated a technique for one-stage repair of hypospadias that is designed to provide adequate esthetic and functional results without compromising normal penile de-

(1–18) Ann. Plast. Surg. 9:81–88, July 1982.

velopment and with a low rate of complications. The goals are perfect correction of the chordee, correction of meatal and distal urethral stenoses, reconstruction of a uniform, hairless urethra reaching the tip of the glans, and normal-appearing cutaneous coverage. The flap procedure is illustrated in Figures 1–10 and 1–11. A Nelaton catheter is left in place for 2–4 days after operation. Micturition is spontaneous after removal of the dressing and catheter.

The one-stage island flap method was used in 753 cases in 1975–1981. Generally, excellent results have been obtained, with good correction of the chordee, adequate neourethral function, and satisfactory final appearance. Although the first patients were operated on only 5–6 years ago, the author is optimistic about the further development of their neourethra. Forty-five patients required a second operation, usually for closure of fistulas. Two required reoperation for reconstruction of the urethra because of necrosis of the intraglandular tract after tunnelization of the glans. No reoperation has been required for stenosis at the anastomotic site; 2–4 urethral dilatations have sufficed.

Fig 1–10.—Delimitation of urethral residues of glans. Rectangular flap of required size is traced on external leaf of prepuce, with longer sides placed transversely. Incision on upper and lateral aspects is made on deeper plane, to reach cleavage plane between two preputial leaflets. Inferior incision is more superficial, just under dermal layer. Care must be taken not to damage fragile superficial vessels of dorsum of penis. (Courtesy of Standoli, L.: Ann. Plast. Surg. 9:81–88, July 1982.)

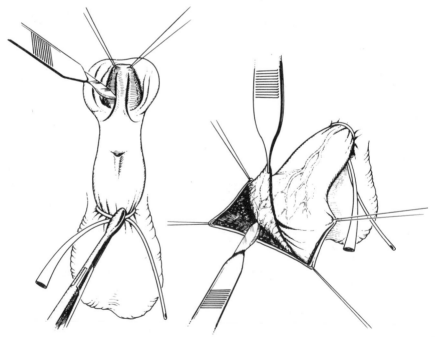

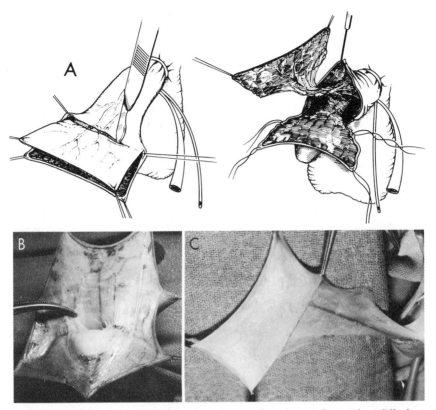

Fig 1–11.—Undermining of island flap along cleavage planes is carried out without difficulty to base of penis. (Courtesy of Standoli, L.: Ann. Plast. Surg. 9:81–88, July 1982.)

This repair should be carried out before school age, but only after sufficient dimensional development of the penis has taken place. Severe meatal stenosis in early infancy is treated by meatotomy. The one-stage island flap repair should be reserved for cases of proximal hypospadias and patients treated many times with unsuccessful results. Glandular hypospadias without meatal stricture is best managed by a modified Mathieu flap procedure. Scrotal hypospadias is repaired in two stages.

▶ [This is a nice technique to keep in mind even though it may not become routine.—R.O.B.] ◀

1–19 **Chordee Without Hypospadias in Children** is a rare anomaly in which an abnormal ventral curvature of the penis coexists with a normally positioned urethral meatus. Stephen A. Kramer, Gazi Aydin, and Panayotis P. Kelalis (Mayo Clinic and Found.) reviewed data on 20 affected boys who underwent surgical correction at a mean age of

(1–19) J. Urol. 128:559–561, September 1982.

8 years. All were followed for a year or longer after operation and 17 for 5 years or longer. Eight of the 9 children with ventral penile curvature secondary to disproportion of the corpora cavernosa underwent excision of dorsal ellipses of the tunica albuginea, and 1 had urethral division with staged urethroplasty. All 8 patients with chordee due to deficiency of the dartos fascia, or skin chordee, underwent lysis by the Allen-Spence method. Two of 3 patients with deficiency of the dartos and Buck's fasciae had urethral mobilization with excision of underlying fibrous tissue and 1 had division of the urethra with staged urethroplasty. All 3 children who also had counterclockwise penile torsion had correction by lysis of the dartos fascia.

No intraoperative complications occurred. No patient in whom the tunica albuginea was excised had a numb glans or impotence postoperatively. Both children with persistent ventral chordee subsequently underwent secondary excision of ellipses of the tunica albuginea, with good outcomes. All patients have had satisfactory cosmetic and functional results, with a straight penis and a urethral meatus positioned distally at the tip of the glans.

Most cases of chordee without hypospadias appear to be due to anomalies of the tissue layers of the penis and can be corrected without division of the urethra. All patients in this series had satisfactory cosmetic and functional results. Excision of anomalous Buck's and dartos fasciae and correction of associated penile torsion are necessary in some patients.

▶ [The overriding burden here is to decide whether the urethra should be lengthened. This cannot be decided until all the other soft tissues have been completely released.—R.O.B.] ◀

1-20 **Z-Plasty for Treatment of Disease of the Pilonidal Sinus** is described by Amir Mansoory and Diana Dickson (Wilmington, Del., Med. Center). Surgical management of pilonidal sinus disease has been dominated by the erroneous concept that epithelial ramifications with tumor-like qualities necessitate wide excision. A pilonidal sinus tends to form from the presence of a deep internatal cleft, overgrowth of local hairs directed toward the cleft, maceration, sebum formation, and friction. A negative suction effect of the cleft facilitates the subcutaneous penetration of fallen hairs. A Z-plasty can eliminate the deep internatal cleft and create a navicular-shaped groove. Local hairs are redirected away from the midline. The procedure is scheduled 5 to 6 weeks or more after incision and drainage of a pilonidal abscess.

TECHNIQUE.—The patient is placed in a semijackknife prone position with general or spinal anesthesia. The sinuses are probed gently. Where sinuses are directed caudally, the Z-plasty is combined with marsupialization of the lower part of the sinus tract. The tracts are excised with a narrow ellipse of skin and the limbs of the Z are cut to form a 30-degree angle with the long

(1–20) Surg. Gynecol. Obstet. 155:409–411, September 1982.

axis of the wound. The original wound is usually about 8 cm and the limbs are about 6 cm long. The flaps are of full-thickness skin and subcutaneous tissue. Dissection is not carried beyond the gluteal fascia. After the flaps are transposed, the tips are trimmed, subcutaneous tissue is tapered thin at the tips, and dead space is obliterated with one or two layers of synthetic absorbable sutures. The table is then flattened to remove tension from the wound edges, and the skin is closed.

This procedure results in a shallow internatal groove that replaces the deep cleft. The operation has been done in 120 patients in the past decade, including 13 with recurrences. There has been one recurrence in primary cases and one in the group of recurrences. Three wound abscesses and two hematomas occurred. There were no wound disruptions, and no flap necrosis occurred. These results represent an improvement over those of other treatments for pilonidal sinus disease.

▶ [Z-plasty will work if the excision is not so extensive that the flaps do not have to fall into a deep cavity.—R.O.B.] ◀

1–21 **Construction of a Rectal Sphincter Using the Origin of the Gluteus Maximus Muscle.** Rectal incontinence after pelvic trauma, surgery, or neurologic disorder has significant medical and social effects. Vincent R. Hentz (Stanford Univ.) reports two cases illustrating the successful use of part of the origin of the gluteus maximus to reconstruct the anal sphincter. Cadaver studies and intraoperative stimulation of the inferior gluteal nerve during closure of pressure sores indicated that the muscle strip remains vascularized and innervated when split parallel with the fascicles to a length adequate for rotation. A low-residue diet is given for several days and a Dulcolax suppository the night before operation.

TECHNIQUE.—With the patient in a jackknife position, mirror-image incisions are made over the midsacrum, descending just inferior and lateral to the ischial tuberosity and on either side of the anus just outside the mucocutaneous junction. About 4 or 5 cm of gluteus maximus is detached (Fig 1–12); as much sacral or coccygeal fascia of origin as possible is harvested. The dissection is just sufficient to permit inferior and anterior rotation to the level of the rectum. A subcutaneous tunnel is made between the incisions, and the dissected muscle fascicles are passed through, their ends being split to make

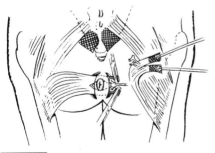

Fig 1–12.—Four to 5 cm of muscle is detached from its coccygeal origin. All available fascia and periosteum about origin are carried with muscle flap. Subcutaneous tunnel must be wide enough to avoid kinking of muscle pedicle. (Courtesy of Hentz, V. R.: Plast. Reconstr. Surg. 70:82–85, July 1982.)

two tails about 4 to 5 cm long. The two ends of one side are passed, one anteriorly and one posteriorly, around the rectum, and the dense fascial origin is sutured to itself with 2–0 absorbable sutures. The muscle from the opposite side is similarly passed and sutured to itself, and more sutures are used to fix the two muscle slings together. The muscle bundles are infiltrated with long-acting local anesthetic. The wounds are closed in layers after suction drains are placed. Broad-spectrum antibiotics are given for 5 days.

Digital stimulation of the new sphincter is begun by the patient 10 to 14 days after operation to initiate a "biofeedback" process. Extensive training, electromyography, and manometric devices have not been necessary. This procedure is thought to have wide application to patients in whom the gluteus muscles are normally innervated. The use of bilateral proximally based gluteus maximus transposition may result in excessive muscular force and difficulty in climbing stairs and walking.

▶ [If the procedure works it might be worth the price suggested by the authors, namely that the patient may have difficulty in climbing stairs and walking.—R.O.B.] ◀

1–22 **Mucosal Reduction for Correction of a Maxillary Double Lip: Report of a Case.** A double or enlarged lip appearing as a congenital or an acquired condition may require correction for esthetic reasons. A simple double lip resulting from submucosal hypertrophy is corrected by intraoral excision of musoca and submucosal tissue. Ira B. Lamster (Fairleigh Dickinson Univ.) describes a method of correcting a double lip resulting from midline hypertrophy of the maxillary mucosa.

Woman, 27, had excess maxillary labial mucosa leading to the appearance of a double lip because of folding of the mucosa on smiling. The hypertrophied mucosa was attached to a broad maxillary labial frenum, which extended coronally to the mucogingival junction at the midline. Three incisions were made, forming an isosceles triangle about the hypertrophied mucosa (Fig 1–13). The base of the triangle was created in the mucosa about 0.5 cm from the mucosal boundary of the vermilion border, and the other incisions included the hypertrophied labial mucosa. The tissue was removed by sharp dissection to a depth of 2 mm, and the borders of the wound were undermined before the arms of the triangle were approximated and sutured to the base

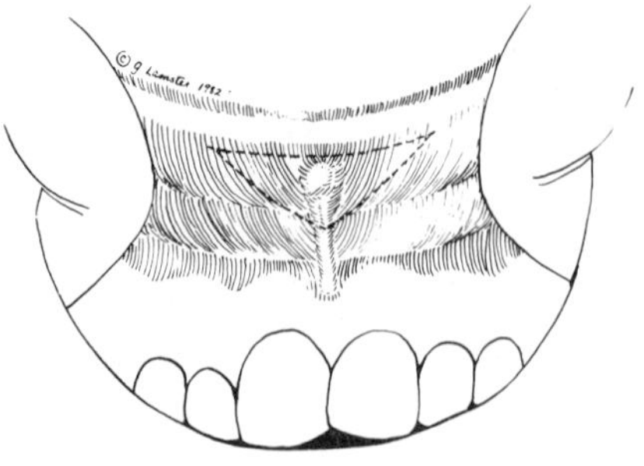

Fig 1–13.—Outline of initial incisions about hypertrophied labial mucosa. (Courtesy of Lamster, I. B.: Oral Surg. 55:457–458, May 1983.)

with 4–0 silk, resulting in a straight-line closure. The sutures were removed after 10 days. The lip was tight for a few weeks. Esthetics were improved postoperatively. Orthodontic therapy was begun about 8 weeks after the operation.

This operation effectively eliminated the maxillary double lip and improved the patient's facial appearance. The maxillary labial frenum was not resected out of concern for excess tissue excision and compromised lip form.

CRANIOFACIAL

1–23 **Longitudinal Orbital CT Projection: Versatile Image for Orbital Assessment.** Radiographic evaluation of orbital disorders has been greatly improved by computed tomography (CT). Jeffrey L. Marsh and Mohktar Gado (Washington Univ., St. Louis) found that an oblique projection, reformatted along a line connecting the orbital apex and the center of the globe, is particularly useful in assessing orbital disorders.

High-resolution axial CT scans of the face were made with the Siemens Somotom II scanner. Scans were made in the axial plane along the orbitomeatal line in 2-mm–thick contiguous slices from the alveolar process of the maxillae to and including the roofs of the orbits. Radiation exposure is equivalent to that from a standard series of skull radiographs. All additional projections are reformatted.

The longitudinal orbital projection graphically shows the relation of the inferior rectus muscle and the orbital floor. Both the degree of enophthalmos and its correction by surgery can be quantified. The size of orbital floor implants can be determined before operation from life-sized CT images in the axial, coronal, and longitudinal orbital planes, and CT may be useful in clarifying the relation between the orbital contents and the anterior cranial fossa and maxillary antrum before performing surgery. The need for orbital floor reconstruction and the magnitude of the reconstruction can be estimated. The globe position in relation to the orbital rims can be quantitated by using a life-sized longitudinal orbital projection. Three-dimensional deformities can be evaluated by multiplanar analysis at a much lower radiation exposure level than is possible with polytomography. In addition, polytome images cannot be manipulated to study bone densities or the effect of dysplasia on the orbital soft tissues.

The longitudinal orbital CT projection is of great value in assessing patients with orbital disorders, and it now is a routine part of CT study of the orbit. Direct measurements of enophthalmos and proptosis can be made before and after surgery. The projection also is useful in combination with other planes of reformation in localizing tumors.

▶ [This sophisticated study is dependent on technology that has already been superceded. In addition, it is unlikely that these methods will replace surgical judgment

---

(1–23) Plast. Reconstr. Surg. 71:308–317, March 1983.

as to what needs to be done. The greatest potential these methods seem to have appears to be in the possibility of estimating orbital volume changes with, for example, the potential for predicting how that volume must be altered in order to correct enophthalmos or exophthalmos. It may also be a study tool for detecting other volume changes.—L.A.W.] ◄

1–24 **Description of a Dry Skull With Crouzon's Syndrome.** Crouzon's syndrome is a rare congenital anomaly characterized by premature craniosynostosis, midface hypoplasia, and exophthalmos. Sven Kreiborg and Arne Björk (Copenhagen) examined a dry skull from a young adult with features of Crouzon's syndrome.

The East Indian subject (probably a female) was judged to be 18 years of age at the time of death. All the calvarial sutures were prematurely fused, and the calvarium was high, short, and pointed in the area of the anterior fontanelle. The glabella and supraorbital ridges were very prominent, but the supraorbital region of the frontal bone appeared depressed. The cranial base exhibited premature fusion of all sutures and of the sphenopetrosal and petro-occipital synchondroses. The anterior and middle cranial fossae were shorter than normal. The optic foramina were compressed vertically, and most sutures in the bony orbit were prematurely fused. The orbital cavities were short, and their axes were deviated laterally; the interorbital distance was increased. Nearly all the maxillary sutures were fused, and the maxilla was short and narrow. The mandible was not markedly malformed. Mandibular overjet and bilateral crossbite were evident.

Extensive synostosis of all calvarial sutures was confirmed in this case of Crouzon's syndrome. The biochemical defect in this syndrome apparently influences both sutures and fibrous cartilage. Involvement of fibrous cartilage may be one of the factors distinguishing complex forms of craniosynostosis from simple forms. Lateral deviation of the orbital axes in Crouzon's syndrome appears to be related to decreased forward growth in the sphenotemporal sutures and perhaps in the sphenozygomatic sutures. Maxillary involvement was moderate in this specimen, but most maxillary sutures showed some degree of synostosis. The malocclusion in the sagittal and transverse planes could be related to the basal disharmony between the jaws.

▶ [This thorough evaluation adds further insight into the etiopathology of the craniosynostosis. In particular, the authors' observation that both sutures and fibrous cartilage are involved in the process confirms previous observations that cranial-based abnormalities are intrinsic to the deformity. Their observations about facial suture synostosis are also relevant and important.—L.A.W.] ◄

1–25 **Morphogenetic Classification of Craniofacial Malformations.** Craniofacial malformations have been difficult to classify because of their many variations. Tessier's system has been widely accepted, but it is a descriptive clinical classification not related to the embryology

(1–24) Scand. J. Plast. Reconstr. Surg. 16:245–253, 1982.
(1–25) Plast. Reconstr. Surg. 71:560–572, April 1983.

of the malformations and does not really enhance understanding of the underlying pathology. J. C. van der Meulen, R. Mazzola, C. Vermey-Keers, M. Stricker, and B. Raphael present a new classification based on embryologic studies and on observations of a large number of patients. A distinction is made between cerebral craniofacial and craniofacial malformations. Craniofacial malformations can be characterized by dysostosis and by synostosis. Dysostosis may be produced by transformation as well as differentiation defects, but synostosis is always caused by a differentiation defect. Both the site of malformation and the time of developmental arrest are specified in the new classification system.

The cerebral craniofacial dysplasias include interophthalmic dysplasia, involving agenesis or underdevelopment of the midline structures of the face and brain, and ophthalmic dysplasia, which may be combined with many of the other dysplasias. The craniofacial dysplasias or dysostoses include sphenofrontal, frontal, frontofrontal, and frontonasoethmoidal. Internasal dysplasia also is known as bifid nose or median cleft nose. The forms of nasal dysplasia include aplasia, aplasia with proboscis, nasoschizis, and nasal duplication. Nasomaxillary dysplasias are encountered laterally and medially. Maxillary dysplasias include the medial and lateral oro-ocular clefts. Other dysplasias involve the maxillozygomatic, zygomatic, zygofrontal, zygotemporal, temporoaural, zygotemporoauromandibular, temporoauromandibular, maxillomandibular, and mandibular regions. An intermandibular dysplasia also is recognized.

Craniofacial malformations with synostosis can be purely cranial or facial, or of a craniofacial nature. The relation between dysostosis and synostosis and the role of each in the production of malformations will have to be specified before an accurate classification of malformations with synostosis will be possible.

▶ [This is a thoughtful approach to the continuing efforts to create order out of the myriad of craniofacial abnormalities. Unfortunately, many of the solutions become those of semantics, and I am not certain that the authors have further clarified the problem. For example, the distinctions made between cerebral craniofacial and craniofacial malformations, and between dysostosis and synostosis, are not always as clear in the patient as one would like.—L.A.W.] ◀

1-26 **Intracranial Pressure in Craniostenosis.** Dominique Renier, Christian Sainte-Rose, Daniel Marchac, and Jean-François Hirsch (Necker Hosp. for Sick Children, Paris) monitored intracranial pressure (ICP) for longer than 12 hours in 92 children with craniosynostosis. An epidural sensor was used. Both preoperative and postoperative recordings were available for 23 of the 58 patients who had an operation. Postoperative recordings were made 15 days and 3 to 6 months after surgery. Seventeen children were studied several years after surgery for craniosynostosis because recurrent intracranial hypertension was suspected. Free flaps and extensive craniectomies

(1–26) J. Neurosurg. 57:370–377, September 1982.

were used in most cases. Fifty-five children had psychometric testing before operation.

The ICP was obviously elevated in one third of the patients and was borderline in another one-third before operation. Waves of increased ICP were recorded during rapid eye movement sleep. The ICP decreased progressively after surgery, returning to normal within several weeks. Pressures in the children with suspected recurrent intracranial hypertension were comparable to those in children who did not have an operation or those studied before operation, indicating the need for further surgery. A significant relation was found between ICP and mental level, the latter being lower at higher ICP levels. Intracranial pressure was found to be maximal at age 6 years and to decline thereafter.

Elevated ICP is observed in one third of the children with craniosynostosis who undergo operation. It is mainly elevated when several sutures are involved. A relationship between ICP and mental level appears likely. The ICP falls progressively after surgery for craniosynostosis. If the ICP can be estimated easily and without risk, it should be done, because the results are of some value in deciding whether surgery should be performed. The progressive fall in ICP that follows surgery may be explained by the resistance of the dura, which is not opened at surgery, and the slow expansion of the brain in the dead space created by the operation.

▶ [This is an extremely relevant study showing the dynamics of intracranial pressure. Subsequent studies will undoubtedly further elucidate the mechanisms and the importance of intracranial pressure dynamics and its influence on craniofacial growth.—L.A.W.] ◀

1–27 **Craniofacial Surgery For Primary Treatment of Craniosynostosis.** Premature synostosis of cranial sutures is a relatively frequent condition of unknown etiology, although hereditary factors usually contribute. One or several sutures may be involved. Growth of the brain is considerable during the first 6–12 months of life. Premature synostosis therefore represents a considerable danger for cerebral development, possibly causing intracranial hypertension which is a source of mental deficiency and blindness if compensatory alterations are not sufficient.

The adaptation of craniofacial surgical principles (osteotomies, remodeling, wiring) has resulted in excellent esthetic and functional results since 1976, in infants as well as in older children. D. Marchac and D. Renier (Paris) have devised a series of procedures to correct the various cranial synostoses, which (with the exception of oxycephaly) are detectable at birth. The basic principle involves the separation of the lower part of the forehead, including orbital edges, from the median and upper segment; these areas are corrected separately for reconstruction of normal anatomical conditions to allow cerebral growth.

(1–27) J. Head Neck Pathol. 2:5–14, 1983.

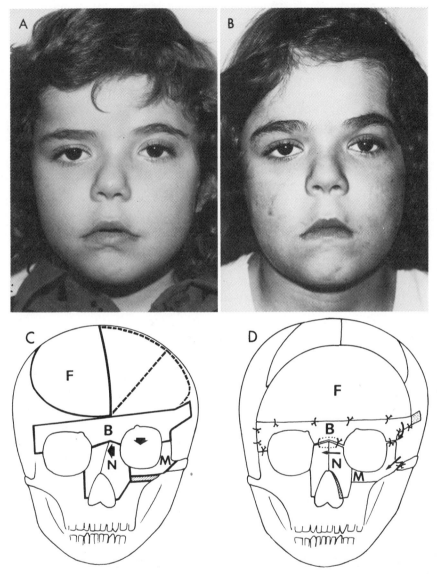

Fig 1–14.—**A,** 8-year-old patient with severe asymmetry; **B,** appearance 4 years after surgical correction; **C,** outline for required osteotomy; and **D,** after mobilization of forehead, left orbit, and nose. (Courtesy of Marchac, D., and Renier, D.: J. Head Neck Pathol. 2:5–14, 1983.)

The plagiocephalies represent unilateral faciocraniostenoses, since the base of the cranium is always involved in the unilateral coronal synostosis. The forehead appears asymmetric; the ocular orbit is higher on the affected side or at times receded, and the nasal root is deviated (Fig 1–14). There is no alteration of the occlusal plane due to a compensatory hypertrophy of the ascending segment of the mandible on the side of the synostosis. Through a series of complex osteotomies it was possible to restore facial symmetry after unilateral correction. In 208 cases currently under observation, remodeling of the forehead did not interfere with the growth process. Early release and advancement of the forehead is effected by the "floating forehead" principle. Results are less satisfactory in Apert's disease because the disease is not merely a morphologic problem.

Frontal remodeling performed during the first few months of life was found to have a favorable influence on facial growth. Early treatment should be performed by a specialized team working in conjunction with the plastic surgeon and the neurosurgeon.

▶ [The authors' extensive experience provides a basis for another valuable contribution. Once again they note the problems with Apert's syndrome and the lack of any adverse effect on growth from operating on the upper face.—L.A.W.] ◀

1–28 **Eye and Orbital Size in the Young and Adult: Some Postnatal Experimental and Clinical Relationships.** The size and shape of the skull are dependent to some degree on the size and shape of the eye and orbit, each of which may influence the other. Bernard G. Sarnat (Univ. of California, Los Angeles) measured orbital volumes in Dutch rabbits and observed an increase in volume from 3.6 ml after 98 days to 5.8 ml after 540 days. After 180 days the volume had nearly peaked at 5 ml and was 25% larger than after 100 days. Ocular volume after 15 days was about 20% of the adult value; after 100 days, about 66%; and after 180 days, about 85%. The adult value was reached after about 300 days. The mean orbital volume and the mean bulb volume were both less after 540 days than after 450 days. A decelerated increase in orbital volume was evident in young rabbits after evisceration, enucleation, or exenteration. The lack of intraorbital mass was directly related to the subsequent lack of orbital development. Addition of a constant-sized implant in the young animal did not enhance orbital growth. Enucleation in adult animals did not alter the orbital volume. Intrabulbar injections of silicone led to an increase in orbital volume in young, but not in adult, rabbits.

Disordered development of the eye and orbit is not corrected by surgical or prosthetic maneuvers, although functional and esthetic improvement may be obtained. When procedures are done to reduce or contribute bulk in a patient who has not reached full skeletal growth, a secondary correction may be necessary in adult life. Much remains to be learned about the growth of and change in the orbit.

▶ [The author has extensive research experience, and once again provides insight into facial growth. He confirms experimentally what has been observed clinically, that is, a normal eye is essential to the stimulation of normal orbital growth.—L.A.W.] ◀

(1–28) Ophthalmologica 185:74–89, 1982.

1–29 **Glabellar Ostectomy and Orbital Craniotomies With Microscopic Control for Correction of Hypertelorism: Preliminary Report of Microcraniofacial Surgery in Two Patients.** David W. Furnas, Don R. DeFeo, and John A. Kusske (Univ. of California, Irvine) used the glabellar ostectomy with microsurgical control to correct orbital hypertelorism in 2 patients. Edgerton's technique was modified by moving the medial and lateral orbital walls independently of each other. A forehead flap was dissected at the subgaleal level as far as the supraorbital ridge and then subperiosteally. After a 360-degree orbital dissection, carried back two thirds of the distance to the orbital apex, transverse osteotomies of the lateral orbital walls and glabellar ostectomies were carried out. The ostectomies extended from the upper limit of the orbital rim to the free border of the pyramidal aperture. In 1 patient a midline segment of bone was left in front of the nasal septum and the crista galli. Excess bone bordering the cribriform plate was then removed, and the orbital cuts were extended to mobilize and approximate the medial orbital walls. A case is illustrated in Figure 1–15.

This "semiopen skull" technique uses microscopic control so that

Fig 1–15.—*Top left,* interorbital distance 48 mm; 50th percentile for her age and sex is 24 mm. *Top right,* dura visible at roof of right orbit, where defect is created by translocation of medial orbital wall. *Bottom left,* split-rib graft has been fitted to dural defect of roof of left orbit. *Bottom right,* patient 3 months after 14-mm translocation on right and about 14-mm translocation on left. (Courtesy of Furnas, D. W., et al.: Plast. Reconstr. Surg. 70:51–63, July 1982.)

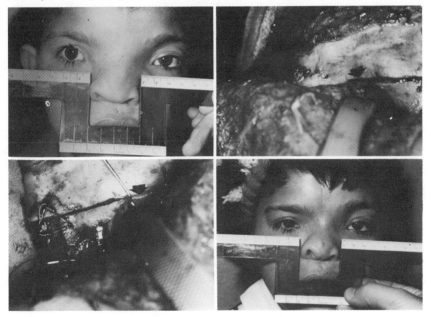

(1–29) Plast. Reconstr. Surg. 70:51–63, July 1982.

the medial orbital walls can be moved precisely by Edgerton's glabellar ostectomy, without need for a formal frontal craniotomy. The lateral orbital walls are cut separately and moved as independent units. The procedures took 10 and 19 hours, respectively, but the 2 patients recovered rapidly without major complications, and blood loss was not marked. This approach is not suitable if full-scale craniotomies are needed to correct deformities of the frontal and parietal bones. It is unnecessary in patients with encephalocele or bony cleft, which in itself provides access.

▶ [Surgery related to hypertelorism should be read in its entirety. The authors present some very excellent results in these very difficult problems. In their article on this subject, Furnas et al. present their technique to avoid an intracranial approach.— R.O.B.] ◀

1–30 **Surgery Related to the Correction of Hypertelorism** is outlined by J. C. H. van der Meulen and J. M. Vaandrager (Rotterdam, Netherlands). Experience with the intracranial correction of orbital hypertelorism in 30 cases has confirmed that the difficulties lie more in correction of associated malformations than in the exaggerated interorbital distance itself. Orbital hypertelorism, with true lateralization of the orbits, should be distinguished from interorbital hypertelorism in which the malformation is limited to the interorbital space and the orbits are not lateralized. A reduction in the interorbital distance may be followed by various deformities, and associated malformations may become more conspicuous after a reduction in the interorbital distance. Medial dislocation and correction of the position of the orbital aperture is not so much obtained by a linear as by a rotatory movement, the nature of which depends on how far the medial orbital walls can be displaced medially.

Canthal drift is probably the most significant deformity produced by the operation, and is difficult to correct, despite effective medial canthopexies. The major cause appears to be the stress created after medial dislocation of the orbit and the anterior projection of its lateral wall. It is helpful to perform the osteotomy behind an intact ligament after careful mobilization of the periorbita, and to reduce lateral pull by recessing the medial orbital wall. Enophthalmos can be prevented by recessing the medial orbital wall and closing residual skeletal defects. Permanent ptosis may result from a loss of support of the upper lid by the anterior projection of the orbital frame. Shortening of the palpebral fissure and temporal depression are other operative effects that have been observed.

Ectopic hair patches may have to be resected, and eyebrow irregularities corrected. Caudocranial divergence of the orbits and sagittal arching of the maxilla can be corrected by medial faciotomy, as shown in Figure 1–16. Medial canthal dystopia following reduction of the interorbital distance is an indication for disinsertion of the ligament

---

(1–30) Plast. Reconstr. Surg. 71:6–17, January 1983.

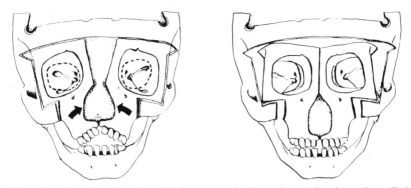

Fig 1–16.—Correction of caudocranial divergence of orbits and sagittal arching of maxilla by medial faciotomy. (Courtesy of van der Meulen, J. C. H., and Vaandrager, J. M.: Plast. Reconstr. Surg. 71:6–17, January 1983.)

and canthopexy. A reduction in the interorbital distance may be followed by a reduction in exotropic strabismus or its conversion to the esotropic form. Abnormalities of the nasolacrimal apparatus may be present. Shortness of the nose usually is overcome by wide dissection of skin and mucosa and implantation of an iliac bone graft to the nasal bridge.

1–31 **Frontofacial Advancement With Bony Separation in Craniofacial Dysostosis** is discussed by H. Anderl, W. Mühlbauer, K. Twerdy, and D. Marchac. Simultaneous advancement of the frontal bones, orbit, and face can lead to infection from opening the anterior cranial fossa to the nasal cavity. Such infection can be avoided by performing a two-stage procedure, protecting the nasal mucoperiosteum, and maintaining the bony structure of the entire anterior cranial base with the supraorbital bar intact during the advancement or shaping, or both, of the front, orbit, and midface.

The authors make a horizontal osteotomy just above the supraorbital nerves after dissecting the soft tissues, and then they remove the frontal bone plate. The small supraorbital bar with the adjacent anterior part of the orbital roof is left in place. After a LeFort III osteotomy and midfacial advancement and stabilization of the maxilla, the forehead is fixed in advanced position. The bony defect left in the area of the supraorbital bar and glabella can be corrected by onlay bone grafts from the cranium or rib. It also is feasible to shift the previously removed frontal plate toward the glabella and the lateral frontozygomatic cut of the LeFort III osteotomy. The supraorbital rim then is shaped by bone excision. If necessary, additional bone grafts can be used in the nasal dorsum and lateral orbit to further improve the external skeletal framework.

This approach was used successfully in a patient with Crouzon's syndrome and one with Apert's syndrome. In the former case the de-

(1–31) Plast. Reconstr. Surg. 71:303–306, March 1983.

fect in front of the frontal bar was filled with a strip of calvarial bone, and a small dead space between the bone graft and supraorbital bar was filled with a mixture of bone dust and fibrinogen glue. In the latter case a minimum of onlay grafting was necessary. This approach should minimize the risk of infection arising from the nasal sinuses and cavities in patients having frontofacial advancement surgery for craniofacial dysostosis.

▶ [A major source of infections in elective and traumatic craniofacial surgery is due to contamination from the nasal cavities. Anderl's technique to minimize this seems successful but requires a two-stage procedure. Perhaps the careful dissection of the tissue planes and the use of autogenous soft-tissue may allow for a watertight seal between the nasal cavity and cranium.—S.H.M.] ◀

1–32 **Harmonization of the "Long Face Syndrome." Two Cases in the Same Family.** Myotonic dystrophy, also known as Steinert's disease, is a hereditary and slowly evolving muscular disorder. Dysfunction of the facial muscles results in a long, dull, expressionless appearance known as the "long face syndrome." Maxillofacial orthopedic surgery allows correction of the facial dysmorphosis by harmonizing the three levels of the face, although correction frequently neglects the rigid and inexpressive appearance of the patient. V. Smatt, P. Der Agopian, and G. Apap (Paris) present data on 2 members of the same family with myotonic dystrophy of different morphologic and functional severity. The surgical procedure was established by the degree of facial deformation and the particular wishes of the patient.

The surgical correction takes place at the level of the hyperplastic maxillary alveolar processes, following the methods described by Bell et al. (1977) and Epker et al. (1980). This technique involves resecting the frontal maxillary process by a Lefort I "down-fracture" technique, focusing either on the maxillary plateau or the superior alveolodental arch, respectively. Each technique has its particular indications, advantages, and inconveniences in terms of possible diminution in volume of nasal fossae and morphologic alterations of the palatal arch.

Early preoperative diagnosis is important. Consideration of anesthetic management must include the possible aggravation of the myopathy that results from operative stress. Although preferable, local anesthesia is not always possible and during general anesthesia curarization it should be avoided. Halothane is equally contraindicated for reasons of enzymatic disturbances. Respiratory depressants must also be used with caution, and respiratory assistance must be maintained during operation. Subsequent facial muscular exercise will reinforce the results.

1–33 **Muscle Reorientation Following Superior Repositioning of the Maxilla** was investigated by Stephen A. Schendel and Lewis W.

(1–32)   Ann. Chir. Plast. 27:350–358, 1983.
(1–33)   J. Oral Maxillofac. Surg. 41:235–240, April 1983.

Williamson (Honolulu). Total maxillary osteotomies are done to correct the long face syndrome with vertical maxillary excess. Although reliable results have been obtained with the LeFort I and multiple segmental techniques, the postoperative soft tissue structure occasionally is suboptimal because of spatial reorientation of the facial muscles.

The authors recommend a V-Y advancement-closure of the horizontal maxillary vestibular incision to avoid undesired effects in the perioral area after superior repositioning of the maxilla. The alar base is reoriented just before closure of the V-Y vestibular incision. Skin hooks are used to adjust the tissues to produce a symmetric, esthetically pleasing appearance. Occasionally other muscles may be suspended as the alar bases are reoriented. In the aging face, a combination of individual muscle suspension and a V-Y advancement can be helpful.

Review was made of 10 total maxillary surgical procedures in which vertical height was reduced and the soft tissues were closed by the present approach. Average follow-up after operation was 4 months. Average superior maxillary repositioning was 6.3 mm as measured at the maxillary incisor. Average lip measurement was 22.6 mm before operation and 22.8 mm afterward. The lip decreased vertically an average of 0.4 mm after operation in relation to the cranium, not a significant change. The vermilion decreased an average of only 0.2 mm. The nasal tip was elevated an average of 2.4 mm. There was no change in lip form after surgery. Average change at the widest area of the ala was + 0.9 mm in the 8 patients evaluated. The change at the junction of the alae and nasal floors averaged + 0.6 mm. Preoperative and postoperative alar widths did not differ significantly.

These findings clearly support the reliability of muscle reorienting surgery after superior repositioning of the maxilla. A V-Y advancement is necessary in conjunction with nasal suturing to maintain nasal width. Other facial muscle reorientation, as is appropriate in individual cases, can also be carried out.

1–34 **Results Following Simultaneous Mobilization of Maxilla and Mandible for Correction of Dentofacial Deformities: Analysis of 100 Consecutive Patients.** John P. LaBanc, Timothy Turvey, and Bruce N. Epker reviewed the results of simultaneous mobilization of the maxilla and mandible for correction of dentofacial deformities in 100 consecutive patients treated at two centers in 1976–1981. The 76 women and 24 men had a mean age of 22.4 years. Fifty-six patients had class II skeletal, and 26, class III dentofacial deformities; 10 had facial asymmetries, and 5 had class I deformities. Three were unclassified. A large majority of class II cases had vertical maxillary excess and mandibular deficiency. All patients but 3 had LeFort I osteotomy,

(1–34) Oral Surg. 54:607–612, December 1982.

generally with segmentalization, and bilateral ramus osteotomies, generally a modified sagittal split. Three patients had a LeFort III midface osteotomy with simultaneous mandibular ramus osteotomy. Simultaneous genioplasty and mandibular subapical osteotomy was done in 22 and 8 cases, respectively.

One patient had diplopia after a LeFort III advancement that resolved incompletely. No patient had significant airway compromise postoperatively. Excellent short-term stability could be expected from a well-executed operation that included the use of proper skeletal stabilization and sufficient posterior bony stops to the maxilla to prevent telescoping. Immediate relapse can occur when the posterior maxillary bony interphases are inadequate or nonexistent. Intraoral skeletal stabilization can prevent relapse in these cases. Early relapse during fixation will occur when the condyles are not properly seated in the fossae, when inadequate stabilization is used, or when there are inadequate posterior maxillary bony interphases, or when all 3 instances occur. The cause of delayed relapse is not clear. In some cases as large as 5 mm of condylar height have been lost, with a resultant class-II open bite occlusion.

Simultaneous mobilization of the jaws appears to be associated with relapse more often than single-jaw procedures, and should not be done without consideration of specific indications. The procedure can be done with few adverse sequelae and complications in selected cases with careful treatment planning, meticulous surgery, and optimal supportive anesthesia and postoperative care.

1–35 **Inappropriate Antidiuretic Hormone Syndrome in Craniofacial Surgery.** Michel F. Brones, Henry K. Kawamoto, Jr., and Justin Renaudin (Univ. of California, Los Angeles) report 3 cases of inappropriate antidiuretic hormone secretion after craniofacial surgery. Three of 65 patients operated on intracranially for correction of craniofacial malformations had the syndrome, which is characterized by progressive thirst, hypertension, excitability and disorientation, seizures, coma, and death. The symptoms can closely mimic those expected in the postoperative period. The laboratory features include hyponatremia, serum hypo-osmolality, continued renal excretion of sodium, urinary hyperosmolality, and an increased plasma ADH level. Fluid restriction usually leads to improvement. Two girls aged 9 years and a boy aged 10, who were treated for Apert syndrome, telorbitism, and plagiocephaly, were affected. All 3 patients improved when fluids were restricted, but 1 with increased intracranial pressure required decompressive craniotomy.

No specific reasons for inappropriate ADH secretion in these cases could be found. Retraction of the brain during surgery or postoperative brain edema, or both, may trigger the osmoreceptors of the hypothalamic-neurohypophyseal system in a susceptible patient. Subtle

(1–35)   Plast. Reconstr. Surg. 71:1–5, January 1983.

postoperative changes must not automatically be attributed to the normal recovery process. The present patients had an altered neurologic status and a decreased serum sodium level within 24–48 hours after surgery. Careful fluid and electrolyte monitoring is necessary during this period.

Fluid restriction is the hallmark of management. Seizures are treated with anticonvulsants, furosemide, and infusion of 3% hypertonic saline solution. Chronic and refractory cases can be treated with demeclocycline or lithium carbonate. However, demeclocycline can produce phototoxicity, and the use of a sunscreen should be considered. Lithium carbonate is not recommended because it may produce hyperpyrexia with impaired consciousness and eventual death.

1–36 **Comparative Study of Wire Osteosynthesis vs. Bone Screws in the Treatment of Mandibular Prognathism.** Bone screw fixation after surgery for mandibular prognathism requires a shorter period of intermaxillary immobilization, and relapse may be less frequent, although pain and reduced temporomandibular joint (TMJ) function may result. G. W. Paulus and E. W. Steinhauser (Erlangen, West Germany) compared the tendency to relapse, mandibular nerve dysfunction, and TMJ changes after the use of wire osteosynthesis and bone screws in 221 patients treated for mandibular prognathism. Sagittal-split surgery was used in 146 cases, and a vertical osteotomy in 75. Bone fixation was maintained with wire osteosynthesis in 117 cases and with bone screws in 104.

After sagittal-split osteotomy the tendency to relapse was less after bone screw fixation. A change of more than 1 degree in the SNB angle was observed in 53% of sagittal-split osteotomy and wire osteosynthesis cases and in 37% of bone screw cases. The anterior facial height increased by more than 1 mm in 63% and 30% of cases, respectively. In vertical osteotomies, relapse was slightly more frequent after bone screw fixation. A change in the SNB angle was similarly frequent in the two methods of fixation, but an increase in anterior facial height was more frequent after wire fixation. Long-term disturbance in mandibular nerve function was comparably frequent in the two fixation groups. No major differences in TMJ change were observed. Pain in the TMJ area was reduced postoperatively in both treatment groups.

The decreased tendency toward relapse and the significant shortening of the time of intermaxillary fixation make the use of bone screws in sagittal and vertical osteotomies preferred to treat mandibular prognathism. The tendency to relapse is minimal when bone screws are used, and no important increase in TMJ problems occurs when compared with use of wire osteosynthesis.

▶ [The authors' study is an important comparison, emphasizing the advantage of

(1–36)   Oral Surg. 54:2–6, July 1982.

bone screws in comparison to wires. This is a consideration of increasing importance to plastic surgeons who perform osteotomies.—L.A.W.] ◀

1–37 **Mandibular Retrognathia with Marked Incisor Supraocclusion. Treatment by Sagittal Osteotomy of the Mandibular Body.** D. Heron and J. Delaire (Nantes, France) present data on 3 patients treated by sagittal osteotomy of the mandibular body. The surgical technique, illustrated in Figures 1–17 and 1–18, varies with the presence or absence of extraction. The exclusively cortical vestibular osteotomy is performed by means of a surgical fraise.

Indications for this procedure are precise and limited. It is suggested for cases in which surgical correction must act on the anterior segment of the mandible, with conservation of satisfactory molar relationships, and when absence of excessive height of the lower region of the face contraindicates a segmental osteotomy designed for reduc-

Fig 1–17.—Illustration of surgical technique showing (**A** and **B**) incision and mucoperiosteal detachment, (**C**) vestibular osteotomy line, (**D**) lingual osteotomy line, and (**E**) anteroposterior separation. (Courtesy of Heron, D., and Delaire, J.: Rev. Stomatol. Chir. Maxillofac. 84:43–49, 1983 Masson, S. A., Paris.)

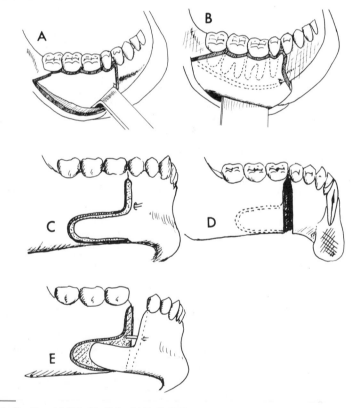

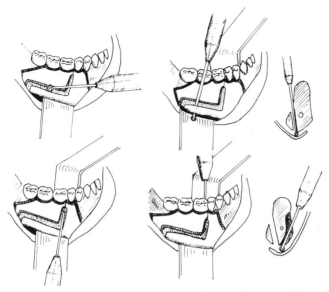

Fig 1–18.—Illustration showing details of surgical technique. (Courtesy of Heron, D., and Delaire, J.: Rev. Stomatol. Chir. Maxillofac. 84:43–49, 1983 Masson S. A., Paris.)

tion of the anterior dentoalveolar section. This technique allows modification of incisor relationships and moderate elongation of horizontal mandibular segments without the application of a graft.

1–38 **"Functional" Genioplasty.** V. Plenier and J. Delaire (Nantes, France) examine the value of genioplasty as a treatment method for the long face syndrome. Genioplasty is viewed as a "functional" intervention when it contributes to the establishment of the osteodentomyocutaneous equilibrium of the lower part of the face. The procedure is planned on the basis of preoperative teleradiographic exploration, which allows a rather precise prognosis regarding the position of the inferior portion of the chin. The surgical technique is that outlined by Michelet et al. (1974), which features the fashioning of a tenon and mortise joint via osteotomies. Postoperative teleradiographic control will confirm the new position of the osseous chin. This procedure is simple and benign, and postoperative complications are rare.

Such "functional" genioplasty was performed (1) in association with maxillary or mandibular osteotomy, or both, in adult patients, and allows stabilization of postoperative dental occlusions; (2) within the context of treatment for the sequelae of cleft palate and harelip, in which bilabial contact is facilitated; (3) in association with a partial anterior glossectomy; or (4) frequently as a corrective measure for

(1–38)   Rev. Stomatol. Chir. Maxillofac. 83:54–61, 1983.

ineffective orthodontic treatment. Moreover, "functional" genioplasty, when performed early enough, may help to avoid the development of significant maxillofacial disequilibrium observed at the conclusion of growth, and thus the necessity of major surgical intervention.

► [The authors describe an interesting technique. Since they are dealing with membranous bone, which maintains its volume and growth potential so well, it is questionable whether the procedure has any advantages over a simple sliding genioplasty.—L.A.W.] ◄

1–39 **Mandibular Protrusion: Results Following Resection of Mandibular Body or Angle.** J. Lachard, J. L. Blanc, J. P. Lagier, and G. Le Retraite (Marseille) focus on the significance and causal aspects of recurrence of maxillary malformations after surgical treatment, particularly mandibular protrusion. The report is based on the analysis of teleradiographic investigations both before and after operation, repeated 1 year after resection. The study involved 5 patients who had resection of the mandibular body and 10 patients who had angle resection of the mandible. The most remarkable finding was the stability of clinical results; only 2 cases of early recurrence were observed, caused by delayed consolidation in angle resection. One was treated by a grinding procedure, the other required reintervention.

The resection of the mandibular body has little effect on the position of the ascending rami, whereas angle resection usually results in parasitic movements in this region. The preoperative position was practically always reestablished after follow-up of 1 year. Following shortening of the body, there is an almost constant drop in the symphyseal region. These movements are apparently caused by the activity of masticatory and suprahyoid muscles; the tongue plays an accessory role.

► [This is an interesting study of the dynamics of the mandible following resection of the body and angle.—L.A.W.] ◄

1–40 **Contribution of Condylectomy in Treatment of Hypercondylia** is discussed by J. Delaire, A. Gaillard, and J. F. Tulasne (Nantes, France). Numerous authors have considered condylectomy as the preferred treatment for the management of hypercondylia in cases where the asymmetry and unilateral mandibular hypertrophy are not too severe. When the facial deformation is more accentuated, the current tendency has been to replace this procedure systematically by combined mandibular and maxillary osteotomies, to achieve in a single surgical session complete spatial normalization of mandibular symmetry and the occlusal plane. This operation was generally postponed until after the conclusion of natural growth. Although these combined procedures have given excellent results, they do impose excessive suffering on the patient, particularly after considering the good results achieved in most cases with condylectomy alone. This procedure, when implemented during the period of growth or young adult-

(1–39) Rev. Stomatol. Chir. Maxillofac. 84:34–42, 1983.
(1–40) Ibid., pp. 11–18.

hood, can considerably modify facial skeletal structures and can make it possible to avoid more complex interventions. If necessary, a simple complementary surgical intervention several months later will assure anatomical symmetry and the desired functional equilibrium.

After a review of data on 6 patients, condylectomy was recommended for practically all instances of unilateral hypercondylia in which it is necessary to obtain equal lengths of condylar units, an essential condition for good mandibulofacial morphogenesis. Condylectomy is associated with postoperative intermaxillary elastic traction. It is worn permanently for 1 month, and then only at night for 2 months. It is capable of normalizing facial skeletal structures integrally, particularly when implemented in the prepubertal period and before conclusion of pubertal growth. Equally good results may be obtained in the young adult, provided mandibular and maxillary deformation is not too severe.

In the more severe cases that are treated later in life, it might be necessary to include an elongating mandibular osteotomy of the opposite side, as well as an osteoplasty of the basilar edge and chin on the affected side. Maxillary osteotomies are only rarely indicated in cases of unilateral hypercondylia. In bilateral forms, maxillary osteotomy may be required in association with shortening mandibular osteotomies of the ascending rami. Even in these cases, however, a bilateral condylectomy might be the better solution, particularly in the presence of mandibular prognathia with supraclusion.

▶ [The authors recommend the use of condylectomy as an essential component in treating the problem. This is an important step in understanding the treatment process since other mandibular or maxillary osteotomies might be considered.— L.A.W.] ◀

1–41   **Mandibular Condyle Hyperplasia** is discussed by D. Jacquemaire and J. Delaire (Nantes, France). Mandibular condyle hyperplasia is typically characterized by hypertrophy and accelerated growth of one of the mandibular condyles, with exceptional bilateral involvement. The homolateral descent of the molar occlusal plane leads to generalized adaptive alterations of the maxilla and the entire facial skeleton, which justifies prepubescent condylar surgery. Clinical and radiologic aspects will vary according to unilateral or bilateral involvement and extent of skeletal malformations. The most frequent unilateral form is characterized by asymmetry of the lower portion of the face, associated with augmented height of the face on one side, hypertrophy of the mandibular angle, lowering and convexity of the basal edge, collapse of the labial commissure, and occasional contralateral deviation of the chin. Palpation confirms osseous hypertrophy of the mandible, predominantly involving the condyle, the mandibular angle, and the basal edge. Mandibular movement is frequently unhampered and free of pain, although some patients do have pain in

(1–41)   Rev. Stomatol. Chir. Maxillofac. 84:5–10, 1983.

the temporomandibular articulation and discomfort and articular "cracking" when opening the mouth. Dental occlusion is generally disturbed to various degrees, which are determined by the extent of mandibular alterations.

The bilateral variety is much less frequent and seldom perfectly symmetrical. The facial malformations are characterized, not only by bilateral hypertrophy of the condyles and ascending mandibular segment and the concave aspect of the basilar edge, but also by the particular mandibular prognathism resulting from the hypertrophy. This prognathism is of a "skeletal" type, frequently with considerable alveolodental compensation.

Hyperplasia of the mandibular condyle rarely appears before 10 years of age, becomes more distinct during pubertal growth, and stabilizes in adulthood. Early diagnosis is certainly desirable, and should be based on a thorough knowledge of these clinical signs.

▶ [This is a sound review of the problem and its natural history.—L.A.W.] ◀

1–42 **External Ear, Mandible, and Other Components of Hemifacial Microsomia.** Alvaro A. Figueroa and Samuel Pruzansky (Univ.

Fig 1–19.—Superimposition of tracings from oriented tomograms. Shaded mandible is ipsilateral to microtic ear. (Courtesy of Figueroa, A. A., and Pruzansky, S.: J. Maxillofac. Surg. 10:200–211, November 1982.)

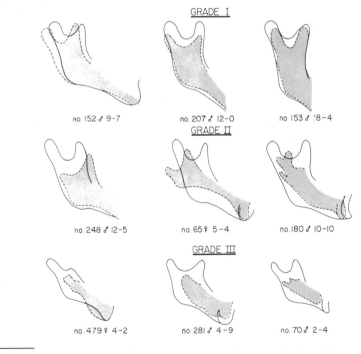

GRADE I

no. 152 ♂ 9-7   no. 207 ♂ 12-0   no 153 ♂ '8-4

GRADE II

no. 248 ♂ 12-5   no. 65 ♀ 5-4   no. 180 ♂ 10-10

GRADE III

no. 479 ♀ 4-2   no 281 ♂ 4-9   no. 70 ♂ 2-4

(1–42) J. Maxillofac. Surg. 10:200–211, November 1982.

of Illinois, Chicago) analyzed data on 100 cases of the unilateral form of hemifacial microsomia (HFM) in patients without other apparent craniofacial or extracranial malformations. An otocentric approach was used, with the external ear being the reference organ. Analysis was based on a three-level gradation of severity of the otic and mandibular deformities that results in 9 different combinations. The gradings are illustrated in Figure 1–19.

In these patients the external ear was more severely deformed than the mandible. Eighty patients had grade II or grade III otic malformations, but only 23 had mandibular malformations of this severity. There appeared to be a relation between the severity of the ear malformations and that of the jaw malformations, but precise correlation between the various grades of deformity was not evident. An imprecise relation between the ear and jaw malformations is explicable on the basis of Poswillo's concept of a vascular accident with randomized effects on the developmental field. Most patients had grade II otic malformations combined with grade I mandibular changes. Only 4 patients had grade III jaw malformations.

Despite the lack of precise correlation between the severity of the ear and jaw malformations in HFM, the likelihood of a more severe mandibular malformation being present increases when the external ear is markedly affected. There is a direct relation between the mandibular deformity and the status of the masticatory muscles. A more precise correlation has been established between the severity of the defect in the mandible and the malleus and incus on the same side, and between the external ear deformity and ossicular abnormalities.

▶ [This carefully done study adds important understanding to the correlation between the severity of the visible defects and the functional problems of mastication and hearing.—L.A.W.] ◀

1–43 **Indications for Simultaneous Mobilization of the Maxilla and Mandible for the Correction of Dentofacial Deformities** are discussed by Bruce N. Epker, Timothy Turvey, and Leward C. Fish. Simultaneous mobilization of the maxilla and mandible must be considered in about 10% of patients with class III dentofacial deformities. An AP skeletal deformity of more than 12 mm must be so considered. When adverse esthetic and cephalometric features coexist with a large AP discrepancy, isolated midface advancement or mandibular setback will have an esthetically poor result. In patients with class III open-bite deformity, vertical maxillary excess, and an anteroposteriorly excessive mandible, the excessive vertical anterior facial height can mask the true AP skeletal and occlusal deformity. The maxilla is treated to correct the vertical and transverse skeletal deformities; the mandible, to correct the AP deformity. Some patients with class III deformity and vertical maxillary deficiency should have

(1–43) Oral Surg. 54:369–381, October 1982.

simultaneous inferior maxillary repositioning and mandibular setback surgery.

Some class II patients also warrant consideration for simultaneous two-jaw surgery. This may be true for patients with vertical maxillary excess and transverse maxillary deficiency, as well as vertical maxillary deficiency, which is a rare accompaniment. Simultaneous mobilization of the jaws may be warranted in class I dentofacial deformities with vertical maxillary excess and malocclusions or bimaxillary protrusion.

Some facial asymmetries cannot be corrected only in the mandible. They basically are asymmetries that result in an adult dentofacial complex with combined vertical, transverse, and AP deformities in both jaws and compensatory canting of the maxilla to an esthetically displeasing degree. Examples include deviate prognathism, condylar hyperplasia, condylar hypoplasia, and hemifacial hypertrophy.

▶ [This paper should be studied in its entirety. Some of these facial deformities can only be corrected by simultaneous osteotomies of the maxilla and the mandible after careful preoperative planning with the use of dental models and pretreatment with cephalometric analysis.—R.O.B.] ◀

1–44 **Mandibular Vestibuloplasty: Clinical Update.** The mandibular split-thickness skin graft vestibuloplasty with lowering of the floor of the mouth is an excellent procedure when adequate mandibular denture function is severely compromised by inadequate residual alveolar bone or poor soft tissue contours. Alan Samit and Larry Popowich (VA Med. Center, Philadelphia) have, on the basis of experience with more than 80 cases, developed several modifications of the traditional technique that have reduced operative and postoperative morbidity without compromising the vestibular extension. The procedure is simplified; operating time averages 75 minutes. Postoperative hospitalization also is significantly shortened. The results have been very satisfying, and patient acceptance is high. Meticulous preparation of the recipient periosteal bed, with removal of all hyperplastic tissue, and close adaptation of the graft to underlying periosteum remain essential to a good outcome.

Vestibular extension can be obtained without use of a stent, which saves much time and avoids jeopardizing graft survival through poor adaptation of the stent. Direct labial suturing of the graft has led to graft survival approaching 100%. The graft is fenestrated after its superior aspect has been sutured to the crestal gingiva, so that the graft can be expanded to cover the labial periosteum and the recipient site can be covered by a smaller graft. Cannulation of the submaxillary salivary ducts can prevent duct obstruction and sialoadenitis. Controlled mental nerve manipulation results in predictable, transient anesthesia and less postoperative pain. Dexamethasone is introduced by intraoperative infiltration into the floor of the mouth rather

(1–44) Oral Surg. 54:141–147, August 1982.

than by intravenous injection. The labial and lingual flaps are ligated with 2-0 chromic gut sutures. Prophylactic antibiotics are omitted unless a specific indication is present. A dermal graft can be used to decrease healing time and scarring at the donor site. If regression is unacceptable, an epidermal graft is used and donor site healing is facilitated by the use of various dressing materials or by meshing part of a large graft with an expander and then replacing the graft at the donor site.

Partial procedures have been completed in some cases. Vestibular deformities after trauma and tumor resection have been corrected. Procedures have been performed in partially edentulous patients in whom the teeth were preserved as overdenture or partial denture abutments.

▶ [It would appear that these authors are applying the graft directly over the periosteum without the use of a stent.—R.O.B.] ◀

1–45 **Anesthesia for Craniofacial Osteotomies** is outlined by Duncan J. M. Ferguson, John Barker, and Ian T. Jackson (Glasgow, Scotland). Single-stage craniofacial reconstruction now is widely carried out to correct deformities such as those seen in Crouzon's and Apert's syndromes, hypertelorism, and craniosynostosis. Only fit patients undergo this surgery.

Tracheostomy is avoided unless intubation is not possible. The fiberoptic endoscope has been most helpful. A nasal route for intubation is mandatory for intermaxillary fixation, but the oral route may be selected initially in some procedures involving change to the nose after mobilization of the maxilla and nasal surgery. The lungs are ventilated artificially throughout operation to maintain a Pa_{O_2} just above 100 mm Hg and a Pa_{CO_2} of 30–35 mm Hg.

Intracranial procedures may require an osmotic dehydration agent, drainage of cerebral spinal fluid, or administration of cerebral metabolic depressant drugs. Drugs are used as needed to provide a passive circulation and a good operative field. Close monitoring of blood loss and adequate replacement are essential. Temperature control and humidification of inspired gases also are important. Antibiotic coverage is used routinely for 2–3 days after operation. Patient monitoring is essential.

Neostigmine and atropine are used to promote rapid return of protective reflexes after surgery. Patients are kept in intensive care for 24–48 hours after operation. Humidified air enriched with 40% oxygen is administered. A lumbar subarachnoid drain may be left in place to control the intracranial pressure. Careful monitoring of vital signs and measurement of losses through drains should prevent oligemic shock. Fluid balance is maintained on the basis of urine output and estimated basal requirements. Opiates are used to relieve postoperative pain. Anxiolytic drugs may also be necessary. Good nursing

(1–45) Ann. Plast. Surg. 10:333–338, April 1983.

care includes attention to drains, intravascular catheters, and incisions, as well as proper care of the eyes, lips, mouth, and pressure areas. A full bladder and constipation should be avoided.

▶ [In spite of what the authors say, tracheostomy is sometimes desirable. The principles they outline, however, are sound and appropriate.—L.A.W.] ◀

1–46 **Psychosocial Impact of Craniofacial Deformities Before and After Reconstructive Surgery.** Arlette Lefebvre and Susan Barclay (Toronto) assessed changes in body image, adjustment, and psychologic functioning after operation in 250 patients aged 6 weeks to 39 years with severe craniofacial deformities. Major congenital deformities were present in 178 patients; the other 72 had tumors or other late-onset deformities. Parents and patients were interviewed separately where appropriate. Deformities were rated by the Hay's Standardized Rating Scale of Appearance and, where appropriate, the Piers-Harris Self-esteem Inventory.

Patients with congenital disorders generally rated their preoperative appearance as more imperfect than those with acquired disorders. The difference was not significant, however, although the actual appearance in the congenital group was much more abnormal. Most tumor patients rated their appearance as poor. Most young patients other than early adolescents rated their appearance more positively than did their parents. Mothers and fathers provided identical ratings in most cases. Improvement in self-ratings after operation were comparable in the congenital and acquired deformity groups. Improvement in parental ratings was less marked. A large majority of the patients evaluated postoperatively had subjective emotional improvement, were more comfortable in public, and felt that they were more appealing to others. Objective improvement in academic or work performance and heterosexual activities was evident in fewer than half of the subjectively improved patients. Several families reported increased friction among family members.

The most significant predictive factors in psychosocial improvement after operation for craniofacial deformity appear to be patient age, preoperative expectations, and origin of the decision to operate. Operation generally provides both physical and psychosocial improvement, especially when patients are actively involved in the decision-making process, but unrealistic preoperative expectations or unilateral decisions to operate can lead to family tension and patient disappointment after correction.

1–47 **Total Reconstruction of the External Ear** is outlined by Radford C. Tanzer (Hanover, N.H.). A framework for ear reconstruction should consist of autogenous cartilage. Any soft tissue used to supplement existing skin in the auricular region should consist of free grafts. No visible scarring should be created other than that essen-

(1–46) Can. J. Psychiatry 27:579–584, November 1982.
(1–47) Ann. Plast. Surg. 10:76–85, January 1983.

tially on or behind the reconstructed ear. The simultaneous production of the auriculocephalic angle and construction of the conchal wall are impractical. The logical solution is to bring the antihelix-scaphahelix unit out into proper position like a valise handle, leaving the conchal wall deficient and later reconstructing it from adjacent retroauricular tissue. A wide auriculocephalic angle is not necessary; reconstructed ears are less conspicuous if set reasonably close to the head.

The first operation is intended to relocate any usable auricular tissue in proper position, but protuberances in the region of the anterior helix are left alone at this stage. Patterns of the whole ear and of the part to be reproduced in cartilage, prepared from a plaster model of the opposite ear, are used. The next step involves fabrication and insertion of the cartilaginous framework. The preparation of costal cartilage is shown in Figure 1–20. The skin is fitted closely to the underlying cartilage. After 4 months the ear is brought away from the head and the superior, posterior, and inferior conchal walls are constructed in three stages. The first two stages are done 2 months apart, and are separated in the interest of a viable blood supply. The final step is to form the tragus and the conchal floor. A modification of Kirkham's method is used to roll the integument of the conchal floor

Fig 1–20.—*(A)* Surgical approach to costal cartilage; *(B)* surgical pattern is laid out on sixth and seventh costal cartilages overlying synchondrosis and extending almost to seventh costochondral junction; *(C)* method of attaching helix to antihelix-scapha unit with wire suture; *(D,E)* diagrammatic detail of method. (Courtesy of Tanzer, R. C.: Ann. Plast. Surg. 10:76–85, January 1983.)

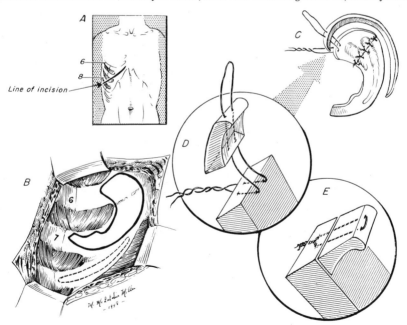

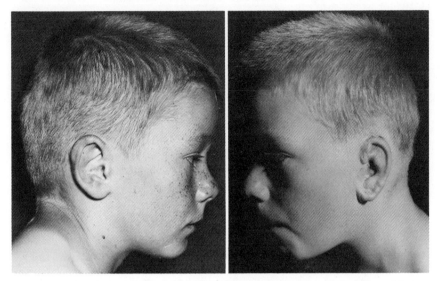

Fig 1–21.—Final view of 5-year-old patient after construction of conchal cavity and tragus. (Courtesy of Tanzer, R. C.: Ann. Plast. Surg. 10:76–85, January 1983.)

under itself. The conchal cavity is deepened, and the conchal floor is lined with a full-thickness graft from the opposite auriculocephalic sulcus. The outcome in 1 case is illustrated in Figure 1–21.

Experience in 2 cases would indicate that this approach is applicable to several types of microtia, and adaptable to at least some degree to partial or total traumatic loss of the auricle. The procedures can be safely completed in 1 year. The method of constructing the cartilage assembly from costal cartilage has been used in 4 other unfinished cases with gratifying results.

▶ [This is a reprint of Dr. Tanzer's original impressive presentation for total reconstruction of the ear which was published in 1959.—R.O.B.] ◀

1–48 **Congenital Unilateral Pseudoptosis of the Upper Eyelid.** Pseudoptosis has been described in conjunction with blepharochalasis and as a state resulting from inadequate posterior support, as after enucleation. It is commonly seen in Orientals who lack a palpebral fold in the upper lid. George S. Pap (Rockford, Ill., School of Medicine) reports an unusual unilateral upper lid deformity associated with absence of a palpebral fold in a Caucasian.

Boy, 12, was seen with overhanging skin of the right upper eyelid that interfered with vision and created an asymmetric appearance (Fig 1–22). The patient could raise both upper lids voluntarily. Hiraga's "double eyelid" operation was used. True herniation of a lobule of fat was found in the lateral region between the orbicularis muscle and the orbital septum, and it was resected. There appeared to be redundant skin laterally, but no skin was

(1–48)   Plast. Reconstr. Surg. 70:483–484, October 1982.

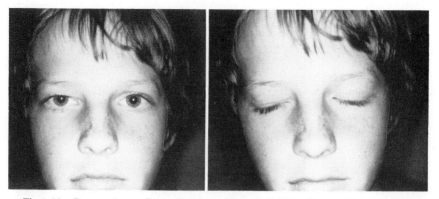

Fig 1–22.—Preoperative condition. (Courtesy of Pap, G. S.: Plast. Reconstr. Surg. 70:483–484, October 1982.)

removed. A lag was noticed on active lid opening 1 month after operation, but at 4 months the lids were symmetric and the palpebral fissures equal.

This case is in the group of pseudoptoses that occur in association with blepharochalasis, when the palpebral folds overhang the lid margin. The deformity was corrected by conventional blepharoplasty.

1–49   **Complications of Ptosis Surgery** are reviewed by C. E. Iliff. Undercorrection is encountered more often in surgery for congenital ptosis when insufficient aponeurosis and levator are resected, tight horns of Whitnall's check ligaments are not recognized, or all the tissues are so abnormal that only partial correction can be obtained. A poor lid crease postoperatively can be corrected by making an incision through the skin where the lid fold should be. Overcorrection, if slight, should be managed by massage for 2–3 months. If necessary, Berke's tarso-aponeurosis tenotomy through the tarsal plate gives good results. A peaked lid may be present after a frontalis sling operation, and usually can be relieved by grasping the lid margin at the site of the peak and pulling to reset the arms of the rhomboid. Peaking after a levator shortening procedure may result from excision of too much tarsus, or from uneven tension on the sutures between the shortened aponeurosis and the tarsus. If corneal staining persists, a recheck for dry eye syndrome is indicated. If this is found, temporary occlusion of the puncta is done.

Infection along the fascial tracts may complicate the frontalis sling procedure for ptosis. Irrigation of the tract with gentamicin may help avoid the problem. A sterile abscess at the site of a fascial tie is less frequent if a single tie rather than a square knot of fascia is used. Ectropion is a rare complication of ptosis surgery, which can be managed by incising through the skin at the lid fold and cutting away subcutaneous scar tissue. Entropion is corrected by opening the skin

(1–49)   J. Pediatr. Ophthalmol. Strabismus 19:256–258, September–October 1982.

along the lid fold and dissecting upward for 1 cm and downward to the cilia base to excise partially the pretardal muscle. True entropion requires complete rebuilding of the lid; usually some skin and subcutaneous tissue must be resected. Loss of lashes is a rare complication with current ptosis operations. The use of paste-on lashes often is preferred to lash grafting from the brow.

1–50   **Reconstruction of the Periocular Mucous Membrane by Autologous Conjunctival Transplantation.** Conjunctiva has been used for corneal re-epithelialization after ocular chemical injuries. David W. Vastine, William B. Stewart, and Ivan R. Schwab (San Francisco) have used large autologous conjunctival grafts to reconstruct the conjunctiva after severe radiation and chemical burns, trauma, tumor resection, excision of pterygium, and in repairing congenital abnormalities. The most common indication in this series of 14 cases was degenerative disease. After complete excision of disease and the release of conjunctival restrictions to ocular or lid movement, normal conjunctiva was taken from the ipsilateral or, where extensive reconstruction was necessary, the opposite eye. The superotemporal bulbar conjunctiva was preferentially used. Donor sites were dissected under high-loupe magnification or microscopic control, taking care to harvest only the mucosal conjunctival surface. Donor patches were fixed to the conjunctival edges and the episclera, most often with 10–0 nylon or 8–0 chromic collagen sutures.

All patients had an uncomplicated postoperative course. None of the grafts failed. Clinical repair was accomplished in all cases. One graft retracted slightly. Topical steroids were used in all cases for 2–3 months to minimize inflammation. Care of patients requiring massive resection of host conjunctiva was much easier than would have been the case after graft repair. All patients with tear function and ocular surface abnormalities had improvement in the tear film and increased corneal clarity after surgery. Two patients with recurrent pterygium and two with active advancing pterygium had excellent esthetic results and improved visual acuity.

Free conjunctival grafting is significantly preferable to the use of buccal mucous membrane grafts in patients with unilateral abnormalities from alkali burn and irradiation injuries, tumor, degenerative disease, and trauma. Autologous conjunctival transplantation is the best method of periocular mucous membrane replacement when suitable donor sites are available.

1–51   **Results of Surgery for Nasal Dermoids in Children.** Congenital midline nasal dermoids can be present at any point from the root of the nose to the base of the columella. Early excision is recommended, if possible before school age, because of progressive expansion leading to distortion and destruction of the nasal bones and cartilages. P. J.

(1–50)   Ophthalmology (Rochester) 89:1072–1081, September 1982.
(1–51)   J. Laryngol. Otol. 96:627–633, July 1982.

Bradley (Liverpool, England) reviewed the results of excision of nasal dermoids in 32 children from 1960 to 1979. There were 17 epidermoid and 15 "true" dermoid lesions. Most epidermoid lesions were at the root of the nose, and most of the true dermoids were on the nasal bridge. Eighteen patients were more than age 12 years when evaluated. All patients had definitive excisional surgery. "Simple" lesions were excised without disruption of the deeper nasal structures. In some "complex" cases, excision of the cyst or fistula, or both, required outfracturing of the nasal bones.

All patients who had excision of an epidermoid lesion at the root of the nose had acceptable wounds and satisfactory surgical results. Sixteen of 22 patients who had surgery through a vertical midline nasal incision had an acceptable scar. Five of the 6 with unacceptable results had true dermoid lesions. Twenty patients in all were satisfied with the outcome of surgery. Four were dissatisfied because of recurrence of the nasal dermoid. Only 2 patients complained of nasal deformity after surgery; both had complex true dermoid lesions. All patients with recurrent lesions had true dermoids.

In complex cases of nasal dermoid, the histologic findings are predictive of the results of surgery. All nasal cartilage and bone removed during excision of these lesions should be preserved and used to fill any defect. Use of a composite graft to replace missing tissue prevents contraction and scarring of the nose. If nasal deformity is present after excision of a nasal dermoid, definitive reconstruction should be delayed until after puberty.

1–52 **Electrothrombosis as a Treatment of Cirsoid Angioma in the Face and Scalp and Varicosis of the Leg** was evaluated by Yutaka Ogawa and Kunio Inoue. Cirsoid angiomas are abnormal communications between the arteries and veins, arising congenitally or after trauma and found most often in the face and scalp. The most common treatments have been ligation and excision of the regional vessels, but problems of recurrence and bleeding persist. Electrothrombosis was evaluated in rabbits and then in patients. Usually general anesthesia was used. Beryllium-copper needles 0.2 to 0.3 mm in diameter were employed. They were passed into the target vessels either directly or through a guide tube. Up to 30 to 40 electrodes were necessary in extensive cases. Commonly used safe doses range from 0.3 to 5.0 mamp and from 30 to 60 minutes in duration.

Boy, 8, had had soft, irregular masses in the left side of the forehead and frontoparietal region since birth, consisting of markedly dilated, pulsating vessels combined with hemangioma simplex (Fig 1–23). Three dark-red vascular growths were present on the left eyelid. Bruits were heard over the superficial temporal area. Electrothrombosis was carried out at age 6, leading to disappearance of the tortuous masses and of the pulsations. The residual hemangioma simplex and the angiomatous eyelid nodules were removed sur-

(1–52) Plast. Reconstr. Surg. 70:310–318, September 1982.

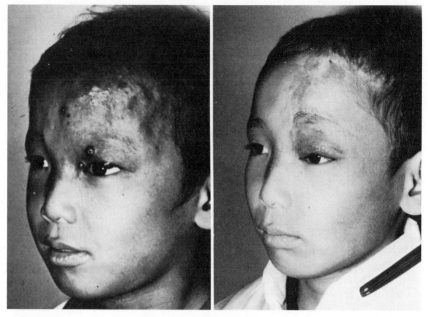

Fig 1-23.—*Left,* arteriovenous malformation with hemangioma simplex before treatment. *Right,* three years after electrothrombosis and excision of medial part (2 cm in width) of forehead. (Courtesy of Ogawa, Y., and Inoue, K.: Plast. Reconstr. Surg. 70:310–318, September 1982.)

gically 2 years later, without marked bleeding. A laterally based flap was raised on the left side of the forehead with the hemangioma simplex in its distal third, and the defect was repaired with an advancement flap. No recurrence has developed in the past 3 years.

Seven patients with cirsoid angioma of the head and neck and 2 with varicosis of the leg were treated by electrothrombosis. Six patients required no further treatment; 3 with angiomas required further operations to reduce the mass to normal size. Prior use of electrothrombosis reduced bleeding significantly in these patients. Electrothrombosis is a simple method that leaves only indistinct scars and imposes much less stress than operation. Accurate electrode placement can be difficult in cases of deep-seated cirsoid angioma. Care is needed to prevent distant embolization

► [An interesting concept. Is it as successful and safe as intravascular embolization? Can it be used in conjunction with intravascular embolization?—S.H.M.] ◄

1-53 **Plastic-surgical Therapy of the Large Facial Port-Wine Stain.** In contrast to true hemangiomas, which are vascular tumors, port-wine stains are vascular malformations consisting of mature telangiectatic vessels in the dermis and the adjacent subcutis. In the case of large facial port-wine stains, no series of patients treated with consistently good results has so far been reported. L. Clodius (Univ. of

(1–53) Schweiz. Med. Wochenschr. 113:274–280, Feb. 26, 1983.

Zürich) treated 50 patients by means of subtotal excision of the nevus flammeus and covered the resultant defects with carefully selected full-thickness skin grafts. Technical difficulties included achievement of complete accretion of the full-thickness skin graft and correct selection of the graft regarding color and texture. The retroauricular and supraclavicular areas are preferred for use in skin grafting. In the 50 patients in this study, 135 full-thickness skin grafts were necessary (2.7 per patient).

The port-wine stain appears clinically as a conspicuous area of red skin of arbitrary size and irregular boundary. The surface becomes elevated and may bleed from slight injuries. When the nevus flammeus involves the upper lip, male patients require, not only normal color of the skin, but also the normal growth of beard (Fig 1–24). A preepilated scalp transplant was used to cover the upper lip defect, which made the bilateral retroauricular skin available for full coverage of the cheek and temple regions.

For the past 14 years, laser therapy has been used and, with the correct light dosage, healing is established without scars. However, the treatment is painful and repeated local anesthetics can be a problem especially for the younger patient. After 40–60 required treatments of larger port-wine stains, significant improvement can be

Fig 1–24.—A, 45-year-old patient with increasing extrusion of vessels of port-wine stain. Excision and reconstruction were accomplished with bilateral retroauricular skin and preepilated scalp. **B,** condition of patient 1½ years after surgery. (Courtesy of Clodius, L.: Schweiz. Med. Wochenschr. 113:274–280, Feb. 26, 1983.)

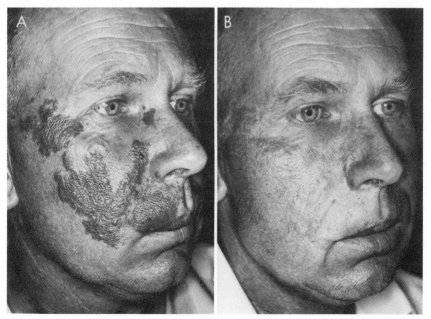

shown, but complete disappearance cannot be obtained. Disadvantages of surgical treatment are general anesthetic, skin transplants and closure of the donor areas, possibility of scars, infection, and mismatching of skin. Hospitalization is also necessary with surgical treatment, whereas the laser treatment can be accomplished on an outpatient basis. Laser and surgical treatments can complement each other; smaller marks can be made satisfactorily lighter by means of laser treatment, whereas the larger nevus flammeus may be treated more successfully with surgery, especially in patients younger than 15 years of age.

Maximal cooperation between physician and patient must be obtained in regard to particular details, such as removal of the affected area, the skin donor areas, the interval between treatments, and type and duration of bandage.

▶ [The use of laser therapy and partial surgical excision in treating these lesions appears to be of benefit. Our experiences with laser therapy are similar, in that it is not the panacea for all port-wine stains.—S.H.M.] ◀

1-54 **Treatment of Capillary-Venous Malformations by Using a New Fibrosing Agent.** Capillary-venous anomalies often are found in the cervicocraniofacial region, usually in the trigeminal distribution. They are low-flow malformations, and embolization does not totally obliterate the anomalous channels. Total excision usually is not possible without sacrificing vital structures. M. C. Riche, E. Hadjean, P. Tran-Ba-Huy, and J. J. Merland (Paris) evaluated the direct percutaneous injection of a new fibrosing material, Ethibloc, a prolamine mixed with ethanol, amidotrizoic acid, and oleum papaveris, in 16 patients aged 6–35 years with capillary-venous malformations.

All but one of the malformations were in the cervicocephalic area; 10 were well-localized lesions. One patient had a diffuse low-flow malformation of an upper extremity. Preliminary angiography usually was not performed. The transverse facial or facial arteries were catheterized superselectively in most cases of cervicofacial malformation. After the artery was temporarily occluded with tiny pieces of dura mater and autogenous clot, the malformation was directly punctured with a No. 21 angiocatheter for injection of the fibrosing material. Usually no more than 1 ml of Ethibloc mixed with 10% alcohol and Duroliopaque was injected at a given site, but 3–4 injections often were necessary to completely fill a malformation. Indomethacin was given for 6 days after the procedure.

The malformation became swollen and hard immediately after the procedure. No skin necrosis or local nerve damage occurred. Excision was delayed for 10–12 days because of the inflammation and swelling (Fig 1–25). Ten lesions were excised, and remarkable delineation of the malformation usually was observed. Chronic inflammation surrounded eosinophilic foreign material within the vessels of the mal-

(1–54) Plast. Reconstr. Surg. 71:607–614, May 1983.

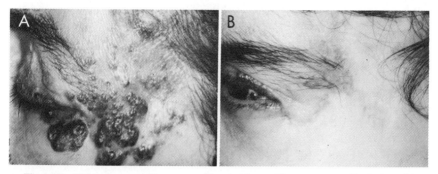

Fig 1–25.—Thirty-five-year-old woman with extensive capillary-venous malformation of fore-head, upper eyelid, and malar region. **A,** before treatment. **B,** 6 months after arterial embolization with dura mater, direct injection of Ethibloc, and excision. (Courtesy of Riche, M. C., et al.: Plast. Reconstr. Surg. 71:607–614, May 1983.)

formation, and numerous thromboses were present. In 6 patients who did not have excision the swelling resolved within 3 weeks of treatment, and further improvement ensued. No long-term skin problems have developed in patients followed up for more than 1 year.

This early experience with the use of Ethibloc to treat capillary-venous malformations by direct injection has been encouraging. Several patients have not required resection. Only low-flow-type malformations should be managed in this way. Radiographic monitoring of the cannula position and the use of external compression are important in insuring that the material solidifies within the malformation. The slow rate of solidification of the material is its chief disadvantage.

▶ [This had exciting potential, but we will await further reports from these authors.—S.H.M.] ◀

1–55 **Surgical Implications of Klippel-Trenaunay Syndrome.** Peter Gloviczki, Larry H. Hollier, Robert L. Telander, Bruce Kaufman, Anthony J. Bianco, and Gunnar B. Stickler (Mayo Clinic and Found.) reviewed the findings in 40 patients seen from 1956 to 1981 with Klippel-Trenaunay syndrome, or osteoangiohypertrophy-type "Klippel-Trenaunay." The term is reserved for limb hypertrophy and varicosity associated with hemangiomas or lymphangiomas, but without arteriovenous (AV) fistula. The 20 males and 20 females had a mean age of 16.8 years when admitted for treatment, 13 were affected at birth. The initial finding was hemangioma in most. The mean length of follow-up was 4½ years. No evidence of genetic transmission of the disease was established. The lower extremity was involved in 38 patients and the upper extremity in 6. All affected extremities were increased in length. Hemanigoma was present in all patients but 1. Five had both hemangioma and lymphangioma. A typical port wine-

(1–55) Ann. Surg. 197:353–362, March 1983.

colored, flat, cutaneous hemangioma was the most frequent finding. Varicosities were marked and significant. Arteriography ruled out AV fistula in the 9 patients examined.

Thirteen patients were treated surgically, 6 having orthopedic procedures. Good functional and esthetic results were obtained in 5 patients. Of the 27 patients managed nonoperatively, 21 presently are in good condition, 4 are in fair condition, 1 is in poor condition, and 1 died of a progressive form of the disease.

The cause of Klippel-Trenaunay syndrome is not known. Treatment is mainly symptomatic, including elastic compression and, in selected patients, varicectomy or transection of fibrous bands. In the future, venous reconstruction may become available for hypoplasia or aplasia of the deep veins. Most patients do not require definitive surgical treatment, but some require surgery to inhibit extreme overgrowth of the affected extremity. Epiphysiodesis or tibial osteotomy should be considered when a marked leg length discrepancy is present.

▶ [While there remains no satisfactory treatment for the underlying pathology of Klippel-Trenaunay syndrome, continuing advances in radiographic techniques and microvascular surgery hold promise for correction in infancy or early childhood, thus avoiding secondary growth aberrations.—F.J.M.] ◀

2. Neoplastic, Inflammatory, and Degenerative Diseases

2–1 **In Favor of Healing by Secondary Intention After Excision of Medial Canthal Basal Cell Carcinoma.** Various reconstructive measures have been used in the management of basal cell carcinoma of the medial canthal region. Rony Moscona, Alon Pnini, and Bernard Hirshowitz (Haifa, Israel) have for 3 years treated tumors of the medial canthus by wide excision only. Eighteen patients with an average age of 45 years were managed in this way. No patient had altered lid function or impaired lacrimal drainage, although there was some postoperative cicatricial change in the shape of the lid, chiefly in younger patients who had wide resections.

Complete extirpation is particularly important in cases of basal cell cancer of the medial canthal region. Hypoxia occurring during lengthy operations can lead to complications in older patients, and sedatives and other premedicants also may add to the risk. Immediate reconstruction should not be attempted when excision has been incomplete or frozen-section histology cannot be obtained, as when bone is involved. Adequate results can be achieved by excising the tumor and permitting the wound to heal by secondary intention. The skin over the medial canthal area is not adherent to subcutaneous structures and is relatively mobile, enhancing wound contraction and formation of a smaller final scar. In young patients with lesions near the lid margins, a relative shortage of skin may predispose to cicatricial ptosis, but this is rare in elderly patients with redundant skin in the region.

▶ [This same philosophy has been successful in several anatomical areas and is most often used by physicians employing Moh's or "fresh tissue chemosurgery." The major disadvantages are the discomfort associated with the open wound, the need for frequent dressing changes, and unsightly scars and irregularities usually requiring reconstructive surgery.—S.H.M.] ◀

2–2 **Statistical Data on Malignant Tumors in Cryosurgery: 1982.** Gloria F. Graham (Univ. of North Carolina, Chapel Hill) reviewed experience with more than 2,500 skin cancers treated by cryosurgery in the past 15 years. The cumulative cure rate was 96%, and the cure rate for new basal cell carcinomas now is approaching 98%. These results are attributed to improved cryosurgical technique, use of a better monitoring system for determining the depth of cold, and bet-

---

(2–1) Plast. Reconstr. Surg. 17:189–195, February 1983.
(2–2) J. Dermatol. Surg. Oncol. 9:238–239, March 1983.

ter patient selection. Lower cure rates have been obtained for tumors more than 2 cm in size and those in the medial canthal region and the nasolabial fold area. The cure rate for tumors of the eyelid in 1980 was 91%. Use of a double freeze for more difficult, deeper cancers and most recurrent cancers has given a cure rate of 94.4%. The cure rate in 58 cases of squamous cell cancer, including six recurrent lesions, was 89.6%. Some of these patients had extensive epidermoid cancers and were referred for palliation.

▶ [This is a modality used by increasing numbers of dermatologists and ophthalmologists. Critical to the success of this method is the size of the lesion and its lateral and horizontal extent; the temperature achieved; the duration of freezing and thawing; and the location. As with other modalities, a successful cure causes tissue necrosis and produces a scar which may or may not be esthetically acceptable.— S.H.M.] ◀

2–3 **Optimal Resection Margin For Cutaneous Malignant Melanoma.** David E. Elder, DuPont Guerry, IV, Richard M. Heiberger, Donato LaRossa, Leonard I. Goldman, Wallace H. Clark, Jr., C. Jean Thompson, Isabel Matozzo, and Marie Van Horn examined the relation between surgical margins and the outcome in a series of 105 patients with histologically confirmed primary malignant melanoma, seen prospectively in 1977. The median follow-up was 3 years. The presence of satellites, or discontinuous tumor deposits within 5 cm of the primary tumor, and of in-transit tumor present beyond 5 cm but still regional, were observed along with the site and time of all recurrences. The modal age group was 40–44 years, and the male-female ratio was 3:2. Forty-four of the 109 primary lesions were intact at presentation. Most primary lesions were of the superficial spreading type. Excision with grafting was done 90 times, and excision with primary closure in 14 cases. Five patients had amputation of a digit. Twenty-eight patients had prophylactic node dissections and 5 had dissection of clinically abnormal nodes.

The crude survival rate after 3 years was 87%, and the disease-free survival rate was 78%. All 16 patients who died of melanoma had documented visceral metastases. No patient had locally recurrent disease; 19 had regional recurrences. All 6 of those with in-transit metastases had minimal operative margins of excision larger than 30 mm. Four of these 6 patients had abnormal nodes. None of the primary tumors were less than 2.15 mm thick, and all tumors were level III or greater. Only 1 of these patients with progressive disease lived beyond 3 years. Satellitosis was found in 5 wide-excision specimens. Four of the primary lesions were of the nodular type and were at Clark level III or greater. All were more than 2.25 mm thick. Three of these 5 patients died, whereas 2 were alive without disease after 3 years.

Survival of these patients with primary malignant melanoma was not dependent on the width of surgical margins. Satellitosis and in-transit cutaneous metastasis occurred only in patients with primary tumors more than 2 mm thick. The findings provide a rationale for wide excision of "thick" melanomas. More modest local treatment seems appropriate for thin cutaneous melanomas.

2–4 **Self-Healing Squamous Epithelioma: A Family Affair** is discussed by Ian T. Jackson, J. O'D. Alexander, and C. N. Verheyden (Glasgow, Scotland). Self-healing squamous epithelioma of the skin was first described by Smith in Glasgow in 1934. It is a familial condition identified in Scottish families and apparently is a heterozygous autosomal dominant condition due to a single autosomal mutation. Cases reported from the United States, Canada, and Australia probably are due to the migration of members of involved families. A total of 80 proved cases are known; 11 families have been shown to be involved.

The first lesion often occurs in adolescence. The sexes are equally affected. Patients have an average of 20 to 25 lesions, but up to 100 have been identified. All stages can be seen in a given case. The face and extremities tend to be involved. Lesions can appear and then resolve for many years. They develop as small red papules, ulcerate, and then heal over several months, leaving a deeply scarred pit. Scars resulting from lesions around the nose and on the ears can be quite disfiguring. A well-differentiated squamous carcinoma is found histologically. The cells appear malignant, but mitoses are infrequent. Invasion of subcutaneous fat and perineural lymphatics is occasionally observed. Metastasis has not been described, and no patient has died of the disease. The tumors can arise from the pilosebaceous follicles or the epidermis, or both. Early excision of the lesions is advisable to obtain the best possible cosmetic results. If subsequent lesions develop near previously healed ones about the nose, mouth, and ears, more extensive reconstructive procedures may become necessary.

This condition is undoubtedly a distinct entity, separable from keratoacanthoma on both clinical and histologic grounds. The similarities to squamous carcinoma are striking except for the multiplicity of lesions, familial features, and absence of metastases. Studies for autoimmune mechanisms have not shown consistent abnormalities.

2–5 **Vascularized Omentum for Facial Contour Restoration.** The use of various free flaps for facial soft tissue augmentation has been limited by difficulties in adequately molding and contouring the flap to fit the defect. Omentum usually is present in sufficient quantity to reconstruct these defects and it can readily be molded to fit a deformity. Marcus Walkinshaw (Univ. of Washington, Seattle), H. Hollis Caffee (Univ. of Florida, Gainesville), and S. Anthony Wolfe (Univ. of Miami) used vascularized omentum for soft tissue facial augmentation in 7 patients in the past 2 years. Four patients had hemifacial

(2–4)   Br. J. Plast. Surg. 36:22–28, January 1983.
(2–5)   Ann. Plast. Surg. 10:292–300, April 1983.

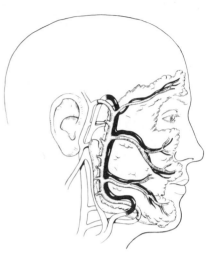

Fig 2–1.—Omental flap sutured in position. (Courtesy of Walkinshaw, M., et al.: Ann. Plast. Surg. 10:292–300, April 1983.)

atrophy, 1 had a variant of hemifacial atrophy known as scleroderma morphia, 1 had a large postablative defect after resection of mandibular fibrosarcoma, and 1 had hemifacial microsomia. Mean follow-up was 8 months.

No major complications occurred in these cases. The technique described by Upton et al. was used to transfer vascularized omentum, except that subcutaneous tunnels were not used for graft fixation. Whenever possible, two vascular pedicles were used, with anastomosis of one end of the pedicle to the facial vessels and of the other to the temporal vessels. Every attempt was made to anastomose more than one vein. Multiple-suture fixation was used, as shown in Figure 2–1. Early postoperative results appear to be quite favorable.

Although a laparotomy is necessary to obtain omentum, most patients requiring the operation are young and have not had previous abdominal surgery. The donor-site deformity is minor. The vascular pedicle of the omentum is quite reliable. Both ends of the vascular pedicle can be used for better graft vascularization. The graft can be trimmed and shaped to adapt to almost any facial defect. It is readily carried to the temporal region, the cheek area, and even down into the neck, all simultaneously. The omentum moves with the mimetic musculature and does not impede normal facial expression. The facial texture over the reconstruction is nearly normal.

▶ [The authors again report the use of omentum, which in spite of their results, has disadvantages. There are other less complex ways of achieving the same results without the disadvantages of the omental free flap.—L.A.W.] ◀

2–6 **Use of Mucosa-Lined Flaps in Eyelid Reconstruction: New Approach.** J. C. van der Meulen (Erasmus Univ.) evaluated the use

(2–6)   Plast. Reconstr. Surg. 70:139–146, August 1982.

of mucosal grafts without cartilaginous support in patients with less than two thirds of the eyelid rim remaining after tumor resection. Grafts are taken from the buccal sulcus, and flaps are raised from the upper to the lower eyelid. Reconstruction of the lower lid with a bipedicled flap from the upper lid is an excellent method. When used in combination with a mucosal graft inserted under some tension, the flap will not curl on itself and sag. A variation consists of reconstruction of the upper eyelid with a mucosal graft and a bipedicled flap from the lower lid. The skin defect in the lower lid is closed with a skin graft from the contralateral upper eyelid. Also effective is reconstruction of lower and upper lids with mucosa-lined monopedicled flaps. These flaps appear to be well vascularized, and healing of the mucosal graft has not been a problem. Cartilaginous support is not needed if the graft is inserted under some tension.

These techniques seem to be preferable to various methods such as transposition of a mucosa-lined flap raised in the area lateral to the outer canthus in reconstruction of the lower lid. This is an elaborate procedure, and rotation may be difficult and requires excision of a skin triangle below the defect. Addition of a Z-plasty to facilitate rotation creates scarring near the lid rim. The tarsoconjunctival flap covered with a skin graft or flap has been abandoned. Composite flap operations may give satisfactory results in experienced hands and in patients with surplus conjunctiva, but contracture may occur in either the donor eyelid or the receptor lid. The simpler methods have restricted reconstructive problems to patients who have been irradiated and those in whom defects in both eyelids must be closed.

▶ [For smaller horizontal defects of the lower eyelid we have favored the use of a composite flap from the upper eyelid. Otherwise, our experiences are similar to the author.—S.H.M.] ◀

2–7　**McCord Procedure for Ectropion Repair.** Some horizontal laxity is present in most ectropion repairs. It usually occurs at the lateral canthal tendon and resection of normal tarsus places more stress on diseased tissue. Ralph E. Wesley and John W. Collins (Vanderbilt Univ.) have used the McCord procedure for ectropion repair, involving an incision at the lateral canthus away from the central margin, resection of the diseased tendon, and adjustment of the position of the lateral canthus with a permanent tarsal periosteal suture.

TECHNIQUE.—After local infiltration of 2% lidocaine with epinephrine and hyaluronidase and corneal anesthesia, a lateral canthotomy is performed as shown in Figure 2–2. Generally, 2 to 3 mm of the full-thickness of the lateral part of the lid is excised. Methylene blue is used to outline the excision. A permanent suture of 4–0 coated polyester is placed as a vertical mattress stitch through the tarsus and through the periosteum inside the orbital rim; the knot is buried internally. The skin is closed with 7–0 silk sutures. If further tightness is necessary postoperatively, the suture can be removed and replaced with local anesthesia.

(2–7)　Arch. Otolaryngol. 109:319–322, May 1983.

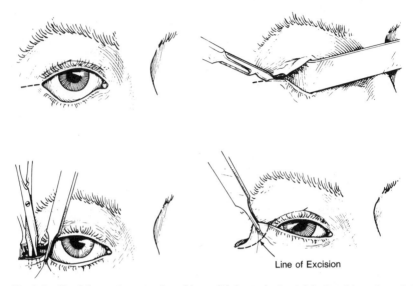

Line of Excision

Fig 2–2.—*Top left,* sagging ectropion of lower lid due to horizontal laxity of lateral canthal tendon. Broken line shows incision. *Top right,* lateral canthotomy performed down to oribital rim periosteum. Malleable retractors are used to protect eye. *(Bottom left,* scissors are used to cut rest of attachments of lower lateral canthus tendon from oribital rim. *Bottom right,* lid is stretched tight to determine amount of lateral part of lid to be resected. (Courtesy of Wesley, R. E., and Collins, J. W.: Arch Otolaryngol. 109:319–322, May 1983; copyright 1983, American Medical Association.)

This operation was done on 85 eyelids in 77 patients, who were followed for 6 to 34 months. A tight lid appearance has not been permanent. Four patients had granuloma formation from the permanent stitch. A permanent suture must be in place for about 2 to 3 months while the tarsoligamentous sling heals. One patient with severe vascular compromise of the face from a previous injury had infection around the stitch; the ectropion did not recur after removal of the stitch. Revision operations were done in 3 patients with artificial eyes; no sagging of the lid followed the second tightening procedure.

This operation is especially useful in patients with an artificial eye who require strong lower lid support. Complications have not been frequent. The procedure is contraindicated in ectropion due to medial canthal tendon laxity.

▶ [This procedure involves an incision at the lateral canthus, resectioning the diseased lateral canthal tendon, and repositioning the lateral canthus to the periosteum at a slightly elevated position. This serves to tighten the lid and position it at a higher level. It appears to be a very nice operation for horizontal laxity of the eyelid with no shortage of tissue.—R.O.B.] ◀

2–8 **Transposition of the Temporalis Muscle into the Anophthalmic Orbit** is described by P. Tessier and D. Krastinova (Suresnes, France). An anterior strip of temporalis muscle is placed in

(2–8) Ann. Chir. Plast. 27:213–220, 1982.

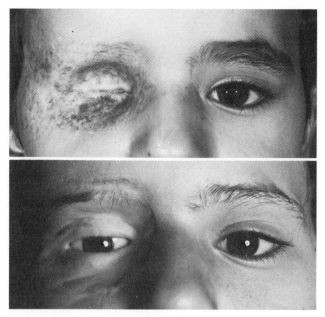

Fig 2–3.—*Left,* Surgical anophthalmia after enucleation and radiotherapy for tumor in 6-year-old patient showing palpebral radiodystrophy and complete atresia of the conjunctival sac without true micro-orbitism. *Right,* same patient after transposition of temporalis muscle showing full-thickness skin graft on both eyelids, skin graft of conjunctival sac, and eyebrow and eyelash graft, with bone graft of zygoma and superciliary arch. (Courtesy of Tessier, P., and Krastinova, D.: Ann. Chir. Plast. 27:213–220, 1982.)

the anophthalmic orbit through a hole drilled in the lateral orbital wall. The temporal muscle flap, applied to the orbital apex, advances the retracted muscle cone, the conjunctival sac, and the eyelids. The outcome in one case is shown in Figure 2–3.

The procedure has been done only in the fairly infrequent cases in which retraction of the muscle cone, conjunctival sac, and eyelids precludes retention of a prosthesis. The procedure is indicated only where these conditions prevent movement of the prosthesis and lid, or when a prosthesis large enough to offset the absence of sclera or an implant is needed. Such conditions are found in patients who have had enucleation some time before, in childhood, for removal of a tumor, and also after radiotherapy.

▶ [This is a clever solution for a difficult problem.—S.H.M.] ◀

2–9 **Treatment of Cranio-Orbital Fibrous Dysplasia** is discussed by Ian T. Jackson, T. Armstrong H. Hide, Patricia K. Gomuwka, Edward R. Laws, Jr., and Keith Langford. Fibrous dysplasia of the skull and orbit may cause progressive facial disfigurement and visual impairment. The condition is believed to represent anomalous bone devel-

(2–9) J. Maxillofac. Surg. 10:138–141, August 1982.

opment. In the cranio-orbital area the process is chiefly fibro-osseous, with predominant bony trabeculae. Spherical masses of bone surrounded by proliferating spindle cells may simulate a psammomatous meningioma. The disease may be monostotic or polyostotic and classically occurs in the first two decades of life, with retarded progress in adult life. Fronto-orbital involvement occurs in 20% of patients. Radiographs generally show opaque areas with a few scattered lucent sections in these cases.

All 4 patients with cranio-orbital fibrous dysplasia had conservative treatment that failed to halt the progress of the disease, even after the first 2 decades of life. All had increasing esthetic deformity, and 2 had functional visual involvement due to encroachment of disease on the optic canal. In 1 patient a previously placed acrylic plate was completely covered by dysplastic tissue. Two patients had forward and lateral displacement of the involved orbit to produce true orbital hypertelorism. The displacement was a result of expansion of the sphenoid and ethmoid sinuses. The gross appearances were due to the nonuniform occurrence of fibrous tissue, bone formation, and hemorrhagic, gelatinous lakes.

These cases suggest that fibrous dysplasia of the cranio-orbital region is an entity distinct from fibrous dysplasia of the maxilla and mandible. Permanent eradication requires total resection of involved tissue, followed by immediate reconstruction. Good results have been obtained without significant complications.

▶ [The authors describe some of the variations of cranial orbital fibrous dysplasia, but its differences appear to be more that of the anatomical location than of the pathologic process itself.—L.A.W.] ◀

2–10 **Steeple Flap Reconstruction of the Lower Lip.** M. F. Stranc and G. A. Robertson (Univ. of Manitoba, Winnipeg) developed a method of lower lip reconstruction as an alternative to nasolabial flap reconstruction to avoid the dog-ear and delayed healing at the flap tip. A full-thickness cheek island flap was designed. The defect is converted to a rectangle with the long border marking the length of excised lip and the short side indicating the height of lip resection (Fig 2–4). A Doppler probe is used to locate and mark the facial artery and its labial branches. When the artery enters the flap at a low point, cheek tissues are tumbled into the lip defect with mucosa along the lateral border cut to excess for reconstruction of the vermilion border. When the artery enters the flap at a high point, the cheek tissues are slid into the lip defect; the mucosa along the medial border of the island is used for reconstruction of the vermilion border.

Six cases were reviewed; 5 patients had lip loss from malignancy, whereas 1 had a gunshot wound. The range in age was 33–80 years. The patients with malignancy had reconstruction as a primary procedure immediately after resection. The only complication was

(2–10) Ann. Plast. Surg. 10:4–11, January 1983.

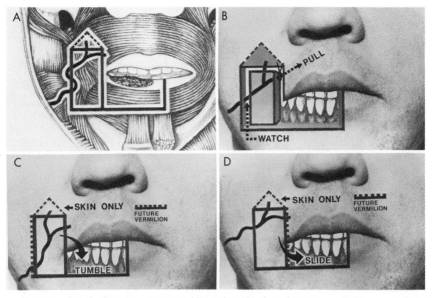

Fig 2–4.—Steeple flap reconstruction of lower lip: **(A)** plan of surgery, and **(B)** maneuver for safe identification of the facial artery. Translocation of the island flap and planning of future vermilion: **(C)** artery enters flap low and cheek tissues are tumbled into lip defect with mucosa along lateral border used for vermilion reconstruction; **(D)** artery enters flap high and cheek tissues are slid into lip defect with mucosa along the medial border used for vermilion reconstruction. (Courtesy of Stranc, M. F., and Robertson, G. A.: Ann. Plast. Surg. 10:4–11, January 1983.)

slightly delayed healing in an 80-year-old patient. Significant microstomia did not develop in any patient during follow-up for 2–27 months. Three patients had a 50% or greater recovery of sensation. All patients had evidence of motor activity after clinical examination, which increased during the follow-up interval. Dribbling of fluids was a definite problem in the oldest patient. All patients except 1 were pleased with the appearance of the reconstructed lip. Slightly delayed healing at the junction of the two steeple flaps produced an irregular contour in this instance.

This simple method of lower lip reconstruction permits total lip reconstruction in one stage. Like other methods using locally available tissues, it is unsuitable for use in simultaneous lower lip resection and reconstruction when nodes in the neck have to be taken in continuity.

▶ [Further studies in more patients will be necessary in order to evaluate this technique. Although microstomia did not seem to be a problem, oral continence was a problem in 4 of 6 patients.—S.H.M.] ◀

2–11   **Reconstruction of the Lower Lip.** Resection of part or all of the lower lip often is necessary for squamous carcinoma. Even modified

---

(2–11) Br. J. Plast. Surg. 36:40–47, January 1983.

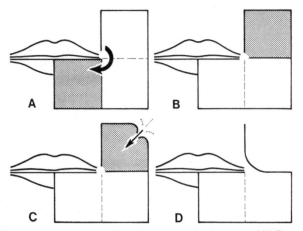

Fig 2–5.—Schematic drawing of modified single fan flap. (Courtesy of McGregor, I. A.: Br. J. Plast. Surg. 36:40–47, January 1983.)

forms of the Bernard procedure tend to leave a tight lower lip and a redundancy of the upper lip. Ian A. McGregor (Glasgow, Scotland) has used a modification of the classic Gillies fan flap to reconstruct full-thickness defects of the lower lip.

In this procedure the defect is designed almost as a square (Fig 2–5) and usually consists of half of the lip. A vertical full-thickness cheek flap is outlined just lateral to the lip defect. The part of the rectangle outlined on the cheek corresponds to the back cut of the classic flap. The narrow pedicle of the rectangular flap contains the superior labial vessels. The pedicle stays in place as a pivot point around which the rectangle is rotated 90 degrees to fill the lip defect. The flap is sutured in position in layers, and the secondary defect is closed by bringing its upper outer angle downward and medially toward the angle of the mouth. A "lip-shave" can also be carried out where there are premalignant changes in the vermilion. A red margin is best created by using a tongue flap.

This approach can be applied to defects of the entire lower lip. It is most successful when a well-marked nasolabial fold is present. Like the classic fan flap, the flap is denervated. This disadvantage has been eliminated by the neurovascular fan flap of Karapandzic. Considerable functional reintegration is, however, possible with the present approach. A minor cosmetic defect may result from a tendency toward development of a slight convexity. The chief advantage of the method is the freedom provided the surgeon to carry out a prophylactic lip shave when premalignant changes are present in addition to a focus of frank carcinoma. Defects of the whole lower lip can be reconstructed by this method.

▶ [This technique borrows tissue from a similar donor area, as does the Stranc paper. In large defects, microstomia still results. The tongue flap appears to have been taken from the dorsum of the tongue and is not as esthetically pleasing as mucosal replacement from the sides of the tongue. The return of motor function in some of these flaps is heartening.—S.H.M.] ◄

2–12 **Paralysis of the Mandibular Branch of the Facial Nerve** is discussed by John Conley, Daniel C. Baker, and Robert W. Selfe (New York). Damage to the marginal mandibular branch of the facial nerve leads to inability to draw the lower lip down and laterally or to evert the vermilion border. When smiling, the paralyzed side of the lower lip is pulled up and flattened, and inwardly rotated by the elevator muscles of the upper lip. Tumors arising in the area of the nerve or its regional muscles nearly always require sacrifice of the facial nerve. Large benign tumors, inflammatory disease, and severe trauma also place the nerve at risk. When paresis occurs unexpectedly after operation, most cases are best managed by observation in the hope that the nerve has merely been traumatized and movement will return spontaneously. Complete regeneration follows total lysis of the mandibular branch in only about 15% of cases. Surgical treatment consists of transposing the tendon of the subdigastric muscle into the lower lip with an intact nerve and blood supply to the anterior belly of the muscle, which remains attached to the inner aspect of the mandible. A submandibular approach is used. The two strips of split tendon are sutured to the orbicularis oris at its middle or inferior border.

Thirty-six patients had this operation in a 10-year period; 22 had an immediate procedure and 14 after a delay. Thirty-three patients had a satisfactory result, with an effective antagonistic counterbalance in the lower lip against the pull of the elevator muscles of the upper lip. The best results were obtained in 6 patients in whom only the depressors on one side were paralyzed. The results in patients having immediate operation after resection of the main lower division of the facial nerve or its mandibular branch compared favorably with those obtained in patients having segmental nerve grafting or segmental transposition of the masseter muscle.

Transfer of the anterior belly of the digastric muscle and its tendon is a direct, simple means of rehabilitating patients who have had resection of the mandibular branch of the facial nerve. The transfer should be done as part of the primary operation in ablative resections. In esthetic procedures or when the status of the nerve is not specifically known, a delay of 3–6 months is appropriate to seek spontaneous return of function.

► [An excellent addition to the armamentarium of the surgeon.—S.H.M.] ◄

2–13 **Mandibular Osteotomy in the Surgical Approach to the Oral Cavity** is discussed by Ian A. McGregor and D. Gordon MacDonald (Glasgow, Scotland). Improved stability from the combination of K-

(2–12) Plast. Reconstr. Surg. 70:569–577, November 1982.
(2–13) Head Neck Surg. 5:457–462, May–June 1983.

wire transfixion of a mandibular osteotomy and direct wiring has made it possible to use a straight, rather than a stepped, bone cut and to avoid dental extractions in some instances. In addition, the osteotomy can be made just anterior to the mental foramen, allowing mandibular swing after division of the mucosa and the mylohyoid muscle only. This approach is best combined with a modified lip-splitting incision.

A better cosmetic outcome is achieved if the incision follows the contours of the lip and chin. The incision begins in the center of the lip and stops in the hollow just above the chin prominence, then follows the curve around the base of the prominence to the submental region. The osteotomy is made in the body of the mandible immediately behind the insertion of the anterior belly of the digastric muscle. The mucosa and the mylohyoid muscle are divided to "swing" the mandible laterally. The genioglossus, geniohyoid, and digastric muscles are left intact.

The exposure provided by this osteotomy is virtually the same as that provided by symphyseal osteotomy, and the two sites are equally easy to stabilize by the combined interosseous wire–K-wire transfixion method. Relatively little soft tissue damage is produced. A stepped osteotomy adds to the overall stability of the reconstructed bone, but the addition of K-wire transfixion provides excellent stabilization of the straight osteotomy. The symphyseal site may be advantageous when tumor extends toward the anterior floor of the mouth, but with a more posterior lesion, the alternative site may be preferable.

▶ [In the severely atrophic mandible we have had more success with direct wiring and an external fixation device, using several K-wires inserted on either side of the fracture and secured to each other with cold cure acrylic or methylmethacrylate.—S.H.M.] ◀

2–14 **Bone Repair in the Mandible: Histologic and Biometric Comparison Between Rigid and Semirigid Fixation.** Monty Reitzik and Willem Schoorl (Univ. of British Columbia, Vancouver) undertook such a comparison of internal fixation of the fractured mandible, where a small interfragmentary gap was maintained and maxillomandibular immobilization was not used. A 0.75-mm defect was produced by transecting the mandible of African green monkeys from the retromolar pad to the antegonial notch. The fragments were fixed with .025 mandibular mesh and 5-mm screws of cobalt-chrome alloy. Four screws were used for rigid fixation on one side and two for semirigid fixation on the other.

All 10 fracture sites were grossly healing well at evaluation. Large excrescences of external callus were present on the side of semirigid fixation. The callus appeared quite vascular compared with the surrounding bone. All specimens were refractured through the original

(2–14) J. Oral Maxillofac. Surg. 41:215–218, April 1983.

defect on biometric testing. The rigidly fixed sites were twice as strong as the semirigidly fixed sites. Histologic studies confirmed the presence of much periosteal callus on the side of semirigid fixation, especially medially where interfragmentary movement was greatest. Laterally, movement was restricted to rotation about a transverse axis by the mandibular mesh and less periosteal callus was evident. At sites of rigid fixation, the woven bone filling the cortical defect and marrow spaces was oriented radially at a right angle to the long axis of the bone and was endosteal in origin. The endochondral bone plug was dense, with relatively few vessel spaces present.

Gap healing occurs in cortical and cancellous mandibular bone when rigid fixation is used and there is a very small defect. The cortical bone defect is replaced by mature lamellar bone. Gap healing with endosteal bone is consistently stronger than secondary bone healing, with considerable periosteal bone present at 6 weeks. Reorientation of the "gap bundles" to conform with the rest of the mandible probably is triggered by stress and coincides with the return of the bone to full strength.

2–15   **Oral Implant For Maxillofacial Reconstruction** is described by Harvey Lash, David B. Apfelberg, and Morton R. Maser (Palo Alto Med. Clinic, Calif.). Silicone was used to act as a periodontal membrane in animal studies. Anchorage to bone was provided by ceramic with a 50- to 100-micropore opening. A female sleeve for placement of a dowel pin was used to hold the dental device, whether it was tooth or denture. Vitallium was chosen to comprise the sleeve. Dacron was used for a gingival seal to prevent formation of pockets. The prosthetic socket is illustrated in Figure 2–6. After incising the edentulous gingiva at the crest, appropriate flaps were developed to expose the underlying bone, which was prepared to receive the implant. An exact bony fit is not essential, since stability depends on ingrowth of osteoid material rather than mechanical fixation. The Vitallium sleeve was exposed after 6 weeks, a core of overlying gingiva was removed by a 3-mm punch biopsy, and the dowel pin was placed in position. Impressions were taken, a dowel pin shield was placed on the post, and dental models were poured and articulated. A crown or prosthesis can be produced on the dowel pin, which was cemented into the Vitallium sleeve of the socket.

Patients with a missing mandibular third molar were first chosen for trial of this prosthesis. The first patient in whom a standard preparation was possible was successfully treated, and has used the prosthetic molar for full mastication without difficulty for 30 months. This approach will hopefully prove helpful to patients whose remaining oral structures make adequate anchorage impractical.

▶ [Can these implants be used to replace several adjacent teeth or an entire arch, or can they provide teeth in a bone graft that will replace the mandible?—S.H.M.] ◀

(2–15) Ann. Plast. Surg. 9:278–281, October 1982.

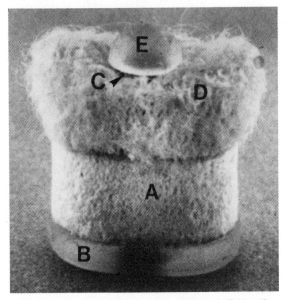

Fig 2–6.—Completed prosthetic socket showing outer ceramic shell *(A)*, silicone shock absorber *(B)*, Vitallium sleeve *(C)*, partially hidden by Dacron cap *(D)*, for attachment of gingiva, and silicone button *(E)*, to protect Vitallium sleeve from ingrowth of tissue until tooth is placed. (Courtesy of Lash, H., et al.: Ann. Plast. Surg. 9:278–281, October 1982.)

2–16 **Lateral Pectoral Composite Flap in One-Stage Reconstruction of the Irradiated Mandible.** John W. Little III, David T. McCulloch, and James R. Lyons (Georgetown Univ.) describe a lateral pectoral composite flap, or pectoralis major-pectoralis-minor osteomusculocutaneous flap, used in reconstructing the irradiated mandible. It is based on the thoracoacromial axis and includes parts of the pectoralis major and minor muscles, a section of the bony fifth rib, and an inframammary skin island. Total division of the pectoralis major muscle is not necessary.

Planning of the incisions is illustrated in Figure 2–7. A sizable paddle is necessary if both lining and cover are absent. Specific tailoring of the island is done at the "fitting in" stage. The skin island is incised down to underlying muscle at all margins. If replacement of the symphysis is necessary, burred grooves are made through the concave cortical rib surface. Skin islands have replaced lining from the hypopharyngeal level to the anterior floor of the mouth, tongue, and cheek. A chest tube is used for larger pleural defects.

This approach has been used to transfer the bony fifth rib to the mandible in 8 patients in the past 2 years. All but 1 of the patients had received large doses of radiation to the head and neck region.

(2–16) Plast. Reconstr. Surg. 71:326–335, March 1983.

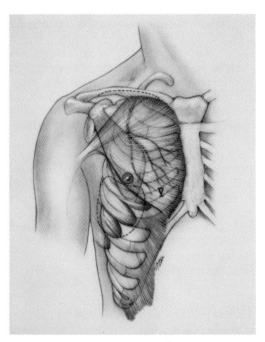

Fig 2–7.—Planned incisions for reconstruction of irradiated mandible. (Courtesy of Little, J. W., III: Plast. Reconstr. Surg. 71:326–335, March 1983.)

Many of the reconstructions followed excisions of massive, often recurrent cancer. Total flap loss in an early case was due to technical error. Another flap had marginal skin loss. In all patients reconstruction was essentially without complications, and a solid, united mandible with good range of motion and residual occlusion was gained. Three patients remain alive without tumor. The patient with total flap loss was 1 of the 2 having total division of the pectoralis major muscle. The others had skeletonized pedicles that spared the overlying pectoralis major.

The pectoralis major can be largely spared with this composite flap approach to mandibular reconstruction. The complication rate has been acceptable despite use of the technique in cases of massive tumor with previous radiation therapy. A thin pedicle has proved as effective as a bulky muscular one in protecting the irradiated carotid artery.

▶ [Both of these techniques offer a means to reconstruct severe orofacial and soft tissue deformities. Please note the careful patient selection in Mr. Taylor's series (see abstract 2–18), and take heed. While Dr. Little's technique might appeal to a larger number of reconstructive surgeons, it is a difficult dissection. A "mock surgery" on cadavers is probably warranted before an attempt on patients.—S.H.M.] ◀

2–17 **New Concept in the Treatment of Osteoradionecrosis.** Pre-

(2–17) J. Oral Maxillofac. Surg. 41:351–357, June 1983.

vious unsuccessful conservative surgical and nonoperative approaches to osteoradionecrosis of the jaws have failed to confront the basic pathophysiology of the condition. An area of irradiated bone and mucosa that breaks down has much greater oxygen and metabolic demands than before injury. Hyperbaric oxygenation has been reported to be an effective adjunctive measure in osteoradionecrosis. Robert E. Marx (Lackland Air Force Base) has developed a program incorporating both hyperbaric oxygen therapy and aggressive surgery and evaluated it in 58 patients with "refractory" osteoradionecrosis of the mandible.

Initially, 100% oxygen at 2.4 atm was given 5 days a week for 90 minutes for a total of 30 treatments. If definite improvement resulted, a course of 30 more treatments was completed. Otherwise a transoral alveolar sequestrectomy was carried out with primary mucosal closure, and hyperbaric treatments were then continued. Patients with wound dehiscence had resectional therapy and stabilization of the mandibular segments by extraskeletal pin fixation or maxillomandibular fixation. Hyperbaric treatments were continued up to a total of 60 or until a healthy mucosal closure was achieved. Subsequently, bone graft reconstruction was carried out from a strictly transcutaneous approach.

All 58 patients responded, with resolution of pain, retention or reconstruction of mandibular continuity, restoration of mandibular function, and maintenance of intact mucosa over all bone surfaces. Follow-up was for at least 18 months. More than two thirds of the patients required resection and reconstructive surgery. These patients received an average of 108 hours of hyperbaric oxygen therapy, including 45 hours of therapy associated with reconstruction. Patients who did not require resection received an average of 90 hours of hyperbaric oxygen therapy.

A progressive regimen of hyperbaric oxygen therapy and surgery is a successful means of treating persistent osteoradionecrosis of the mandible. Antibiotics, irrigation, and nutritional support remain important adjunctive aspects of the care of these patients.

▶ [Does hyperbaric oxygenation add to adequate surgical debridement and coverage of the defects with good blood-bearing soft tissue? Does its use limit the eventual amount of bone loss? Is it cost-effective? This concept sorely needs a controlled animal model or clinical model or both, with measurements of tissue (including bone) oxygen tension levels to demonstrate its true worth.—S.H.M.] ◀

2–18 **Reconstruction of the Mandible With Free Composite Iliac Bone Grafts** is discussed by G. Ian Taylor (Melbourne). A free composite graft of iliac bone with appropriate soft tissue attachments, transferred in one stage by microvascular technique, offers a feasible approach to jaw reconstruction when the bone defect is large or previous procedures have failed. When designing the graft on the deep

(2–18) Ann. Plast. Surg. 9:361–376, November 1982.

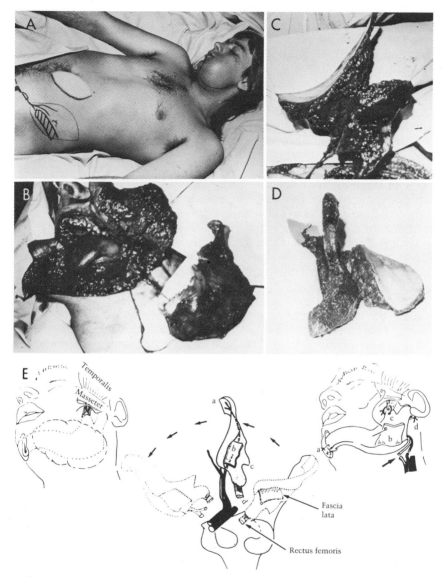

Fig 2–8.—**(A)** Incisions marked on jaw and hip of same side of patient; **(B)** resection of tumor; **(C)** composite graft isolated on deep circumflex iliac vessels; **(D)** graft shaped and prepared for revascularization. **(E)** Diagram of procedure showing soft tissue and bony refinements used to reconstruct the chin *(a)*, to reattach muscles of mastication *(b* and *c)*, and to reconstitute capsule of temporomandibular joint *(d)*. (Courtesy of Taylor, G. I.: Ann. Plast. Surg. 9:361–376, November 1982.)

circumflex iliac vessels, the entire iliac crest and most of the blade of the ilium are available. Experience in 8 cases in which an associated defect of mucosa or skin was present has been encouraging. The ramus and body of the mandible were reconstructed in 5 cases, and in 3 of them the graft was extended across the midline, incorporating a step or wedge osteotomy to reconstitute the chin. In 3 cases the body or central segment of the mandible was reconstructed; in 1 the jaw was replaced from angle to angle. A soft tissue defect was present in all cases. Seven patients had had tumor resection, and 2 had heavy irradiation. In 4 patients, defects were repaired at the time of resection. One patient was treated for hemifacial microsomia.

Grafts ranged as large as 21 × 7 cm in these cases, and skin flaps were as large as 27 × 14 cm. Donor sites were closed with minimal contour deformity of the hip. The ramus of the jaw can be designed from the iliac crest to avoid a wedge or step osteotomy, but this graft provides only a short body segment. The graft is contoured to match a methyl methacrylate model before the vascular pedicle is divided. When necessary, the outer cortex and rim of the iliac crest are removed to provide an exact replica of the jaw. The procedure is illustrated in Figure 2–8.

The free osteocutaneous graft based on the deep circumflex iliac vessels provides a large block of living composite tissue. The bone, lining, external skin, and other soft tissue attachments of the mandible can be repaired in one stage. The subcutaneous pedicle affords considerable flexibility to the skin flap in relation to the underlying bone. The color match is poor, but preferable to scarring of the forehead. The procedure has been reserved for young patients with a good prognosis and those for whom the alternative was discouraging.

2–19 **Maxillofacial Prosthetics** are discussed by Augustus J. Valauri (New York Univ. Med. Center, New York). Prosthetic support is necessary in cases of gunshot wounds of the face with tissue destruction and disorganization. Prostheses are used to maintain facial form and contour and to restore such facial features as the nose (Fig 2–9), auricle, and orbital region when reconstructive surgery is not feasible. Prosthetic restoration of missing parts may be indicated in traumatic deformities when surgery cannot be expected to give satisfactory functional or esthetic results. Skull defects may be restored with a prosthesis when bone grafting is contraindicated. Prostheses often are used temporarily or transitionally before or during surgical treatment to maintain tissues during healing. Either solid or soft, flexible material can be used in fabricating a facial prosthesis. Surgical restoration of the mobile parts of the face is preferred before inserting a rigid type of appliance. Prostheses in the region of the oral or nasal cavity also must rest on a base of healthy tissue.

A facial prosthesis can be removed for postoperative examination

(2–19) Aesth. Plast. Surg. 6:159–164, 1982.

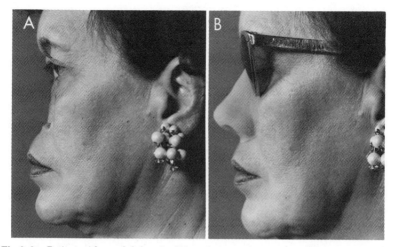

Fig 2–9.—Patient with nasal deformity *(A)*; patient wearing nasal prosthesis made of silicone *(B)*. (Courtesy of Valauri, A. J.: Aesth. Plast. Surg. 6:159–164, 1982.)

of the site. Fitting requires no lengthy hospitalization, and the patient can be made presentable shortly after a surgical deformity is incurred. There is no ideal material for external maxillofacial prostheses, but materials such as silicone rubber and vinyl plastics show promise. Several methods of coloring and tinting have been developed. A combination of rigid and elastic impression materials produces the best results. A dental stone cast is used as the foundation. The flexible prosthesis usually is retained by medical-grade adhesives. Mechanical aids may be necessary in some cases. Patients should be advised on methods of retention. The use of cosmetics may be helpful to some patients. External facial prostheses are expensive, and they tend to deteriorate in time. The possibility of detachment exists, especially with auricular prostheses. When possible, surgical reconstruction is preferable in cases of extensive loss of the nose or ear.

▶ [This paper needs to be read in its entirety. There are situations in which we need to consider prosthetics rather than surgical reconstruction.—R.O.B.] ◀

2–20 **Analysis of Morbidity Following Major Head and Neck Surgery with Particular Reference to Mouth Function.** Eugene David Vaughan (London) reviewed the outcome in 50 patients who underwent major surgery for cancer of the head and neck. Twenty patients had tongue carcinoma, and 5 of them received chemotherapy. Radiotherapy was used in 14 of these cases, generally with a curative dose of 6,000 R or more. All the patients were operated on. Three of 9 patients with carcinoma of the lower alveolus received chemotherapy, and 5, radiotherapy. Full composite resection was done in 7

(2–20) J. Maxillofac. Surg. 10:129–134, August 1982.

cases. Two of 7 patients with cancer of the floor of the mouth had chemotherapy, and 5 received curative doses of radiotherapy before surgery. Four had composite resections without flap repair. Two of 6 patients with cancer of the maxilla and maxillary antrum received chemotherapy, and 4, curative radiotherapy. All had prosthetic replacement after surgery. Two of the 5 patients with malignant tumors of the salivary gland received radiotherapy. There were single cases of maxillary osteosarcoma, mandibular fibrosarcoma, and massive ameloblastoma. Distant pedicle flap reconstruction was undertaken in many cases. Where appropriate, lost tissue was replaced by a prosthesis.

The subjective outcome was one of reasonable satisfaction in 33% of cases. About 25% of patients considered the results to be excellent. The objective results were excellent in 20% of cases, reasonable in 40%, and poor in 40%. Only 46% of patients found oral sphincter incompetence to be a major problem. Taste was severely compromised in 33% of cases. Two-thirds of patients were confined to a liquid diet. Half weighed significantly less than normal and were unable to increase their weight. Nearly 80% of patients had severe difficulty chewing, and 70% had severe disruption of the occlusion. Considerable difficulty in swallowing was experienced in 25% of the patients. Speech was poor in nearly 50% of the cases. Only 10% of patients had evidence of disordered temporomandibular joint function.

Serious problems in oral function and social adaptation follow major surgery of the head and neck. Relatives have a critical role in the psychological rehabilitation of patients. Both disfigurement and speech difficulties tend to isolate the patients. Speech therapy should be an integral part of rehabilitation, along with nutritional care. A maxillofacial prosthodontist also is needed in these cases.

▶ [The purpose of this paper is to quantify social and occupational rehabilitation following head and neck surgery. The failure to adequately demonstrate good masticatory and speech rehabilitation in this small number of patients suggests a need to look more closely at each failure and to modify techniques of reconstruction when possible.—S.H.M.] ◀

2–21 **Cis-Platinum and 5-Fluorouracil as Induction Therapy for Advanced Head and Neck Cancer.** The treatment of advanced squamous cancers of the head and neck region has generally been disappointing, but recent multidrug protocols have produced a significant response in previously untreated patients. Arthur Weaver, Susan Flemming, Julie Kish, Henry Vandenberg, John Jacob, John Crissman, and Muhyi Al-Sarraf (Wayne State Univ.) evaluated induction chemotherapy in 61 patients with stage III and stage IV squamous carcinomas of the head and neck. All had measurable local disease without distant metastases and were candidates for cytotoxic drug therapy. Administration of 12.5 gm of mannitol was followed by

(2–21) Am. J. Surg. 144:445–448, October 1982.

an intravenous bolus of 100 mg of cis-platinum per sq m and then an infusion of mannitol in dextrose-saline with potassium chloride added. The patient then received 1 gm of 5-fluorouracil per sq m daily by 24-hour infusion in dextrose-saline for 120 hours. Allopurinol was also given. Two subsequent courses were given at 3-week intervals or when toxicity subsided.

Nine patients had multiple primary lesions. Many were considered to be inoperable. A complete tumor response occurred in 54% of patients and a partial response in 39%. Three other patients had a minimal response, and 1 had no change. Thirteen patients with a complete response subsequently underwent surgical resection, and 9 of them had no histologic evidence of tumor. Biopsy specimens taken from 8 other patients before radiotherapy showed no residual tumor. Fifteen patients who had subtotal responses underwent resection. Twenty-three patients had radiotherapy only after induction chemotherapy. Toxicity from chemotherapy was acceptable. Four patients had severe and 1 had life-threatening hematologic toxicity. Only 3 patients failed to complete all three courses of chemotherapy.

Over half the patients in this study with advanced head and neck cancers had a complete clinical response to induction chemotherapy with cis-platinum and 5-fluorouracil, and over 90% of the patients had a significant response. Several patients refused operation after their disease disappeared. The results are encouraging, but it is too early to draw conclusions.

▶ [The data presented in this article require further substantiation and a further determination of whether induction or adjuvant chemotherapy increases survival. Preliminary data from our Head and Neck Tumor service at the Veterans Administration Hospital of Portland does not confirm these superb response rates.—S.H.M.] ◀

2–22 **Adjuvant Chemotherapy in Advanced Head and Neck Cancer: Update.** Monica B. Spaulding, Anjum Kahn, Rafael De Los Santos, Douglas Klotch, and John M. Loré, Jr. (SUNY at Buffalo) treated 48 patients, who had previously untreated advanced squamous carcinomas of the head and neck, with cis-platinum, vincristine, and bleomycin. All patients but one had resectable lesions. One patient died of myocardial infarction after the first course of therapy. An infusion of 80 mg of cis-platinum per sq m was given after hydration with dextrose in saline plus potassium chloride and in conjunction with mannitol. Vincristine was given in a dose of 1.4 mg/sq m up to 2 mg, followed by an infusion of 15 mg of bleomycin per sq m daily for 5 days. Chemotherapy was repeated after 3 weeks, and operation was performed 2 to 14 days after its completion. Irradiation was given 2 to 3 weeks after the end of chemotherapy. Forty-three patients were operated on. Four received postoperative radiotherapy, and 4 patients who were not operated on were irradiated.

Eleven tumors disappeared, and 33 others responded partially.

(2–22) Am. J. Surg. 144:432–436, October 1982.

Only one lesion failed to respond. Nineteen patients had stage II disease or better after chemotherapy, and none of them has had a relapse. Nine of the 24 patients who still had stage III or stage IV disease had relapses. Three of the 4 patients given postoperative radiotherapy had relapses. The chemotherapy was well tolerated. Renal impairment was reversible in all instances. There was only one minor episode of myelosuppression, and no pulmonary complications occurred. Twelve patients had recurrent tumor, all within 18 months of initial operation. Twenty-seven patients were without disease for 14 to 42 months after operation. Nine patients had cancers elsewhere.

Dramatic responses of advanced squamous cancers of the head and neck to chemotherapy with cis-platinum, vincristine, and bleomycin have been observed. Whether high response rates will be associated with improved survival remains to be determined. Irradiation apparently need not always be given postoperatively.

2–23 **Head and Neck Cancer in the Elderly.** Moo Young Jun, Elliot W. Strong, Eric I. Saltzman, and Frank P. Gerold (Memorial Sloan-Kettering Cancer Center, New York) reviewed experience with 159 patients aged 80 to 95 years who had head and neck cancer, including 15 with recurrent tumors.

Cancer arising in the oral cavity was the most frequent, followed by laryngeal and pharyngeal cancers. Tumors of the salivary glands, paranasal sinuses, and thyroid also were seen. Epidermoid carcinoma was by far the most common malignancy. Twelve patients also had other malignancies at admission, and 15 had a history of past malignant disease. Six patients developed new primary cancers during follow-up, 2 in the head and neck region. Major medical illness was present in 77% of patients, and 11.3% had incapacitating systemic illness that constantly threatened life.

Resection was the most common management, being performed in 74.8% of cases alone and with radiation therapy in another 7½%. Radiation therapy alone was used in 14.4% of cases. Hospital mortality after surgery was 5.3%. Resections requiring entry into the pharynx carried a relatively high mortality. The rate of local recurrence after resection of primary lesions was 7.5%. About 10% of patients died of malignancy during follow-up. Average survival after surgical treatment alone for primary head and neck lesions was 41 months. Overall average survival of patients treated for primary lesions of the head and neck was 3 years. Patients with earlier stages of disease had significantly better survival than those with more advanced disease.

Many elderly patients with carcinoma of the head and neck region in this series had associated medical illnesses. Frequently the cancers were in advanced stages at presentation. An absolute survival of 36 months for all treated patients and 41 months for all surgically

(2–23) Head Neck Surg. 5:376–382, May–June 1983.

treated patients suggests that surgical treatment is worthwhile in these cases. Careful preoperative staging, evaluation of medical illness, and skillful operative and postoperative management will minimize operative morbidity and mortality. Management must be individualized. There is little reason for a nihilistic attitude, even in elderly patients.

▶ [The patient who has reached the age of 80 has far more chance to live to be 100 than does the patient who is 50. Surgical mortality and morbidity in the elderly can be minimized by attention to detail. With increasing numbers of elderly cancer patients facing certain death from malignant disease, age should not be a contraindication to surgical treatment.—S.H.M.] ◀

2–24 **Breast Esthetics When Reconstructing With the Latissimus Dorsi Musculocutaneous Flap** are discussed by D. Ralph Millard, Jr. (Univ. of Miami). When a latissimus dorsi musculocutaneous flap reconstruction is planned, the mastectomy scar is best placed low and transversely in the inframammary line or in a lateral oblique position running from the axilla into the inframammary line. Ideally, the skin part of the flap is inserted along the axis of the mastectomy scar. The shape of the muscle flap depends chiefly on the shape of the patient's latissimus dorsi muscle. The skin island must be placed far enough posteriorly for the muscle pendulum to swing its island from the fixed anterior humeral attachment and fit easily into the chest

Fig 2–10.—*Top left*, woman, 59, with high, tight, transverse scar after left modified radical mastectomy. *Top right*, latissimus dorsi musculocutaneous flap marked with elliptical skin island showing dart extension. *Bottom left*, skin island has been cut. *Bottom center*, flap has been transposed to breast area with dart in position. *Bottom right*, result after lift and implant on right and areola and half-nipple graft from right to left breast. (Courtesy of Millard, D. R., Jr.: Plast. Reconstr. Surg. 70:161–171, August 1982.)

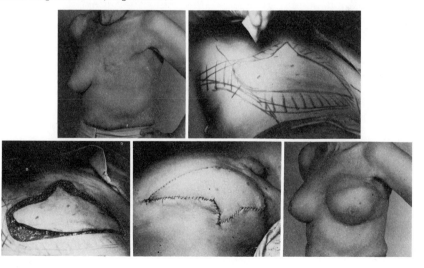

(2–24)   Plast. Reconstr. Surg. 70:161–171, August 1982.

skin defect. Projection is most desirable at the point of the nipple. The author has been reasonably satisfied with the round, gel-filled Mc-Ghan type of implant. A transverse donor scar is most desirable.

If the most desirable mastectomy scars are unavailable, a transverse oblique scar is acceptable since its medial part can be hidden under a brassiere. The midvertical mastectomy scar is less desirable. In some patients in whom the scar is good and the skin slack, the mastectomy scar can be ignored in preference to an inframammary insertion of the skin island. When the vertical scar must be excised, a teardrop diamond shape is best for breast contour with projection at the nipple site. If a high transverse mastectomy scar is unacceptable and the opposite breast is lacking in projection, a simple elliptical skin island may be best. If projection is desired, a diamond-shaped skin island is helpful. In some high, tight transverse scars the upper or lower edges of the wound may be unusually tight, threatening a crease, and an ellipse or diamond with a dart may aid breast shaping (Fig 2–10). If a transverse scar is excellent and the skin reasonably slack, inframammary insertion of the skin island may be advantageous, but its shape might be better as a flat pie wedge than as an ellipse, depending on the projection of the opposite breast.

▶ [Refinements such as those described here may be helpful; however, placement of back skin and a scar that is high on the breast can be distressful for some patients.—S.H.M.] ◀

2–25 **Self-Inflating Tissue Expander.** The ability to induce excessive full-thickness skin or mucosal development adjacent to a defect holds much promise for the reconstructive surgeon. Eric David Austad and Gregory L. Rose (Univ. of Michigan) developed a device that self-inflates with extracellular water via an osmotic gradient. It consists of a sealed, semipermeable membrane "shell" that envelops a substance (e.g., sodium chloride) that can create an osmotic gradient across the implant wall. The silicone shells of testicular prostheses were used in initial studies. The effects of sodium chloride on the rate of inflation are shown in Figure 2–11, and the relationship between membrane thickness and inflation rate in Figure 2–12. Histologic studies were done in guinea pigs using an 18-cc implant containing a saturating load of NaCl. No significant inflammatory response was provoked by the implants, and a thin, fibrous "capsule" was formed. There were no dysplastic or metaplastic changes. No increase in epithelial mitotic activity was noted in up to 18 weeks of observation. Hair follicle morphology remained normal.

Two patients underwent implantation of self-inflating tissue expanders. A girl aged 15 with iatrogenic left breast agenesis and moderate hypertrophy of the right breast, who had very taut skin over the left hemithorax, received a 300-cc implant containing an isotonic level of NaCl on the left. The partially filled implant was removed 12 weeks

(2–25) Plast. Reconstr. Surg. 70:588–593, November 1982.

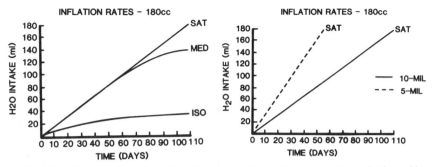

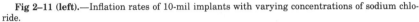

Fig 2–11 (left).—Inflation rates of 10-mil implants with varying concentrations of sodium chloride.

Fig 2–12 (right).—Inflation rates are inversely related to membrane thickness.

(Courtesy of Austad, E. D., and Rose, G. L.: Plast. Reconstr. Surg. 70:588–593, November 1982.)

later and replaced by a standard gel-filled prosthesis; reduction mammaplasty was done on the right side. The final result was relatively good. In a girl aged 12 years with a large soft tissue defect in the left lateral thigh incurred in an accident 3 years earlier, two implants 250 cc in size containing saturating loads of NaCl were placed in subcutaneous pockets superior to the defect. After 14 weeks the implants were fully inflated and tissue quality was excellent. Primary closure of the entire defect was possible. After 1 year, more than 90% of the defect was eliminated, representing a net gain of about 64 sq cm of apparently normal surface area.

This method offers potential advantages over percutaneously inflated devices. Clinical results to date have been encouraging, but a more permeable membrane would hasten inflation of the implant and reduce the NaCl requirement.

▶ [A thoughtful and interesting study applying a new approach to the Radovan and other expander devices. One wonders whether recent FDA strictures on implants will dampen efforts such as these in the future.—R.J.H.] ◀

2–26 **Soft Tissue Reconstruction of the Breast Using an External Oblique Myocutaneous Abdominal Flap** is described by Donald R. Marshall, E. John Anstee, and Murray J. Stapleton (Melbourne). The latissimus dorsi myocutaneous flap technique is occasionally indicated in breast reconstruction, but practical difficulties preclude its routine use. The external oblique muscle is a possible carrier for flap transfer. Cadaver dissections indicated that it is technically feasible to carry skin and subcutaneous tissue of the lower part of the abdomen to the breast region via a subcutaneous tunnel lying over the ribs, using an external oblique myocutaneous flap. The circulatory competence of the flap can be confirmed by a number of routine abdominal lipectomies in which the skin and fat are left as an island attached to the muscle flap, which is temporarily developed up to the

(2–26) Br. J. Plast. Surg. 35:443–451, October 1982.

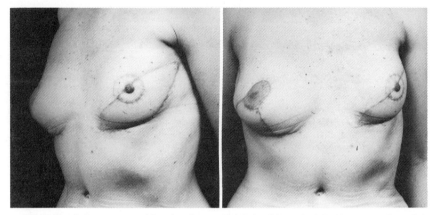

Fig 2-13.—*Left,* appearance after detachment of pedicle of flap, which has been turned into left breast to augment volume further. Right breast has been reduced and nipple uplifted along with nipple reconstruction on left side. *Right,* same patient showing satisfactory symmetry. Fullness over left rib cage is no longer evident. (Courtesy of Marshall, D., et al.: Br. J. Plast. Surg. 35:443–451, October 1982.)

rib cage. It is later replaced, the skin is excised, and the lipectomy is completed in the usual manner. The muscle defect seems unlikely to be a problem if the underlying muscles are undamaged.

The results obtained in a patient requiring breast reconstruction, in whom all elements of the external oblique myocutaneous flap were employed, are shown in Figure 2–13. No prosthesis was used in this patient. The method has been successfully used in 5 patients. One failure resulted from flap necrosis, due to compression in the subcutaneous tunnel, in an elderly, obese patient. An incision through the overlying skin of the tunnel might have prevented vascular compression.

Breast reconstruction using only skin and fat of the lower part of the abdomen obviates the disadvantages of a prosthesis. The contour of the abdomen is improved, and the donor scar is in an acceptable position. The procedure causes minimal blood loss and is relatively nontraumatic to the patient. A prosthesis may be necessary in an extremely thin patient. The soft tissue method is also suitable for patients who have complications related to use of a prosthesis, after either total or subcutaneous mastectomy, or augmentation mammaplasty on one or both sides.

▶ [This paper is another clever variation on the use of abdominal tissue to create a breast mound. Again, caution must be exercised, as one out of five flaps failed. Additionally, indications to use this or any flap should not be stretched when subpectoral placement of an implant can provide a satisfactory result.—S.H.M.] ◀

2–27 **Transverse Abdominal Island Flap:** *—Part I. Indications, Contraindications, Results, and Complications*—are discussed by Michael

(2–27) Ann. Plast. Surg. 10:24–35, January 1983.

Scheflan (Med. College of Virginia, Richmond) and Melvyn I. Dinner (Cleveland Clinic). The transverse abdominal island flap, based superiorly on one rectus abdominis muscle, is a suitable reconstructive method for patients with marked skin deficiency, altered chest wall coverage, or denervated pectoralis muscles after modified radical mastectomy, as well as for those with large or extensive soft tissue deficiencies. The deep superior and inferior epigastric vessels interconnect within the substance of the rectus abdominis, and the superficial epigastric system joins the deep system with the contralateral superficial epigastric system across the midline. The myocutaneous branches of the deep system are in the medial part of the musculofascial component. Three to 5 large and several smaller myocutaneous vessels penetrate the skin and fat at and below the umbilicus. This vascular pedicle permits tension-free transposition of the flap to the chest wall and the coverage of extensive defects.

Sixty-five consecutive breast reconstructions were done using the transverse abdominal island flap, which has almost completely replaced the latissimus dorsi myocutaneous flap in suitable patients. Contraindications include an age of older than 60 years, obesity, severe irradiation injury of the chest wall, heavy smoking, and lower abdominal scars. All but 2 of the 65 operations, performed in 60 patients, were done using the ipsilateral rectus abdominis. Ten patients had had chest wall irradiation. Silicone breast implants were necessary in 3 patients. Flap necrosis occurred in 7 cases. Five patients had an abdominal wall hernia, and 1 had fat necrosis. One had myalgia paresthetica. No patient had infection, deep vein thrombosis, or pulmonary embolism. Two patients had near-total flap necrosis; 1 was massively obese, and 1 had delayed diagnosis of a large underlying hematoma. These complications are preventable, and are chiefly attributable to a relative lack of experience with the technique.

2–28 **Transverse Abdominal Island Flap:** *—Part II. Surgical Technique—*is outlined by Scheflan and Dinner. Patients begin a program of 30 sit-ups a day 45 days before transverse abdominal island flap surgery.

TECHNIQUE.—The contralateral portion of the flap is elevated first, with progressive dissection of the skin and fat flap from lateral to midline in a plane just above the external oblique fascia. The ipsilateral side of the flap constituting the myocutaneous part of the ellipse is raised in a similar plane up to the lateral edge of the rectus abdominis muscle. The anterior abdominal wall then is progressively dissected to above the subcostal and xiphoid margins. The anterior rectus sheath is incised midway between the midline and the lateral edge of the rectus muscle, and the medial and lateral leaves of the sheath are dissected before delivering the rectus muscle caudally from between the rectus sheaths. The deep inferior epigastric pedicle is ligated before flap transposition. The old mastectomy scar can be opened, although a new incision in the inframammary fold is preferable. A large tunnel is made to

(2–28) Ann. Plast. Surg. 10:120–129, February 1983.

accommodate the flap comfortably. A tension-free transfer should permit the flap to easily reach the clavicle. Direct approximation of the anterior rectus sheath usually is possible with the abdominal wall completely relaxed. It is best to reduce the size of the flap and place a breast prosthesis beneath it, when appropriate, rather than attempting to use questionable parts of the flap to achieve an autogenous mound.

Ancillary procedures generally are done at the same time as the reconstruction. Nipples are reconstructed 1 to 5 months after the initial procedure.

No flap loss has occurred in 34 recent procedures. Presently the authors prefer to use a flap based on the contralateral rectus abdominis muscle when the abdominal wall is unscarred. The muscle is rotated 90 to 120 degrees into the defect, rather than 180 degrees as with the use of ipsilateral muscle, and there is no torsion or rotation of the flap pedicle. Synthetic mesh is being used more liberally to close the rectus sheath defect below the arcuate. It is useful to transect the umbilical stalk and treat the umbilicus as a free full-thickness graft.

▶ [These two papers summarize the large experience these authors have had with the RAM flap. The flap is tricky and the number of complications reported, 14 out of the 65 patients, is significant. We have seen significant loss of the umbilicus in one patient and loss of the central skin of a flap based on the contralateral rectus in a smoker who had been irradiated. Reports of late fat necrosis, suggesting recurrent tumor, have been reported and are troublesome. The technique appears to be a worthwhile addition to our armamentarium, but not to the total exclusion of other methods.—S.H.M.] ◀

2–29 **Psychologic Reactions to Prophylactic Mastectomy Synchronous With Contralateral Breast Reconstruction.** The breast remaining after mastectomy for cancer occupies a somewhat equivocal position in the hierarchy of the women's body image. It is a powerful source of support to the psyche as a persisting symbol of maternal nurturing and femininity, but it most often goes unused in any way and is an awkward impediment in dressing and in sports.

Marcia Kraft Goin and John M. Goin (Univ. of Southern California) evaluated the psychologic reactions of 10 women who had breast reconstruction after mastectomy for cancer and who elected to have simultaneous prophylactic mastectomy and immediate reconstruction of the remaining breast. In each case, the Breast Reconstruction Interview questionnaire was used. Most women were seen 2 and 4 weeks and 6 months after surgery and then annually. Total mastectomies were done, with immediate reconstruction by using subpectoral silicone gel or double-lumen implants. The nipple-areola complex was reconstructed by areola-sharing at the time of breast reconstruction, or later with skin and composite grafts. The women were aged 38 to 54 years.

Four women first learned of the risk of cancer developing in the

(2–29) Plast. Reconstr. Surg. 70:355–359, September 1982.

remaining breast during talks with the plastic surgeon, and this came as a frightening revelation to them. All women anticipated a deep sense of loss with removal of the "other" breast. All patients had some anxiety about the original cancer and the possibility of cancer in the remaining breast. Two patients were pleased by the prospect of a prophylactic mastectomy because of their large pendulous breasts. Although most of the women had strongly negative feelings about the prospect of a mastectomy, their pleasure with the results of reconstruction was not less for the immediate reconstruction than for the breast that had a delayed reconstruction.

The fear of cancer and concerns about loss of the remaining breast are more or less inextricably intertwined in these patients. Several of the present women expressed a strong wish that immediate reconstruction had been done at the time of the first mastectomy. There would appear to be no psychological benefit from delaying breast reconstruction, and immediate reconstruction seems to be quite helpful in easing some of the pain of a necessarily difficult experience.

▶ [We need to explore further our recommendation for therapy to the "other breast" by defining rigidly the indications and remaining cognizant that man-made is rarely as acceptable as God-made.—S.H.M.] ◀

–30 **Phantom Breast Syndrome in Young Women After Mastectomy for Breast Cancer: Physical, Social, and Psychologic Aspects.** Phantom breast syndrome (PBS) is characterized by a sensation of the continued presence of a breast after mastectomy. K. Christensen, M. Blichert-Toft, Ulla Giersing, C. Richardt, and J. Beckmann (Odense, Denmark) examined the occurrence of PBS among 35 consecutive women, aged 45 years or less, who underwent mastectomy and partial axillary dissection for breast cancer in 1978 and 1979. The patients were assessed physically, psychologically, and socially 6 to 21 months after operation. Thirty-one were examined, and 28 of them agreed to psychosocial assessment.

Eleven patients (35.5%) had PBS postoperatively, most during the daytime only. Six had a sensation localized to the nipple region, whereas 5 described diffused sensations in the whole breast region. The occurrence of PBS could not be related to age, marital status, occupation in or outside the home, early or late postoperative sequelae, or radiotherapy. Body image was moderately or severely impaired in 45% of the women with PBS and in 18% of the others. Sexual identity was affected in comparable numbers. Sexual function was more often impaired in the group with PBS. Affective disorders were comparably frequent, but anxiety was more frequent in the women without PBS. Emotional dissociation from close relatives was identified in 2 women with PBS and in 3 without.

Phantom breast syndrome occurred in about a third of these young mastectomy patients. It is not always a minor disturbance, and it

(2–30) Acta Chir. Scand. 148:351–354, 1982.

seems to mask deep psychologic problems of a complex nature. The appearance of PBS should be interpreted in the context of a patient's overall psychologic reaction to mastectomy. Jamison et al. reported that women with PBS used more tranquilizers than others. Phantom breast syndrome can involve intense pain.

▶ [It would be very interesting if a psychosocial assessment could be carried out in 2 age-matched groups of patients before mastectomy, and then 6–12 months postoperatively. If half of the group then chose to be reconstructed and the other half did not, psychosocial testing 6–12 months postreconstruction could again be performed and compared between the 2 groups to see if the syndrome was time-related and if it could be alleviated by reconstruction.—S.H.M.] ◀

2–31 **Toxic Shock Syndrome From Infected Breast Prosthesis.** Toxic shock syndrome (TSS) initially was associated with the use of tampons by young menstruating women. Andrew Barnett, Elliott Lavey, Robert M. Pearl, and Lars M. Vistnes (Stanford Univ.) report data on a case of TSS secondary to an infected breast prosthesis.

Woman, 32, had had bilateral subglandular breast augmentation elsewhere. Bilumen prostheses were used, with Solu-Medrol in the outer lumen. The right-sided prosthesis became mildly displaced inferiorly, with tissue atrophy, and it was removed after 6 months and then replaced after steroid was removed from the outer lumen. No antibiotic prophylaxis was used. Watery diarrhea, myalgias, rash on the extremities, sore throat, and fever to 39 C developed 4 days after operation. The rash subsequently spread, and 7 days after operation cephalosporin was given. Her menses began and a tampon was inserted. The patient was seen later that day in extremis. On admission to Stanford she had fever of 39.5 C and blood pressure of 80/40 mm Hg. A confluent macular rash was present on the chest and upper extremities. Gentamicin and nafcillin were given empirically, but the patient became progressively more toxic and required ventilatory support as well as vasopressor therapy. Renal function deteriorated, and anuria was briefly present.

Findings at exploration of the right breast at an outlying hospital had been reported as negative. Nevertheless, the prosthesis was removed, and 20 ml of purulent material was noted around it. The left prosthesis was removed later the same day; it was found to be free of infection. The white blood cell count rose to 45,000 the next day and the platelet count fell to 10,000. Chest films showed mild adult respiratory distress syndrome. The patient then began to improve. Culture of the right periprosthetic fluid yielded penicillin-resistant *Staphylococcus aureus*. A confluent bullous lesion developed on the chest and upper extremities. The patient was discharged 19 days after operation.

Features of TSS include fever, hypotension, erythroderma, hyperemia of the conjunctivae or mucosae of the oropharynx or vagina, and involvement of at least three systems. Local signs of infection generally are minimal. The only organism implicated has been *S. aureus*. Diagnosis of TSS remains a clinical one. Toxic shock syndrome should be suspected in the presence of postoperative fever with watery diarrhea and erythroderma. β-Lactamase-resistant antibiotics should be given prophylactically when there is a risk of infection. Treatment

(2–31) Ann. Plast. Surg. 10:408–410, May 1983.

for TSS is chiefly supportive; the bacterial focus must be eliminated and antibiotics administered.

▶ [This has got to be an exceptional case.—R.O.B.] ◀

2-32 **Necrotizing Fasciitis: Preventable Disaster.** Necrotizing fasciitis (NF) is a serious soft tissue infection characterized by fascial and subcutaneous tissue necrosis and eventual involvement of the skin and muscle. Thomas M. Rouse, Mark A. Malangoni, and William J. Schulte (Med. College of Wisconsin, Milwaukee) reviewed 28 cases of NF in 27 patients, seen in 1969–1981. The 20 men and 7 women had a mean age of 61 years. The diagnosis was based on findings during surgery of a spreading liquefactive necrosis of the fascia and subcutaneous tissues. Twenty patients had associated chronic diseases such as diabetes and atherosclerotic cardiovascular disease. The most common causes of fasciitis were perineal disease, postoperative infection, and chronic skin ulceration. Postoperative cases developed 3 to 14 days after initial intra-abdominal surgery.

Twelve patients had a single operative debridement, whereas 15 had more than one debridement. A colostomy was performed in 6 cases, and 1 had a suprapubic cystostomy. Two patients had drainage of an intra-abdominal abscess, 2 had orchiectomy, and 1 each had hip disarticulation and left colectomy. Mortality was 73%. Death was attributed to persistent wound sepsis in 9 cases, systemic septic complications despite apparent local control of infection in 9, and myocardial infarction in 2. Eight patients had nosocomial infection. Five of 12 patients whose NF was controlled by a single debridement survived. The predominant organisms were *Bacteroides, Escherichia coli, Enterococcus,* and *Clostridia.* At least 1 species of *Streptococcus* was isolated in 23 cases.

Operative debridement remains the key treatment for NF, and should not be postponed. Perirectal abscess and infected skin ulcers must be recognized as early manifestations of NF. Necrotizing fasciitis can be prevented by the prudent management of causative infections. Antimicrobial therapy should be directed against anaerobes as well as aerobes. After NF is controlled, the risk of development of antibiotic-resistant infection must be considered.

2-33 **Anoplasty For Anal Stricture.** Anal stricture is a distressing problem. Although a true anatomical stricture due to loss of anal tissue often does not respond to nonoperative treatment, a surgical increase in size of the anal canal is effective. Changyul Oh and Joel Zinberg (Mt. Sinai Med. Center, New York) have developed a relatively easy technique that minimizes skin necrosis and provides uniformly good results. High colonic irrigation is performed preoperatively unless the anal canal is too narrow, and intravenous antibiotics are given. After dilation of the anal canal, if necessary, with use of a

---

(2–32) Surgery 92:765–770, October 1982.
(2–33) Dis. Colon Rectum 25:809–810, November–December 1982.

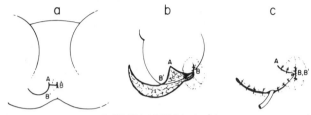

C-ANOPLASTY (Author's)

Fig 2–14.—Method of C-flap anoplasty; *(a)* anal skin is incised from dentate line to anal verge *(AB)* and a C-shape incision is made at distal end of original incision; *(b)* anal canal is dilated to a width of 4 finger-breadths and the C-flap is undermined; *(c)* anal defect is covered with C-flap as it is drawn into dentate line *(BB́)*. (Courtesy of Oh, C., and Zinberg, J.: Dis. Colon Rectum 25:809–810, November/December 1982.)

radial lateral incision from the dentate line to the anal verge, a C-shaped incision is made at the distal end of the radial incision (Fig 2–14), and involved scar is excised. The C-flap is undermined through full-thickness skin. The flap is approximated loosely after being drawn into the anal canal, and each side of the anal canal wound is approximated with 2-0 chromic sutures. The external wound is loosely approximated with 4-0 nylon by undermining the opposite skin. Tension is avoided at all suture lines. Only water is given for 2 days. The drain is removed after 3 days. Bacitracin ointment is applied over the wound.

Twelve patients with an average age of 50 years had C-anoplasty in 1976–1981. Ten had an anal stricture due to previous hemorrhoidectomy. Fistulectomy had been done in 1 case, and fissurectomy in another. All patients had been treated conservatively for 4–22 years without obtaining reasonable relief. All the surgical wounds were healed within 2 months, and 11 patients were satisfied with the outcome. One had a restricture that responded to 3 anal dilatations. No flap necroses or infections occurred. Most patients were able to resume normal activities about 3 weeks after surgery.

The C-anoplasty extends the pedicle without compromising the vascular blood supply. Suture-line tension can be controlled by extending the incision. The size of the graft is readily adjusted to anal size.

► [Anoplasty for anal stricture could also be handled by Z-plasty.—R.O.B.] ◄

2-34 **Multiple Glomus Tumors: Special Reference to Radiologic Findings.** Multiple glomus tumors (MGT) are a benign, autosomal dominant skin disease, characterized by small bluish intradermal tumors (Fig 2–15). They resemble cavernous hemangiomas clinically, but are distinguished by the intraluminar presence of glomus cells. The condition is rare; only 1 family with MGT has previously been reported in Scandinavia. Igor A. Niechajev (Malmö, Sweden) reports 4 cases of MGT, 3 hereditary familial cases and 1 sporadic case. The

(2–34) Scand. J. Plast. Reconstr. Surg. 16:183–190, 1982.

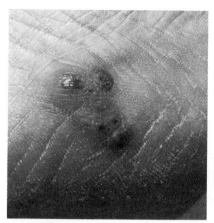

Fig 2–15.—Conglomerate of intradermal bluish MGT lesions on heel of left foot. (Courtesy of Niechajev, I. A.: Scand. J. Plast. Reconstr. Surg. 16:183–190, 1982.)

only skeletal change was a short fifth metacarpal in 1 patient. Angiography showed a conglomerate of tortuous vessels resembling a cavernous hemangioma at the site of a palpable tumor in 1 of the 2 patients examined. The tumor was supplied chiefly by a radial artery branch. Repeated angiography, done because of recurrence, showed small vessels with irregular walls as the only abnormality. Venography and thermography were not diagnostically helpful in these cases.

Brachymetacarpia and skeletal hypoplasia probably are common components of the MGT syndrome. Since both MGT and brachymetacarpia are genetic disorders with autosomal dominant transmission patterns, both traits may be coded in the same chromosome, and linkage may exist among the aberrant genes. Routine radiography is recommended in cases of MGT.

2–35 **Perichondrial Wrist Arthroplasty: Follow-Up Study in 17 Rheumatoid Patients.** Wrist involvement is frequent in rheumatoid arthritis. Patients may adapt to slowly evolving wrist lesions by progressive modification of gestures, resulting in poor habits that can become true deformities, contributing to the overall imbalance in the wrist and contiguous joints. Paolo Pastacaldi (Pisa, Italy) performed arthroplasty with autologous perichondrial grafting in 17 patients with severe rheumatoid disease in the wrist. The age range was 38–64 years. In 10 patients the operation was done on the dominant hand. Postoperative follow-up ranged from 6 to 50 months. Complete dorsal synovectomy was done after resecting the head of the ulna, and the distal part of the tip of the radius then was resected. The osteotomy is done perpendicular to the axis of the radius after remolding the volar crest to support the carpus. The perichondrial graft is taken from the sixth and seventh ribs and placed as shown in Figure 2–16.

(2–35)   Ann. Plast. Surg. 9:146–151, August 1982.

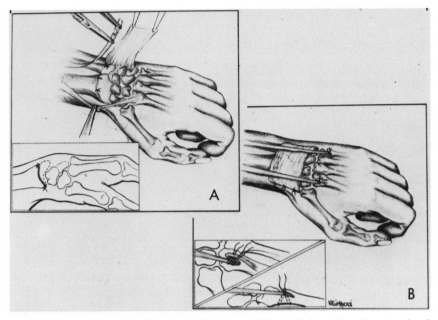

Fig 2–16.—A, the perichondrium is positioned on radial end. B, the retinaculum is replaced under tendons and the extensor tendons of the carpus reinserted under tension. (Courtesy of Pastacaldi, P.: Ann. Plast. Surg. 9:146–151, August 1982.)

Pain initially was regularly present on daily activities, and in 9 patients it prevented most active movement. All reported loss of strength. Pronation-supination averaged 86 degrees before surgery. Flexion-extension clearly improved postoperatively, and pronation-supination averaged 140 degrees; the chief improvement was in supination. Only 2 patients had slight pain after the operation. Improvement in pain led to better function, and all patients reported improved strength. Joint swelling occurred in 5 patients preoperatively and in only 1 after operation. No clinical relapse of joint inflammation was observed.

Persistent functional improvement was obtained after perichondrial wrist arthroplasty in these patients with severe wrist involvement by rheumatoid disease. All patients had stable improvement in hand motion and in ability to perform daily activities. No symptoms of synovial inflammation were present after arthroplasty, and there was no recurrence of osteoarticular deformity on follow-up for up to 4 years.

▶ [It is hoped the author will provide long-term reports that will support his interesting successes to date.—F.J.M.] ◀

2–36 **Hoffman Procedure in Ulcerated Diabetic Neuropathic Foot.** In some diabetics, complicated ulcerative lesions occur on the plantar

(2–36) Foot Ankle 3:142–149, Nov.–Dec. 1982.

surface of the forefoot that fail to respond to conservative treatment or resection of a metatarsal head. Richard L. Jacobs (Union Univ., N.Y.) used the Clayton modification of the Hoffman procedure to treat such problems in 12 diabetic patients who had varying degrees of insensitivity of the foot and forefoot ulceration beneath 1 or more metatarsal heads, associated with local abscess formation. The metatarsal heads were amputated by oblique cuts through the necks during constant irrigation by triple antibiotic solution. After removal of dirty granulations and debris with a sponge, a suction drain was placed through a separate stab incision, loose subcutaneous closure was performed, and the skin was closed with nylon sutures. No wires were placed. Systemic antibiotic coverage was continued postoperatively. The patient was kept on flat-foot touch weight-bearing until the wounds healed and drainage ceased.

Woman, 53, after ulceration developed beneath the first metatarsal head, sustained a "spontaneous" fracture of the first metatarsal neck. Increasing deformity of the great toe was evident. A small ulcer beneath the first metatarsal head healed, but a new ulcer developed beneath the second metatarsal head. Infection developed in the forefoot, and an abscess drained spontaneously between the second and third toes. Pulse volume recordings indicated adequate blood flow to the extremity. A modified Hoffman procedure was carried out (Fig 2–17), resulting in good healing, cessation of drainage from the sinus and ulcer, and full weight-bearing with protective shoes a month after surgery.

This operation is extensive, and should be done only if adequate circulation is probable; pulse volume recordings should show some semblance of pulsatile flow. Healing was prolonged in some instances, but all feet operated on healed, and the patients proceeded to full weight-bearing with extra-depth shoes having soft neoprene rubber insoles. This approach may be considered in place of transmetatarsal

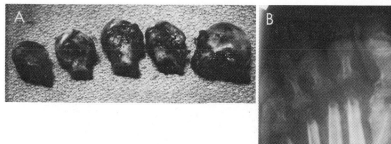
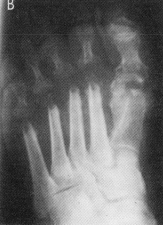

Fig. 2–17.—A, excised metatarsal heads. **B,** postoperative radiograph. (Courtesy of Jacobs, R. L.: Foot Ankle 3:142–149, Nov.–Dec. 1982.)

amputation in some patients having ulceration and abscess formation of the forefoot if the circulation is adequate, or can be made adequate by vascular reconstruction.

▶ [A forthright and courageous attack on a discouraging condition.—F.J.M.] ◀

2-37 **Radical Vulvectomy With Use of Tensor Fascia Lata Myocutaneous Flap.** The most common complications of radical vulvectomy have been wound breakdown, skin flap necrosis, and wound infection. Weldon Chafe, Wesley C. Fowler, Jr., Leslie A. Walton, and John L. Currie (Univ. of North Carolina) used the tensor fascia lata myocutaneous flap to facilitate coverage of vulvectomy defects and reduce postoperative morbidity.

TECHNIQUE.—The fascia lata flaps are dissected with temporary suture of the fascia to the overlying dermis. The flaps are elevated, rotated into place, and sutured with 3–0 absorbable material to create a functional pseudovulva, as shown in Figure 2–18. The urethra is sutured to the inferior fascia of the urogenital diaphragm, and the flap skin edges are joined to the external urethral meatus. Large drains are placed beneath the flaps before they are sutured into the perineum. The donor site is closed primarily; skin grafts are occasionally necessary.

Thirteen patients have had this procedure. A two-team approach was used. Patients were ambulated 1 to 2 days after operation. There

Fig 2–18.—Completed repair with creation of pseudovulva. (Courtesy of Chafe, W., et al.: Am. J. Obstet. Gynecol. 145:207–213, Jan. 15, 1983.)

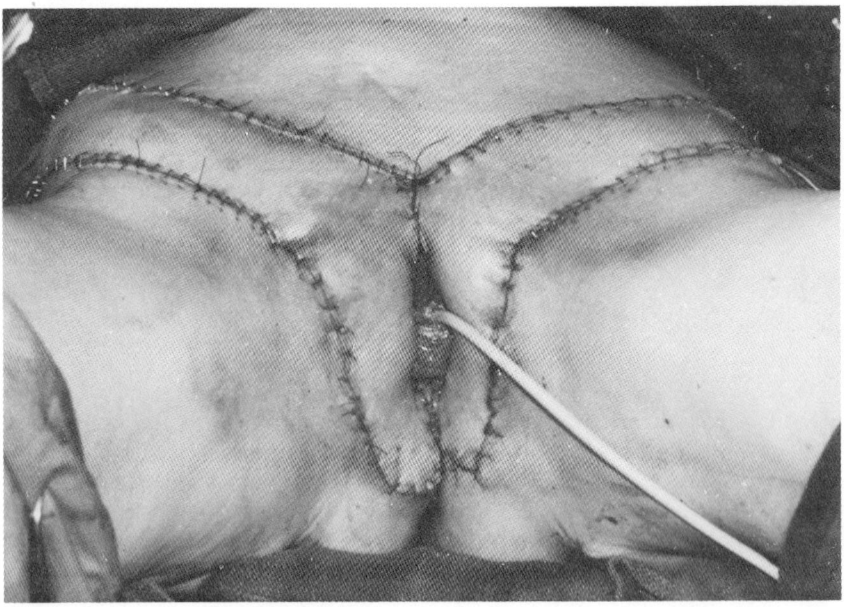

(2–37) Am. J. Obstet. Gynecol. 145:207–213, Jan. 15, 1983.

have been virtually no wound complications. Two early patients required evacuation of hematoma beneath a flap and ligation of bleeding vessels in the flap subcutaneous tissue. Two patients had small areas of flap necrosis. Patient discomfort did not last more than 48 hours after operation. The postoperative hospital stay averaged 10 to 12 days. Three patients received postoperative radiotherapy without wound complications. The functional and cosmetic results have been acceptable. No patient has developed stress urinary incontinence.

Radical vulvectomy and groin dissection with use of tensor fascia lata musculocutaneous flaps to resurface the wound have proved to be a safe, reliable treatment for invasive vulvar cancer. Postoperative wound complications have been markedly reduced. Patients are ambulated and discharged earlier after vulvectomy when this approach is used.

▶ [Coverage after a radical vulvectomy has always been somewhat of a problem and the authors have suggested a very nice procedure.—R.O.B.] ◀

3. Trauma

3–1 Immediate Management of Severe Facial War Injuries is discussed by Sabri Shuker (Basrah, Iraq). Immediate restoration of appearance and function in patients with severe wounds of the middle and lower parts of the face is very important in rehabilitation. The presence of oral surgeons at forward medical installations has resulted in definitive treatment of maxillofacial injuries at the initial operation. The proximal mandibular stumps will be drawn superiorly and medially if not stabilized either by replacement of the lost segment or by intermaxillary traction. Results of late reconstruction of soft and hard tissues in severely wounded men are poor. Treatment methods may have to be modified if adequate dentition is absent or there is mandibular segmental or maxillary loss.

Twenty-four patients have been treated by using Kirschner wires when other means of fixation and immobilization were not available. Use of these wires has proved to be simple, convenient, rapid, and versatile. Adequate stabilization and immobilization are obtained without dead space, and healing has been excellent. Occlusion was maintained in most cases. The horseshoe-shaped wire acts as a spring to keep the mandibular stumps in position. Only 1 case of tissue breakdown occurred; this was due to delayed evacuation. Five patients have had the wire replaced by a bone graft.

Use of a Kirschner wire has proved helpful in the early management of severe facial injuries with an avulsed mandibular segment seen at an early evacuation hospital in a war zone. Immediate restoration of shape and function is possible in cases of both hard and soft tissue loss involving the middle and lower parts of the face. Patients can be rehabilitated early and restored to a socially acceptable existence. The technique helps to preserve soft tissue position and makes use of pieces of denuded bone that otherwise would be lost. Patients having a large segment of the mandibular body and symphysis avulsed without middle-third injury have not required tracheostomy. It is much easier to immobilize the fragments initially in these cases than has previously been thought.

▶ [Should there be extensive soft tissue injury accompanying these injuries, the use of external fixation devices, i.e., Steinman pins inserted on the opposite sides of the fracture stabilized with cold wire acrylic, is another useful technique for maintaining bone position.—S.H.M.] ◀

(3–1) J. Maxillofac. Surg. 11:30–36, February 1983.

3-2 **Use of Small Plates for Facial Osteosynthesis: Experience With 160 Plates Placed During 1 Year.** A. Gary-Bobo, Ch. Merlier, P. Tarot (Montpellier, France) used small screwed plates (Champy's implants) in 85 patients after facial and craniofacial trauma to reduce and stabilize the frontal region and fix associated fractures on other levels in certain complex injuries, to fix external orbital support structures, and to isolate unstable displacement fractures or plurifocal fractures at the mandibular level in order to allow for immediate condylar mobilization or intraoral elastic traction. Four-hole plates were held in place by 7-mm screws in 85% of cases.

Two conditions are imperative in the placement of such plates to avoid the risk of major infection. First, the absence of open wounds at the site of osteosynthesis, and second, total exclusion of the frontal sinuses from drill holes.

The 12% "unjustified" cases of bimaxillary traction constitute the most disputable issue of the series. In effect, osteosynthesis by means of plates should logically make it possible to dispense with traction altogether; however, this has yet to be confirmed. Tolerance of the implants has been good after a follow-up of 1 year, but long-term tolerance will need to be established. Functional status and morphological results in 78 patients available for 1-year follow-up were considered good to satisfactory in 90% of cases.

▶ [The authors describe the use of plates which will probably have increasingly greater application in fractures and osteotomies of all types.—L.A.W.] ◀

3-3 **Current Concepts on Management of Orbital Blowout Fractures** are discussed by Leo Koornneef (Amsterdam). Controversy continues over how to best manage blowout fractures not associated with fractures of the orbital rim. Most orbital blowout fractures produce impaired movement in upward and downward gaze in all directions, as if the inferior oblique and inferior rectus muscles were trapped together. This can be explained by the intricate system of orbital connective tissue (Figs 3–1 and 3–2). Motility problems in case of blowout fracture are currently attributed, not to entrapment of specific muscles, but to dysfunction of the entire motility apparatus in the region of fracture. Restricted motility is due to soft tissue edema, scarring, hemorrhage, or nerve damage to the extraocular muscles. Prolapse into the maxillary sinus involves the connective tissue septa of the muscles in the region of fracture. This can have traction and checking effects on the connective tissue septa of the medial and lateral recti, explaining the severe bizarre disturbances in motility observed.

Conventional surgical treatment with repair of the orbital floor only no longer has a sound theoretical basis. A conservative approach

(3–2) Ann. Plast. Chir. 27:41–47, 1983.
(3–3) Ann. Plast. Surg. 9:185–200, September 1982.

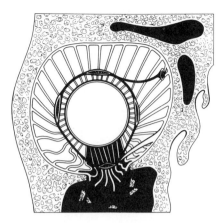

Fig 3–1.—Involvement of connective tissue after fracture in which connective tissue septa in traumatized area are ruptured and surrounded by blood and edema *(dark areas)*. (Courtesy of Koornneef, L.: Ann. Plast. Surg. 9:185–200, September 1982.)

is recommended until microsurgical methods become available for treating the sequelae of blowout fractures at their origin. Although a severely dislocated zygoma, maxilla, or orbital floor with displacement of the eyeball into the maxillary antrum should be replaced before scar tissue forms, a pure blowout fracture is a relatively benign condition. Few patients complain of enophthalmos, and even fewer wish to have anythinng done about it. Early eye-movement exercises can improve the excursions of eye movements, and may even stimulate formation of a partially adequate connective tissue

Fig 3–2.—Representation of how future connective tissue surgery might be performed to free the scar clot from muscle and the fracture area. (Courtesy of Koornneef, L.: Ann. Plast. Surg. 9:185–200, September 1982.)

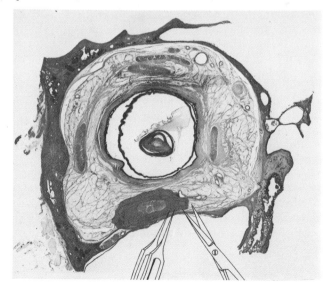

system around the muscles. Surgery should be delayed in cases of pure blowout fracture when no major esthetic deformity is expected. Conventional extraocular muscle surgery is indicated if complete recovery does not take place and the scar clot cannot be treated surgically.

▶ [A worthwhile addition to our knowledge, if confirmed. Can an experimental animal model be developed to help answer the controversy?—S.H.M.] ◀

3–4 **Management of Scalp Injuries.** Scalp avulsion injuries can have serious results in terms of hospitalization, economic loss, and disfigurement with its adverse psychologic effects. Scalp injury is now a major industrial hazard, usually occurring in unskilled persons in an unsupervised setting when the unprotected hair is caught in the exposed moving parts of a machine. V. Bhattacharya, J. K. Sinha, and F. M. Tripathi (Banaras Hindu Univ., Varanasi, India) reviewed 20 cases of scalp injury treated in the past 5 years, excluding scalp defects after ablative surgery and minor injuries to the scalp. There were 14 avulsion injuries, 3 injuries caused by traffic accidents, and 3 injuries from electrical burns. Eight patients were treated within 24 hours of injury, and 7 after more than 3 days. Split-skin grafts only were used in 15 patients. The others had flap repair, a combination of skin grafting and flap repair, or drilling through the outer table followed by skin grafting.

Bleeding may be a severe problem in these cases, but usually can be controlled by a pressure dressing and elevation of the head. Split-skin grafting remains the best and easiest treatment when the pericranium is intact. Ideally, grafting is done immediately after injury. A local flap is used if the defect is over a prominent area or bare bone is exposed. The skin-grafted bald donor area will then be in the least conspicuous site, and may be covered by growing hair. When the periosteum is avulsed or after an electrical burn injury, the outer table of the skull is removed with a chisel, and a flap is rotated in place. A transposition flap or S-shaped double flaps may be used. In a case of exposed denuded bone due to electrical burn injury, multiple perforations were made through the outer table to permit outgrowth of granulation tissue. Relatively thick split-skin grafts are preferred. Recurrent ulceration and breakdown may necessitate replacement by local or distant flaps at a later stage.

▶ [The authors review a broad experience and comment in a generally sound manner on the management of scalp injuries.—L.A.W.] ◀

3–5 **Frontal Sinus Fractures: Therapeutic Attitudes** are discussed by L. C. Merville, C. Brunet, and P. V. Thanh (Suresnes, France). The management of displaced frontal sinus fractures depends on the wall

---

(3–4) J. Trauma 22:698–702, August 1982.
(3–5) Rev. Stomatol. Chir. Maxillofac. 83:206–213, 1982.

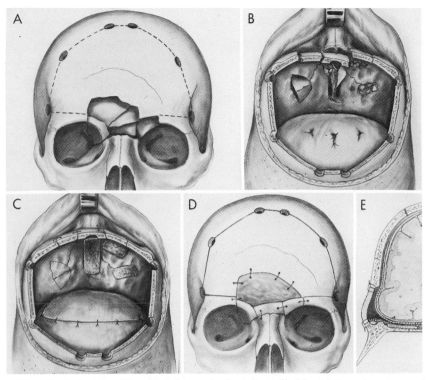

Fig 3–3.—A, fracture with multiple fragments of anterior wall of frontal sinus along course of nasofrontal orbital dislocation showing outline *(broken lines)* of neurosurgical exploration; **(B)** endocranial view; **(C)** resection of posterior wall and medial fronto-ethmoidal osseous graft allowing exclusion of sinus through cranialization; **(D)** satisfactory reconstitution of anterior wall; *(E)* profile view showing cranialization and reconstitution of anterior wall by means of osseous graft. (Courtesy of Merville, L. C., et al.: Rev. Stomatol. Chir. Maxillofac. 83:206–213, 1982 Masson, S. A., Paris.)

affected. A harmonious frontal outline can be achieved by osteosynthesis of the fragments under certain conditions, or by bone grafting. The sinus cavity should be excluded and filled with spongy grafts when an anterior wall graft is inserted. Neurosurgical exploration with cranialization and obturation of the nasofrontal canal is necessary if a posterior wall defect threatens the meninges. Physiologic drainage must be assured for the sinus cavity, especially in cases of inferior wall fracture.

Representative results of treatment are shown in Figures 3–3 and 3–4.

▶ [Many instances of anterior frontal sinus wall displacement may be adequately treated with cranial bone grafts or osteosynthesis of fragments, without filling the sinus cavity. Likewise some simple posterior wall defects do not require that cranialization be done. The principles in this article, however, are for the most part sound.— L.A.W.] ◀

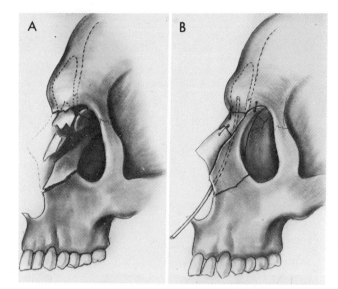

Fig 3–4.—A, fracture of inferior wall of frontal sinus caused by nasofrontal orbital dislocation with depression of nasal spine; **(B)** simple reposition of orbitonasal skeleton allowing reestablishment of nasofrontal permeability by maintenance of adequate dimension for introduction of catheter. (Courtesy of Merville, L. C., et al.: Rev. Stomatol. Chir. Maxillofac. 83:206–213, 1982 Masson, S. A., Paris.)

Fig 3–5.—Side view of patient **(A)** before and **(B)** after reconstruction of frontal vault and anterior floor of cranial base in two stages by autogenous iliac bone graft and homogenous frontal bone graft. (Courtesy of Merville, L., et al.: Ann. Chir. Plast. 27:205–210, 1982.)

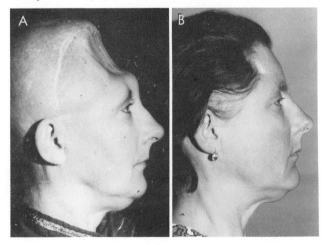

3–6   **Reconstruction of the Frontal Bone and Sinuses.** L. Merville, C. Brunet, and P. Derome (Suresnes, France) describe the management of frontobasal reconstruction when the bone flap is infected after the repair of previous craniofacial trauma. Cranioplasty was performed 12 years after frontobasal trauma with secondary cerebrospinal fluid rhinorrhea. Two unsuccessful rhinologic attempts had been made to close the fistulas, which were finally closed after an episode of meningitis. The frontal bone flap ultimately became infected and had to be removed. After an attempt to find the cause of infection in an opening of the ethmofrontal cavity and the anterior fossa, frontal sinus cranialization was completed, and the base of the anterior fossa was filled in with autogenous cancellous iliac bone. Reconstruction of the cranial vault was performed 6 months later under aseptic conditions, after the bone grafts had taken. A frontal bone homograft was used. Follow-up after 3 years indicates that the procedure was successful (Fig 3–5).

3–7   **Fronto-Orbito-Nasal Dislocations: Secondary Treatment of Sequelae** is outlined by Louis C. Merville, Patrick Derome, and Geoffroy de Saint-Jorre (Foch Hosp., Paris). (Four cases are described in detail.) Fronto-orbito-nasal dislocations must be treated early by maxillofacial and neurosurgical teams. A wide approach is necessary in cases of bone loss to explore not only the anterior fossa but also the upper part of the face. A bicoronal scalp flap is essential. Cerebral and dural injuries are repaired in conjunction with bone grafting of the anterior fossa and fronto-orbito-nasal areas and with ablation of the frontal sinus. Malunions result from either a lack of initial treatment or inadequate treatment. The frontal vault is depressed, the orbital rim is driven down and back, the nose is broadened and deviated, and there may be diplopia, upper eyelid ptosis, anosmia, and rhinorrhea with a risk of meningeal infection.

Simple onlay bone grafting usually is not sufficient to restore function. The malunited fractures must be osteotomized so that the various parts of the fractured region can be replaced in correct anatomical position. Bone gap must be filled with bone graft material. Expansion often is necessary, and bone must be inserted after expansion-advancement surgery. Bone fragments must be stabilized by fixation to sound parts. Reconstruction of the frontal area is particularly important because the inferior orbital and nasal fragments will be fixed to it. An intermediate band is preserved between the fracture and the craniotomy. With medial displacement, the bone is fixed on the lateral pillar. Cranialization is the best means of ablating the frontal sinus if it is exposed by trauma or craniotomy. Bone grafts are necessary when the cribriform plate and ethmoidal cells are opened. Dural lacerations are sutured and closed by a pericranial graft.

(3–6)   Ann. Chir. Plast. 27:205–210, 1982.
(3–7)   J. Maxillofac. Surg. 11:71–82, April 1983.

No sinus or meningeal complications have followed total reconstruction in more than 9 years. One-step reconstruction is preferable to multiple procedures. Lost bone is best replaced with autogenous bone grafts; no foreign material is really suitable. There is a risk of sequestration of the frontal bony vault when the frontal sinuses are not adequately obliterated.

▶ [The authors' extensive experience and excellent results illustrate the soundness of their principles. In spite of this, there are occasions when onlay bone grafting, with attention to the details of mobilization and soft tissue correction, solve problems well and without the need for osteotomies.—L.A.W.] ◀

3–8 **Management of Naso-Ethmoid-Orbital Fractures** is discussed by Raymond F. Morgan, Paul N. Manson, R. Bruce Shack, and John E. Hoopes (Johns Hopkins Hosp., Baltimore). Significant functional and esthetic deformities can result from naso-ethmoid-orbital fractures. Patterns of injury often are complex and do not fit the classic LeFort patterns. The best results are obtained through early assessment and treatment by direct open reduction followed by internal fixation of the body fragments and medial canthal ligaments. A multidisciplinary approach by a neurosurgeon, ophthalmologist, and plastic surgeon is essential.

Man, 46 was admitted with pulmonary contusion and multiple facial fractures after a vehicular accident. Results of an abdominal paracentesis were negative. Oral intubation was performed, and a tracheostomy was done with the patient under general anesthesia. A LeFort II maxillary fracture, a comminuted left zygomatic fracture, and naso-ethmoid-orbital fractures were present without apparent ocular damage. Results of a computerized tomographic study were normal. The naso-ethmoid-orbital fractures were reduced and internally fixed. The canthal ligaments were wired to one another transnasally, and the small nasal dorsum fragments were approximated and secured in place with steel wire. The patient's maxillary and mandibular partial dentures were wired in place, and intermaxillary fixation was provided. Nasal compression plates were applied. The zygomatic fracture was reduced and wired in place 6 days later, and a transfacial Kirschner wire was placed for added support to the comminuted arch. The patient recovered without complications.

Traumatic telecanthus with a rounded medial canthal angle and a depressed nasal dorsum are frequent findings in cases of naso-ethmoid-orbital fracture. Often other, life-threatening injuries are present. An "open sky" approach to the fractured region provides excellent exposure. The medial canthal ligaments must be firmly reattached. External nasal compression plates must be padded. Cerebrospinal fluid rhinorrhea, ocular globe injuries, injuries to the lacrimal drainage system, and other fractures must be recognized early and treated appropriately.

3–9 **Contraindications for Further Oculoplastic Surgery.** Alston Callahan (Birmingham, Ala.) points out that when orbital structures

(3–8) Am. Surg. 48:447–450, September 1982.
(3–9) Ann. Plast. Surg. 10:194–199, March 1983.

have been badly damaged by cancer surgery, trauma, irradiation, or oculomotor nerve paralysis further oculoplastic surgical procedures may not be warranted. These patients may go from one surgeon to another requesting further surgery so as to gain a better appearance. Minor surgery may be warranted where major procedures are contraindicated. Conditions that defy repair include fixation of a seeing eye in extensive scar tissue; destruction or complete loss of function of the levator palpebrae superioris combined with a seeing eye that cannot be moved; and grossly contracted sockets with inadequate lid or mucosal remnants, or both.

A young man presented with an immobilized right eye due to profuse scar tissue after severe injury in a collision. The orbital walls and floor were crushed and the orbital roof was fractured, but the eyeball survived. No further surgery was recommended, but another surgeon was persuaded to operate. Although minor procedures provided some help, an extensive attempt to correct enophthalmos was not helpful.

Another young man was seen after a serious ocular injury and two unsuccessful attempts to repair a blowout fracture with implant material. The left globe was fixed in scar tissue, and ocular motility was limited to a few millimeters at most in two directions. The globe was ptosed downward and was enophthalmic. Three operative stages were used in an attempt to remove scar tissue and elevate the orbital contents, but finally the eye was sealed off as a "reserve" eye.

A woman with marked ptosis and lateral rotation of the left eye from oculomotor nerve paralysis, due to surgery for a brain tumor, repeatedly requested that the eye be straightened and the ptosis corrected. The eye was straightened, but the ptosis was only partly corrected to protect the cornea. The patient subsequently saw other surgeons in an attempt to improve her situation.

A girl who had radiation therapy for retinoblastoma in infancy underwent seven operations to reconstruct the socket of the left eye and had marked fibrosis as a result. There was no vestige of eyelids, and movement of skin flaps had distorted the eyebrow. Corrective surgery was carried out before providing a glue-on prosthesis.

▶ [Sage advice which hopefully will be modified when we can control scar tissue biochemically.—S.H.M.] ◀

3–10 **Dacryocystorhinostomy by the Method of Iliff: Long-Term Follow-Up.** Jens Winther (Univ. of Aarhus, Denmark) performed 41 consecutive dacryocystorhinostomies by the method of Iliff in 36 patients in 1973–1981. Twenty-five primary and one secondary operations were done in 25 patients with idiopathic stenosis of the nasolacrimal duct. Twelve primary and three secondary procedures were done in 11 patients with stenosis due to fracture of the nose, maxilla, and zygoma. The operations were done by 9 different surgeons. The

(3–10)   Acta Ophthalmol. (Copenh.) 60:564–567, August 1982.

lacrimal sac and periosteum were dissected from the lacrimal fossa through a 1.5- to 2-cm incision just below the medial canthal ligament along the orbital rim, and an osteotomy was done in the nasal bony wall with the 8-mm Iliff dacryotrephine. A No. 14 urethral catheter was passed up the nose and out the osteotomy opening. The end of the catheter was placed in the top of the lacrimal sac and fixed with a catgut suture to the sac wall and, with a silk suture, in the wing of the nose. The catheter was removed after 11–28 days.

Thirteen of 20 primary operations for idiopathic stenosis and the secondary operation were patent at a follow-up examination, an average of 4½ years after surgery. The patency rate was 93% in 14 cases in which the catheter had remained in place for 3 weeks or longer postoperatively. Only two of nine primary operations and two of three secondary operations for posttraumatic stenosis were patent at the follow-up examination, an average of 5.8 years after surgery.

The method of Iliff is a simplified form of dacryocystorhinostomy that involves a small incision and no soft tissue damage. The catheter should not be removed for at least 3 weeks after operation. With this modification the procedure is likely to be a reliable means of relieving stenosis of the nasolacrimal duct.

3–11 **Traumatic Enophthalmos** and its management are discussed by Orkan George Stasior and Janet L. Roen (Albany Med. College). Traumatic enophthalmos is encountered in patients with facial fractures, usually including orbital floor fractures, and in those requiring enucleation after globe injury. Enophthalmos may not be evident immediately after injury because of the presence of edema and hematoma. The eye or ocular prosthesis is sunken into the orbit and is slightly ptotic. A deep superior lid sulcus, a pseudoptosis, and a flattened, nearly concave lower lid are noted. These deformities are caused by redistribution of the remaining orbital fat and levator muscle retraction by the superior rectus muscle and lid, as well as by tissue loss itself.

Use of a cosmetic shell may be the simplest measure in anophthalmic patients. Magnifying lenses in front of a nonfunctioning eye or prosthesis may make it appear normal sized. An implant within the muscle cone can provide excellent volume restoration and maintenance of any motility. An alloplastic sphere or a large dermal fat graft can be used. An alloplastic implant should be covered by Tenon's capsule. Subperiosteal implants can be used both in the presence of an eye and in the anophthalmic orbit. Silicone rubber chips may be useful. Enophthalmos that is present after orbital floor fracture can be managed by reducing herniated tissue. Residual enophthalmos may necessitate implant surgery. An alternate approach is to camouflage enophthalmos by creating the illusion of a normally positioned eye. The palpebral fissure can be enlarged vertically or hor-

(3–11) Ophthalmology (Rochester) 89:1267–1273, November 1982.

izontally, or it can be framed with expanded contours. Pseudoptosis can be treated by Müller-conjunctival resections. Superior sulcus deformity can be corrected with implants of fascia lata or dermal fat.

In the future, lysis of fibrosed orbital tissue may advance the management of traumatic enophthalmos.

▶ [The authors discuss multiple solutions to the problem of enophthalmos which would not be accepted by surgeons who have a knowledge of modern craniofacial techniques. Camouflage procedures, silicone rubber chips, and the enlargement of the palpebral fissure are probably rarely necessary. In fact, there is probably never any reason to use silicone rubber chips.—L.A.W.] ◀

3–12 **High-Resolution CT Analysis of Facial Struts in Trauma.—** *Part I. Normal Anatomy.*—Computed tomography (CT) provides a means of simultaneously evaluating both the osseous and soft tissue components of the face. High-spatial-resolution, thin-section CT can accurately depict the thin bony septae of the facial skeleton, enhancing the evaluation of patients with facial trauma. Lindell R. Gentry, William F. Manor, Patrick A. Turski, and Charles M. Strother (Univ. of Wisconsin, Madison) studied the normal anatomy of the face in 6 cadaver heads by using 1.5-mm section, high-resolution CT. The scanner was a GE CT/T 8800.

The face was conceptualized as three groups of interconnected osseous struts, or buttresses, oriented in the horizontal, sagittal, and coronal planes. Coronal and axial scans made at about 90 and 0 degrees, respectively, to the infraorbital-meatal line usually provided the best perspective. Coronal scans revealed areas of sutural discontinuity anteriorly. Sections made in the middle of the face posterior to the body of the zygoma intersect the horizontal and sagittal struts. A coronal scan through the infraorbital canal will show interruption of the orbital floor at this site. Scans made through the most posterior aspect of the facial skeleton will parallel the posterior coronal strut and may demonstrate fractures of the pterygoid plate region.

Inferior axial plane scans of the face roughly parallel the inferior horizontal strut. The middle horizontal strut is difficult to evaluate on axial scans. Axial scans made through the orbit between the middle and superior horizontal struts intersect the sagittal and coronal buttresses.

The coronal plane is the best for evaluating facial trauma. It is perpendicular to both the sagittal and horizontal struts, and the most important soft tissues of the face are best demonstrated in this plane. The facial skeleton can be thoroughly evaluated with fewer sections. Dental fillings may obscure detail. When coronal scans fail to completely show certain osseous or soft tissue structures, a limited direct axial evaluation or axial reformation of the coronal scans may be helpful. Axial scanning is preferable for demonstrating the zygomatic arch, the pterygomaxillary fissure, the posterior walls of the maxil-

(3–12) AJR 140:523–541, March 1983.

lary and frontal sinuses, and the lacrimal crest and lacrimal sac fossa.

Part II. Osseous and Soft-Tissue Complications.—Gentry, Manor, Turski, and Strother have used high-resolution, thin-section computed tomography (CT) to evaluate the osseous and soft tissue complications of facial trauma. Facial fractures were produced in 6 cadaver heads by applying force anteroposteriorly to the anterior maxilla or to the nasofrontal complex, anteroposteriorly or slightly caudocranially, and biplanar thin-section CT was then carried out. The face was conceptualized as a series of horizontal, sagittal, and coronal osseous struts in interpreting the CT findings.

Computed tomography proved to be accurate in detecting and classifying LeFort-type facial fractures. All the specimens had bilateral LeFort I and II fractures, and 5 also had tripod fractures, 2 of which were bilateral. Many secondary and tertiary fractures also were present. In all specimens CT provided more data on the osseous and soft tissue complications than could be communicated by conventional classification schemes.

Changes associated with horizontal strut fractures included dural disruption at the cribriform plate, involvement of anterior cranial fossa structures, optic nerve injury, and involvement of the extraocular muscles. Disruption of the sagittal struts can be associated with nasolacrimal duct injury and changes in the maxillary sinus ostium, the rectus muscles, and soft tissue structures in the superior and inferior orbital fissures. Fractures of the coronal struts can involve the frontal sinus, anterior fossa, lacrimal gland and sac, nasofrontal duct, and the soft tissues of the pterygopalatine fossa.

Study of the injured face by thin-section, high-resolution CT is a useful approach. Coronal sections generally are best for evaluating complications due to disruption of the horizontal and sagittal struts, whereas axial sections are best for studying complications involving the coronal struts. In most instances complications can be detected in either plane of a section.

▶ [CT analysis for facial trauma has been used and described by several plastic surgeons. Its primary indication has been neurosurgical but the addition of facial bone views has been helpful. Should it be used in all patients with maxillofacial trauma? Will its use improve or alter surgical correction of the traumatic injuries?—S.H.M.] ◀

3–14 **Our Experience With Freilinger's Method for Dynamic Correction of Facial Paralysis.** Temporal muscle flaps do not provide unconscious, synchronous smiling in patients with facial paralysis. Cross-face nerve grafting is effective only in relatively recent cases. In 1975 Freilinger proposed a combination of muscle flap transposition and cross-face nerve grafting in which the temporal muscle is denervated 6 to 8 months after the nerve transplantation. Then a flap is dissected out and transposed to the nasolabial area, after which the

(3–14) Br. J. Plast. Surg. 35:483–488, October 1982.

end of the nerve graft is inserted into the muscle fibers of the flap. This method is less time consuming than free muscle transplantation with microvascular anastomosis, and anastomotic thrombosis is not a risk.

J.-P. A. Nicolai, H. M. Vingerhoets, and S. L. H. Notermans (Nijmegen, Netherlands) used Freilinger's method in 8 patients with unilateral facial paralysis of varying etiology and duration. The sural nerve was used for the cross-face nerve transplant at the first operation in all instances. In most cases all fascicles of the graft were buried between muscle fibers at the second operation, without attempting a definitive nerve anastomosis.

All patients obtained movements in the paralyzed cheek, but excursion of the mouth angle always was less than on the unaffected side. All patients produced movements when clenching the teeth, and some showed movement without biting. In no case were the movements convincingly unconscious. Some muscle fibers apparently obtained innervation of the cross-face nerve graft, and others obtained trigeminal reinnervation. Some time was necessary before reinnervation of the flap was apparent; 3 patients showed no flap response at 1 year when the nerve graft or facial nerve was electrically stimulated.

The results in this limited number of patients indicate that Freilinger's method of treating facial paralysis has merits as a principle. Better results may be obtained by using a muscle that is easier to denervate than the temporal muscle and has a greater range of excursion. Possible alternatives are the ventral half of the masseter, the sternocleidomastoid, or a flap from the pectoralis major. With Freilinger's method the graft fascicles reinnervate the flap through neural neurotization in most cases, but the flaps also are partially innervated by the trigeminal nerve.

3–15 **Evaluation of Results in 36 Cases of Facial Palsy Treated with Nerve Grafts.** Grazia Salimbeni-Ughi (St. Chiara Univ., Pisa, Italy) performed nerve grafting in 36 cases of recent facial palsy in the past 3 years. Twenty patients with recent traumatic paralysis in whom the lesion was distal to the stylomastoid foramen had homolateral faciofacial grafting. Sixteen with a lesion proximal to the stylomastoid foramen had faciofacial cross-face grafting. Faciofacial homolateral grafts were done 40 days or less after injury in patients aged 3–59 years. With two exceptions, no loss of nerve tissue was observed. Sural nerve grafts were sutured in place with one or two 10–0 nylon sutures connecting a group of fascicles with each cable graft. In 4 cases in which the wound reached the oral commissure, the distal end of the graft was divided into single fascicles, and each was buried in the muscle tissue. Satisfactory reinnervation and good symmetrical emotional mobility were obtained in this group. No patient required a second operation. The 4 patients with synkinesis con-

(3–15) Ann. Plast. Surg. 9:36–41, July 1982.

tract the nasolabial fold when they firmly contract the orbicularis oculi.

Eleven of the 16 patients who had cross-facial nerve grafting had an intracranial interruption because of acoustic neurinoma surgery. The age range was 15–63 years. A two-stage technique was used in the later cases, but a one-stage method currently is preferred. Three cable grafts are used; one placed superiorly in a subcutaneous tunnel under the eyebrows, and two in a superior lip tunnel. Reinnervation developed slowly and incompletely in these cases, although a good static aspect sometimes was restored to the face. Three cases were failures. In 4 cases only minimal emotional facial movement resulted. Encouraging results were obtained in the most recent cases, which included the youngest patient and the most recently denervated patient. Currently, patients younger than age 50 are operated on as soon as possible after denervation when no spontaneous regeneration is expected. The chief impediment to this method probably is the need for the regenerating fibers to travel a relatively great distance to reach their motor end plates.

3–16 **Electrophysiologic Evaluation of Cross-Face Nerve Graft in Treatment of Facial Palsy.** J. Delbeke and Ch. Thauvoy (Catholic Univ. of Louvain, Brussels) performed a cross-face autogenous single graft in 8 patients with facial palsy. The patients, aged 12–63 years at the time of surgery, were regularly tested for 18–44 months. All had a unilateral facial palsy considered to be irreversible, 5 after acoustic neuroma or its surgical treatment, or after both. A single sural nerve stump was placed in the upper lip and connected on the healthy side with the proximal severed branches of the facial nerve. The other side of the graft was connected with terminal twigs of the heterolateral facial nerve on the paralyzed side via a midfacial incision. No attempt was made to reinnervate the frontal muscles.

The clinical results were disappointing. The only observed recovery could not be ascribed to the graft procedure. Chronaxy was unacceptably long in all muscles of the paralyzed side of the face, even in the cases with the best reinnervation. A blink reflex appeared on the paralyzed side 7 to 21 months after the first voluntary activity of the orbicularis oris. Spontaneous activity generally was limited to a few fibrillations during needle insertion. Voluntary potentials generally remained small. In two instances the graft was not the only source of reinnervation. Conduction velocities in the graft reached about 30 m/second.

The cross-face nerve graft techniques appears to be a failure in patients with facial palsy, and can no longer be recommended. Collateral reinnervation was not effective in the present cases. Muscle degeneration is an important limiting factor, even with intensive

(3–16) Acta Neurochir. (Wien) 65:111–127, 1982.

physiotherapy. It may become possible to bring the graft directly into the paralyzed muscles, avoiding a second suture and the terminal twigs of the paralyzed nerve, which obstruct axonal growth.

▶ [Would a two-stage nerve graft anastomosis, as suggested by Anderl et al. (see abstract 1–31) work better? Were the results as poor when comparing the very young patient with the elderly patient, or when the facial paralysis was of more recent origin? Our experiences suggest that, as with any nerve repair, young patients with a recent onset of paralysis are the best candidates for this type of procedure.

Would the results of combining the cross nerve graft procedure with a masseter of sternocleidomastoid muscle provide a better result? Will either of these methods restore more normal function than can be achieved using muscle transfers alone?— S.H.M.] ◀

3–17 **Alternate Innervations of Facial Musculature.** The several reports of spontaneous return of facial function without grafting or other surgery indicate that there may be alternate pathways of innervation of the facial muscles. Steven M. Parnes, Norman Strominger, Steven Silver, and Jerome C. Goldstein (Albany Med. College, New York) injected selected facial muscles of the rhesus or cynomolgus monkey and cat using the technique of retrograde axonal transport with chromogens tagged to horseradish peroxidase (HRP) to demonstrate CNS representation. In 3 of 10 monkeys the facial nerve was injected directly with HRP. In 2 monkeys the stapedius muscle was exposed and injected with the marker enzyme, and in another study, the chorda tympani was injected. Two animals had the facial nerve transected in the middle ear. The animals were killed 24–48 hours after the injections.

The facial nucleus was identified, showing a topographic arrangement in the CNS. In several specimens nuclear cells of the mesencephalic tract also were stained. This tract is part of the trigeminal system, normally associated with proprioception, whose axons travel with other fifth cranial nerve branches. The trigeminal motor nucleus showed no accumulation of the enzyme marker, which indicated a lack of contamination from facial musculature innervated by the fifth cranial nerve.

These findings indicate that the facial musculature has a nerve supply in addition to the seventh cranial nerve. Mesencephalic cells directly innervate facial musculature in primates, presumably via the trigeminal nerve. Many interconnections exist between the mesencephalic and other aspects of the trigeminal system with the facial nucleus. A direct connection may exist between mesencephalic cells and the facial musculature. A central reorganization may occur in the brain stem so that, when the facial nerve is transected, the trigeminal system compensates by means of these interneural connections. Physiologic studies are needed to support the anatomic findings.

▶ [This is an interesting study emphasizing that the seventh cranial nerve is not the only motor nerve in facial musculature.—L.A.W.] ◀

(3–17) Arch. Otolaryngol. 108:418–421, July 1982.

3–18 **Indications for Open Reduction of Mandibular Condyle Fractures.** Michael F. Zide and John N. Kent (Louisiana State Univ.) point out that although most mandibular condyle fractures are managed by closed reduction, open reduction is absolutely indicated when there is displacement into the middle cranial fossa, inability to obtain adequate occlusion by closed reduction, lateral extracapsular displacement of the condyle, and invasion by a foreign body, as in a gunshot wound.

Relative indications for open reduction exist chiefly in adults with condyles displaced out of the fossa and the associated malocclusion. Edentulous patients with bilateral condylar fractures and no splint available, or in whom splinting is not possible because of alveolar ridge atrophy, can have open reduction, as can those with unilateral or bilateral condylar fractures if splinting is not recommended for medical reasons. Open reduction may be indicated for patients with bilateral condylar fractures associated with comminuted midfacial fractures or with gnathologic problems.

The pathogenesis and severity of an injury are the most important factors in the outcome of treatment. The operative approach is influenced by the position of the fracture, its age, and the amount of edema present. In using a face-lift approach, it must be decided whether to dissect out the facial nerve first or to merely dissect bluntly through the parotid and masseter muscle. Once the condylar fracture is exposed, stabilization can be obtained by complete removal and replacement of the segment, bone plating, direct wiring, using a K-wire or pin, wiring via a drill-guide, or other methods of plating or pinning. Plating with at least two screws in the condylar segment and two in the stable mandible is the only method that routinely permits immediate postoperative mobilization. In cases of recent fracture, the segments can be replaced in as anatomical a position as possible without wiring if maxillomandibular fixation is used.

Twenty-one patients with condylar fractures, or about one fifth of all those seen with such fractures, were treated by open reduction at the authors' institution in 1980. The results were gratifying in nearly all cases, although follow-up is 2 years or less.

▶ [The authors give sound recommendations for reduction of displaced condylar fractures. However, they use an incision that would be unacceptable to most plastic surgeons and call it a face-lift incision when, in fact, it certainly is not because of its anterior and inferior placement.—L.A.W.] ◀

3–19 **Histopathology Associated With Malposition of the Human Temporomandibular Joint Disk.** The pathosis associated with meniscal displacement has an important bearing on mandibular dysfunction and its management. Robert P. Scapino (Univ. of Illinois, Chicago) examined three serially sectioned whole temporomandibular joints (TMJs) as well as menisci removed surgically from 14 consecu-

(3–18) J. Oral Maxillofac. Surg. 41:89–98, February 1983.
(3–19) Oral Surg. 55:382–397, April 1983.

tive patients with internal joint derangement. Two pathologic TMJs were taken at autopsy from men aged 23 and 64 years, and 1 was from a woman aged 75.

In all whole joint specimens the bulk of all the posterior band lay anterior to the condyle. The central part of the disk lay below or just anterior to the summit of the articular eminence, and the anterior band lay well forward of the condyle. In each instance the disk seemed to overlie more of the lateral pterygoid muscle than is normal. The degree of disk deformity varied in these specimens. Disruption of the collagen fiber pattern in the posterior band and in the central part of the disk ranged from slight to considerable. Transverse fiber bundles extended forward into the posterior end of the central part of the disk, disrupting the compact anteroposterior orientation of collagen fibers in the central region. Fibers oriented perpendicularly to the surface sometimes were seen within the central part of the disk.

Arthrograms from 7 of the patients who had meniscectomy showed clear evidence of flexure of the disk. Abnormalities were noted at the junction of the posterior attachment and posterior band. Local areas of progressive and regressive remodeling were present in all the whole joint specimens, but the integrity of the articular tissue covering these sites usually was not obviously affected.

Anterior displacement of the TMJ disk is associated with remodeling of the soft tissues of the joint. The anterior part of the posterior attachment becomes fibrotic. The capsule connecting the anterior band of the disk to the condyle appears to be elongated, and the disk appears to overlie an inordinate part of the lateral pterygoid muscle. Variations in pathologic features may be responsible to some extent for differences in symptoms observed in patients with displacement of the meniscus of the TMJ.

3–20 **Interpositional Cortical Plate Augmentation in the Reconstruction of a Labially Deficient Alveolar Process.** Problems have occurred in using autogenous cancellous bone and marrow grafts in treating alveolar bone defects. Extensive resorption may occur. Cyrus J. Amato and Howard Israel (VA Med. Center, East Orange, N.J.) have used a new technique designed to reduce or eliminate graft resorption and obtain more predictable results. A greenstick fracture is created in the region of the alveolar defect involving the outer cortical plate, and the cortical plate then is contoured to the shape of an ideal alveolar ridge. Cancellous bone and marrow from the ilium are placed in the space. The cortical plate remains attached to the mucoperiosteum and functions as a pedicled graft.

Woman, 23, had an alveolar defect of the right maxilla, due to traumatic avulsion of several teeth and buccal alveolar bone, which prevented fabrica-

(3–20) J. Oral Maxillofac. Surg. 41:185–187, March 1983.

tion of a functional and esthetic fixed bridge. A narrow maxillary right alveolar ridge with deficient buccal contour was observed. A sunken deformity was noted in the region of the right canine eminence. After cancellous bone and particulate marrow were obtained from the left ilium, an incision was made along the alveolar crest, and a cut was made along the ridge through cortical and cancellous bone. A curved osteotome was used to make two vertical cuts through the buccolabial cortical bone on each side of the defect. The cortical plate was expanded by wedging osteotomes into the surgical site before packing the cancellous bone and marrow graft into the surgically created defect. A full-thickness mucoperiosteal flap was elevated by a midline palatal incision, and the periosteum was scored to mobilize the flap and obtain primary closure over the wound. Good wound healing took place. No resorption has occurred 8 months after operation, and the contour of the alveolar ridge has been maintained.

Interpositional cortical plate augmentation may prove valuable in reconstructing the labially deficient alveolar process. The same principles can be used to reconstruct other contour deformities of the face. The procedure is based on sound biologic principles and may offer a technique that minimizes the amount of graft resorption.

▶ [The authors describe an important principle of interposing bone as an inlay graft sandwiched between layers of vascularized bone. This has been recognized for some time as an important principle in maintaining bone volume and avoiding onlay grafts which seem to absorb at a higher rate.—L.A.W.] ◀

3–21 **Occupationally Acquired Vibratory Angioedema With Secondary Carpal Tunnel Syndrome.** Vibratory angioedema has been described as a hereditary form of physical urticaria in a single kindred with autosomal inheritance. Mark H. Wener, W. James Metzger, and Ronald A. Simon observed a patient in whom nonfamilial vibratory angioedema led to intermittent compression neuropathy of the median nerve.

Man, 32, experienced intermittent discomfort of the left hand after 3 years of work as a metal grinder; he used his left hand to hold objects against a revolving grindstone. Symptoms usually developed within 5 minutes of starting to work and lasted for 30 minutes to 2 hours afterward. Swelling often was preceded by pruritus in the hands and fingers, as well as paresthesias of the thumb and the index and middle fingers. Pain in the left palm and wrist occurred with progressively less exposure to vibration. Diffuse erythema and swelling of the wrist and hand developed after minimal vibration or trauma, with hyperesthesia and dysesthesia in the median nerve distribution. Exposure to ice water did not elicit symptoms, and a methacholine skin test yielded negative results. Findings on roentgenograms were normal. The condition was reproduced using a vibrating laboratory vortexer. Nerve conduction velocities were progressively slowed on the affected side. Trials of treatment with antihistamines and nonsteroidal anti-inflammatory drugs failed. When left carpal tunnel release was carried out, mild narrowing of the median nerve was observed. Swelling and pruritus persisted during work but were improved, and normal activities could be resumed without symptoms. Vibration of the forearm still produced angioedema, but nerve conduction

(3–21) Ann. Intern. Med. 98:44–46, January 1983.

velocities remained normal. The plasma histamine concentration increased during vibratory exposure.

Recurrent vibration apparently may predispose to an acquired form of vibratory angioedema. The results of routine measurements of nerve conduction velocity may be normal in patients with compression neuropathies. The presence of transient swelling, pruritus, and paresthesia in persons exposed to vibration should lead to further study to identify acquired vibratory angioedema and secondary compression neuropathy.

▶ [A rare phenomenon nicely reproduced clinically and presented as a case report.—F.J.M.] ◀

3–22 **Two-Stage Reconstruction of Flexor Tendons.** E. Paneva-Holevich (Sofia, Bulgaria) has, since 1965, used 2-stage tenoplasty with a pedicled tendon graft for secondary reconstruction of damaged flexor tendons in the critical zone in 249 patients; the total number of reconstructions was 324. In another 28 patients, 39 two-stage tenoplasties were combined with use of a silicone rod to form a pseudosheath, as suggested by Hunter. Initially, the flexor tendons are di-

Fig 3–6 (left).—Second stage of 2-stage tenoplasty. Release of proximal part of superficial tendon.

Fig 3–7 (right).—Graft is shown in situ in second stage of the procedure.

(Courtesy of Paneva-Holevich, E.: Int. Orthop. 6:133–318, 1982; Berlin-Heidelberg-New York; Springer.)

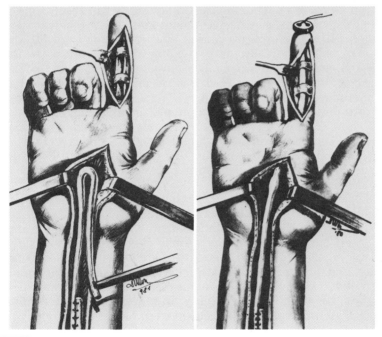

(3–22) Int. Orthop. 6:133–138, 1982.

vided at the level of the lumbrical muscles, and the proximal ends of the superficial and deep flexor tendons are joined end to end. A month later the tendon of the flexor sublimis is divided at the musculotendinous junction and mobilized distally for use as a pedicle graft (Figs 3–6 and 3–7). The silicone rod, when used, is placed in the tendon bed after excising scarred tissue and attached distally to the stub of the profundus tendon. The pedicle graft is prepared 2–3 months later, and its distal end attached to the proximal end of the silicone rod, which is then removed through a small incision at the level of the distal phalanx to pull the graft through the prepared canal. The graft tip then is sutured to the profundus remnant.

The patients, aged 2–56 years at the time of surgery, were followed up for 6 months to 10 years. Of fingers classed as favorable for repair before operation, very good or good results were achieved in 96% as assessed by the distance from the pulp of the fingertip to the distal palmar crease on active flexion. Less satisfactory results were obtained in scarred or stiff fingers. When more than 1 finger was involved, the outcome was not influenced by surgery on another digit. Use of the Hunter technique improved the results, but only slightly when stiffness was present preoperatively. Even a small increase in the range of finger motion often led to considerable improvement in hand function and was appreciated by the patient.

3–23 **Flexor Pollicis Longus Abductor-Plasty for Spastic Thumb-in-Palm Deformity.** Thumb-in-palm deformity can result from spasticity of the adductor pollicis, the thenar muscles, or the flexor pollicis longus (FPL). In deformities caused by spasticity of the FPL, the interphalangeal (IP) and metacarpophalangeal (MP) joints of the thumb are flexed, and the trapeziometacarpal joint is flexed and adducted. Richard J. Smith (Harvard Med. School) managed 7 patients having a palmar clenched thumb caused by FPL spasticity, transferring the FPL to the radial side of the thumb and arthrodesing or tenodesing the IP joint. Five patients had cerebral palsy, and 2 had spasticity as a result of cerebral injury. The 5 males and 2 females were aged 8–35 years at the time of operation. All had difficulty in holding and grasping objects. In 2, previous surgery failed to improve thumb function satisfactorily.

The operative procedure is illustrated in Figure 3–8. The hand was immobilized in plaster for 6 weeks postoperatively, and a C splint was worn for another 6 weeks. On follow-up at 33–55 months, the appearance of all hands was improved. Arthrodesis or tenodesis of the IP joint was uneventful in all instances. One patient refused capsulorrhaphy, and another requires MP joint arthrodesis. Maximum active thumb abduction averaged 54 degrees. Adduction was weak in 1 patient, who required further surgery. In no case did hand dominance change. The limb operated on continued to be used for assistive pur-

(3–23) J. Hand Surg. 7:327–334, July 1982.

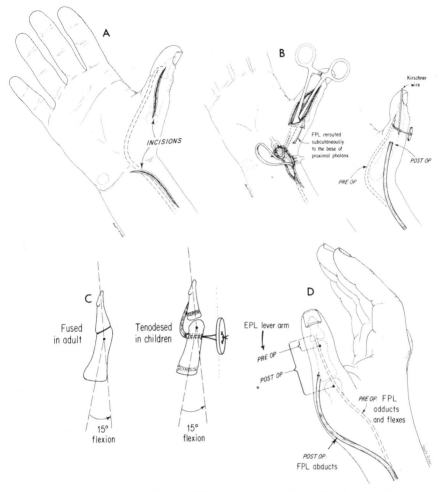

Fig 3–8.—A, incision to radial side of thumb exposes insertion of the flexor pollicis longus (FPL), interphalangeal (IP) joint, and base of proximal phalanx. Second curved incision to radial side of wrist exposes the FPL near its musculotendinous juncture, allowing the tendon to be withdrawn from the carpal canal. **B,** the FPL is transected at its insertion and withdrawn from carpal canal through wrist incision. It is passed subcutaneously to the radial side of the proximal phalanx base. Distal joint is stabilized in slight flexion. **C,** the IP joint of the thumb is arthrodesed in about 15 degrees of flexion in adults. In children with open epiphyses, the distal joint may be tenodesed in about 15 degrees of flexion. **D,** transfer of the FPL to the radial side of the proximal phalanx reduces adduction-flexion deformity and augments thumb abduction by the transferred position of the FPL. Arthrodesis of the IP improves metacarpophalangeal joint extension by increasing the lever arm of the FPL on the metacarpophalangeal joint. (Courtesy of Smith, R. J.: J. Hand Surg. 7:327–334, July 1982.)

poses only. Patients were better able to grasp and release larger objects than before the operation.

In properly selected patients with thumb-in-palm deformity caused by spasticity of the FPL, improved function and appearance can be achieved through IP joint stabilization and subcutaneous transfer of the FPL to the radial side of the proximal phalanx of the thumb. However, there is a danger of overcorrection, with disabling weakness of thumb flexion and adduction resulting. Risks are minimized by performing FPL abductor-plasty only in patients without soft tissue contracture who have active wrist palmar flexion and dorsiflexion, and who exhibit good strength of the thumb adductors, thenars, and extensors.

3–24   **A Staged Technique for Repair of the Traumatic Boutonniere Deformity** is described by Raymond M. Curtis, Robert L. Reid, and John M. Provost. The chronic boutonniere deformity must be splinted initially to stretch the contracted palmar capsule of the stiff proximal interphalangeal (PIP) joint. Full passive extension is a prerequisite for surgery. The first surgical stage is tendolysis of the extensor tendon and freeing of the transverse retinacular ligament. If full extension is not then present, the freed transverse retinacular ligament is sectioned through its length on both sides of the finger just palmar to the

Fig 3–9 (left).—Stage III in repair of traumatic boutonniere deformity consists of lengthening the lateral bands over the middle phalanx or tenotomy of the extensor tendon.
Fig 3–10 (right).—In stage IV, the central extensor tendon is repaired.
(Courtesy of Curtis, R. M., et al.: J. Hand Surg. 8:167–171, March 1983.)

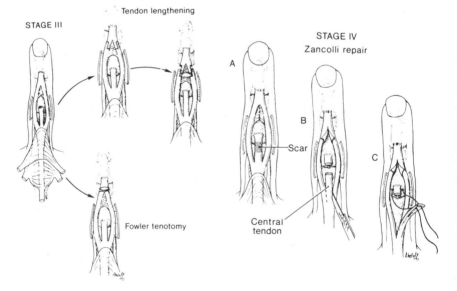

lateral band. If necessary, tendon lengthening of the lateral bands over the middle phalanx is carried out at a subsequent session (Fig 3–9). The final stage is repair of the central extensor tendon (Fig 3–10).

Twenty-three patients aged 17–57 years were treated for chronic traumatic boutonniere deformity. Most of the injuries were caused by laceration with a sharp instrument. Several fingers were splinted in flexion for 4–6 weeks. Six patients required stage IV rather than stage III treatment in addition to the first 2 stages. These patients lacked 55 degrees of extension at the PIP preoperatively, but lacked only an average of 17 degrees postoperatively. The 17 patients who lacked an average of 41 degrees of extension preoperatively lacked an average of 10 degrees postoperatively. All but 3 patients were able to touch or approximate the distal palmar crease postoperatively. The overall average distance from the distal palmar crease was only 1 cm.

The staged approach to chronic traumatic boutonniere deformity often permits a less complex procedure to be carried out in the involved digit, and unnecessary surgery often is avoided.

▶ [This is a systematic, step-by-step surgical approach incorporating separate solutions with each of the principle elements involved in the boutonniere deformity. Each step has previously been described but usually only as the single maneuver necessary for correction.—F.J.M.] ◀

3–25 Arteriovenous Anastomosis as Solution for Absent Venous Drainage in Replantation Surgery. Replantation of amputated digits at the level of the distal interphalangeal joint or further distally is difficult because the vein is not suitable or a venule is too small for microsurgical repair. The survival of "artery only" replantations is much less than that of implants in which both arteries and veins are anastomosed. Arlan R. Smith, G. Jan Sonneveld, and Jacques C. van der Meulen (Rotterdam) attempted to substitute for absent venous drainage by using the contralateral artery in the replanted digit as a venous outflow pole, connected with or without a venous graft to a vein in the proximal stump of the digit. The procedure is illustrated in Figure 3–11. Three patients were managed in this way for distal phalangeal injuries. On follow-up for 1½ years, none had claudication, and no arteriovenous (AV) tumor developed in the replanted part.

It is possible that sudden high arterial pressure results in the mechanical opening of multiple communications already present with the associated vein, creating an AV fistula. Nutrient circulation is essentially bypassed, and hypoxia develops in the region adjacent to the artery and vein. Surgical manipulation of the recipient bed results in trauma, edema, and a change in capillary blood flow, accentuating ischemia and hypoxia. In addition, angiogenesis is stimulated. With AV anastomosis, new venules may develop that provide sufficient drainage. Early postoperative PO_2 measurements in the

(3–25) Plast. Reconstr. Surg. 71:525–532, April 1983.

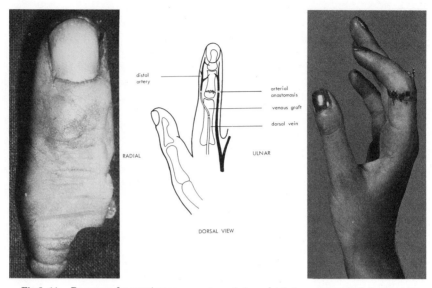

Fig 3–11.—Proceaure for arteriovenous anastomosis in replantation surgery. *Left,* finger at time of injury. *Center,* diagram showing the vascular anastomoses. *Right,* appearance of finger 4 weeks after replantation. (Courtesy of Smith, A. R., et al.: Plast. Reconstr. Surg. 71:525–532, April 1983.)

present patients yielded curves resembling those in replantations with normal inflow and outflow. No significant changes in P_{O_2} were noted 1 year postoperatively. Oxygen levels measured directly after surgery did suggest reduced tissue oxygenation, and thus relative hypoxia.

▶ [This is a fascinating and tantalizing piece of work. The arterial to venous blood flow is easy to accept on a purely hydrodynamic basis, but how does capillary perfusion take place sufficiently to sustain cellular vitality until vascular neoplasia develops to consolidate the viability? Perhaps it is simply back pressure. Whatever the mechanism, it serves no one to argue with success.—F.J.M.] ◀

3–26 **Palmar Arthroplasty for Treatment of the Stiff Swan-Neck Deformity** is described by Frank A. Scott and John A. Boswick, Jr. (Univ. of Colorado). Proximal interphalangeal (PIP) stiffness in extension severely limits the grasping ability of the hand. Flexor tenosynovitis is a major factor in the production of PIP stiffness. A palmar zigzag incision is made under tourniquet control. The membranous part of the flexor sheath between annular pulleys II and IV is incised, elevating a rectangular flap, and tenosynovitis or nodules are removed. The release of palmar plate adhesions is shown in Figure 3–12. The distal and proximal attachments of the palmar plate are preserved. Collateral ligament adhesions can be released by blunt and sharp dissection at the lateral aspects of the condyle. The accessory collateral ligament then is incised in its midportion on each side until

(3–26) J. Hand Surg. 8:267–272, May 1983.

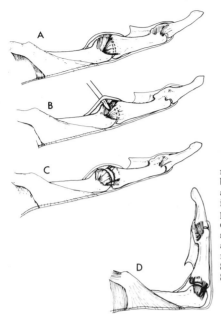

Fig 3–12.—Palmar arthroplasty. **A,** retrocondylar recess is obliterated by adhesions between palmar plate and proximal phalanx. **B,** adhesions are released by means of bilateral incisions on each lateral edge of the palmar plate and blunt dissection beneath it. **C,** collateral ligament contracture is incised sequentially until full passive motion is achieved. **D,** manipulation stretches the remaining dorsal contractures. (Courtesy of Scott, F. A., and Boswick, J. A., Jr.: J. Hand Surg. 8:267–272, May 1983.)

full passive motion is achieved. A superficialis tenodesis can be done to limit the last 15–20 degrees of PIP extension. The sheath need not be closed, but the rectangular flap can, if intact, be laid across the defect. Motion is begun after 24–48 hours, depending on swelling. Extension is limited to −30 degrees with a dorsal extension block splint for 3–4 weeks.

Soft tissue arthroplasty was done through a palmar approach in 47 stiff, extended PIP joints in 14 hands of 9 rheumatoid patients. The average motion ranged from +20 degrees of extension to 9.5 degrees of flexion preoperatively. On follow-up for an average of 2 years, the average range of motion was −7 degrees of extension to 72 degrees of flexion. Postoperative hyperextension was less frequent in later patients. The total arc of motion was improved from 29.5 degrees to 65 degrees postoperatively, and the arc changed from an attitude of hyperextension to one of flexion, producing a more functional range of motion.

Palmar arthroplasty can increase the range of motion in patients with swan-neck deformity from rheumatoid disease. Postoperative monitoring of joint motion is necessary to obtain the best results. This technique also has been used successfully in patients with fractures and tendon injuries, and in those undergoing replantation procedures.

3–27   **A Technique To Facilitate Drilling and Passing Intraosseous Wiring in the Hand** is described by L. R. Scheker (Glasgow). Intraos-

(3–27)   J. Hand Surg. 7:629–630, November 1982.

seous wiring is useful in joint arthrodesis and in the treatment of metacarpal and phalanageal fractures. Considerable dissection is necessary to drill holes in a bone and pass a wire through them. A simpler approach is based on the use of a 19-gauge disposable needle to drill the bone, threading the wire through the needle lumen. The needle tip is bent slightly to maintain needle alignment in the opposite bony cortex. The needle passes through bone as readily as a Kirschner wire does. The wire is introduced after removing bone debris from the end of the needle; the needle is withdrawn, leaving the wire in the bone. The procedure is repeated on the opposite bone fragment using the other end of the wire, forming a wire loop that is tightened for bone fixation.

This technique requires minimal dissection, and the entire loop of wire usually can be placed in less than a minute. The hole is slightly greater in diameter than the wire, but this has not created a clinical problem. Also, the wire sometimes twists, but this can be prevented by introducing it as far as possible into the needle.

▶ [I have also used Doctor Scheker's method in placing anchor wires for canthoplasty in traumatic telecanthus and found it fast, simple, and effective. The wire twisting can usually be traced to the bend in the needle tip partially occluding the lumen and forming a hook.—F.J.M.] ◀

3–28 **Free Nail Bed Graft for Treatment of Nail Bed Injuries of the Hand.** Previous methods of treating the severely crushed or avulsed fingernail bed with an intact matrix have not resulted in normal-appearing nails. Hidehiko Saito, Yorio Suzuki, Keiji Fujino, and Tatsuya Tajima (Niigata, Japan) achieved normal-looking nails by free grafting of a full-thickness nail bed from the lesser toes or from an amputated finger. Using a knife blade, the nail bed is harvested with the matrix in 1 piece, and the donor site is covered with a small split-skin graft from the lateral side of the foot. The graft is trimmed to fit and placed on the finger defect. The hyponychium is first reconstructed in avulsion and amputation injuries. In injuries involving both the nail bed and matrix, the epionychium may have to be reconstructed with local skin flaps.

This procedure was used on 11 fingers of 10 patients having an average age of 29 years. All injuries were traumatic, and the nail matrix was intact in all patients but 1. All 4 patients with type I injury (i.e., localized to the nail bed) regained normal-appearing nails (Fig 3–13). The 2 with type II or avulsion injuries regained a normal nail and a nearly normal nail, respectively. Repair of 3 type III (amputation) injuries resulted in nearly normal-appearing nails, and the outcome in a fourth such injury awaits final evaluation. The 1 patient with a type IV injury involving both the nail bed and matrix regained a smooth, relatively good-looking nail. No donor site difficulties occurred.

Excellent results can be obtained in patients with severely crushed

(3–28) J. Hand Surg. 8:171–178, March 1983.

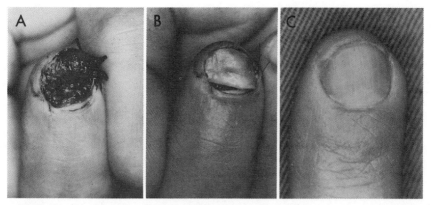

Fig 3–13.—Type I injury to the fingernail localized to the nail bed with only minor injury to surrounding structures. **A,** cortex of the distal phalanx is exposed in center of the defect. **B,** nail shown after application of the graft (proximal portion is the nail matrix). **C,** nail appearance 10 months postoperatively. (Courtesy of Saito, H., et al.: J. Hand Surg. 8:171–178, March 1983.)

or lost nail beds but an intact nail matrix using free full-thickness grafts of nail bed from the lesser toes or an amputated fingertip. The procedure can be used when restoring the length of the tip in fingertip amputations in conjunction with local skin flaps. One of the present patients had a good result from free grafting of both the toenail bed and matrix.

▶ [The authors have performed a service not only in describing their technique but just as importantly in emphasizing the desirability (to patients) of nail restoration.— F.J.M.] ◀

3–29 **The "Antenna" Procedure for the "Hook-Nail" Deformity** is described by Erdogan Atasoy, Alan Godfrey, and Michael Kalisman (Univ. of Louisville). The hook-nail deformity (Fig 3–14) frequently follows distal fingertip amputation with loss of part of the distal pulp, phalanx, and nail bed. The deformity may be of cosmetic importance to some individuals, or may be disabling to those with certain occupations. Four patients with the hook-nail deformity who were managed by an "antenna" procedure involving multiple Kirschner wires were followed up for 1–4 years. The nail plate is elevated from the nail bed along its full length, the part distal to the lunula discarded, and the pulp skin incised and reflected out to a normal contour. Scar tissue may have to be removed from the deep surface and margin of the pulp. The full-thickness nail bed is elevated from the distal phalanx back to the point at which it is straight and splinted there with two or three Kirschner pins inserted into the dorsum of the distal phalanx. The defect is covered by a cross finger flap from the dorsum of the adjacent finger, which is divided after 2 weeks. The Kirschner pins are left in place for 3 weeks.

(3–29) J. Hand Surg. 8:55–58, January 1983.

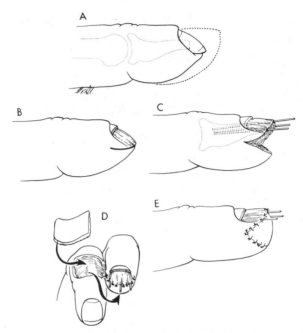

Fig 3–14.—Correction of hook-nail deformity. **A,** hook-nail deformity compared with normal fingertip contour *(dotted line).* **B,** nail plate is removed and pulp skin incised along hyponychium. **C,** pulp is reflected and full thickness of nail matrix is elevated; 3 small Kirschner wires resembling antennae are used for splinting; **D,** defect is covered with cross finger flap; **E,** appearance of repair after flap is divided 2 weeks postoperatively. (Courtesy of Atasoy, E., et al.: J. Hand Surg. 8:55–58, January 1983.)

The antenna procedure supports the nail bed, and the cross finger flap reconstructs the lost pulp and relieves the deforming tension. The viability of the elevated nail bed is not compromised as long as its continuity with the remaining proximal matrix and paronychial skin fold is not interrupted.

▶ [The results shown by the author are impressive. I can't wait to try it.—F.J.M.] ◀

3–30 **Restoration of Finger Extension by Free Transfer of the Tensor Fascia Lata Muscle.** In cases where extrinsic muscular loss makes conventional tendon transplants impracticable, tensor fascia lata muscle can be used in a free neuromuscular transfer to correct the functional deficit. The tensor fascia lata lends itself naturally to replacement of digital extensors due to the strength of its contraction and short tendon course, and its wide fascia allows easy division. One additional advantage is the large cutaneous flap, which simplifies the procedure.

M. Brice, G. Fiévé, and J. Xenard (Nancy, France) report the case of a crush injury of the forearm with Volkmann's syndrome, in which

(3–30) Ann. Chir. Plast. 27:267–271, 1982.

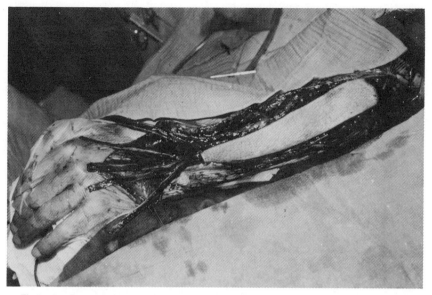

Fig 3–15.—Preoperative view showing 5 tendon strips. (Courtesy of Brice, M., et al.: Ann. Chir. Plast. 27:267–271, 1982.)

necrosis had destroyed all the extensor muscles and a great part of the anterior group. Restoration of wrist and finger extension was achieved by the free transplant of a myocutaneous flap using the tensor fascia lata muscle, which was vascularized by the anterior interosseous artery. Innervation was supplied by the motor branch of the radial nerve. The tendon was divided into five strips attached to the extensor tendons (Fig 3–15). Complete digital extension was possible after 8 months. After 2 years and a supplementary tendon transplant of the flexor digitorum profundus the patient was able to resume manual work.

▶ [This is a real contribution to the restoration of finger extension in a discouraging problem. Flexion might also be provided in the same way with limited excursion in a useful range. As Bunnel was fond of saying, "When you have nothing, a little bit is a lot!"—F.J.M.] ◀

3–31   **The Forearm Flap** is described by Wolfgang Mühlbauer, Eugen Herndl, and Wolfgang Stock (Munich). Free forearm flaps have been used by Song in China to release burn contractures. The flap has potential as a reliable, technically easy free or island flap that can provide good, pliable skin with a thin layer of subcutaneous fat and sensation. The free neurovascular forearm flap is an axial-pattern free flap based on the radial artery, 1 or 2 forearm veins, and 1 or 2 cutaneous nerve branches of the forearm. The vessels are large, with long

(3–31)   Plast. Reconstr. Surg. 70:336–344, September 1982.

pedicles and consistent anatomy. The donor site is closed directly when a long elliptical flap is used; otherwise, it is closed with a split-skin graft. The flap is raised by following the course of the radial artery proximally. The fascia of the forearm is included in the flap. The deeper arterial branches to muscles and tendon sheaths are ligated, as are the venae comitantes. The radial artery is reconstructed immediately by interposing a reversed vein graft from the same arm or a leg.

This type of flap was used in reconstructing a burn contracture of the neck, a heel defect that developed after replantation of the foot, and a forearm that sustained a crush injury. The only complication was venous thrombosis in latter patients. The flap provides skin of excellent quality in relatively large amounts along with a thin layer of subcutaneous fat not requiring defatting and relatively large nutrient vessels. Adequate drainage is obtained with a single venous anastomosis. The sensory supply is excellent. The only real disadvantage is the need to skin graft the donor site in many instances.

Song points out that the forearm flap differs from the classic axial-pattern free flap, and that its proximal border can be extended safely beyond the level of the elbow as far as the lower fourth of the upper arm. The forearm flap can be used as a pedicle island flap in reconstructing the thumb or resurfacing the denuded palm.

▶ [An impressively versatile flap with minimal donor site debilitation and excellent quality provided to the recipient area. Dr. Song's technical observations in the discussion, which follows the article (*Plast. Reconstr. Surg.* 70:336–344, September 1982), are instructive.—R.J.H.] ◀

3–32 **Restoration of Elbow Flexion by Pectoralis Major and Pectoralis Minor Transfer.** Use of the pectoralis major alone to substitute for the biceps muscle involves a difficult dissection. Tsu-Min Tsai, Michael Kalisman, John Burns, and Harold E. Kleinert used both the pectoralis major and pectoralis minor muscles to restore elbow flexion. Four patients with brachial plexus injury were treated, none of whom had significant active flexion preoperatively. The pectoralis muscles are dissected as a single mass, protecting the neurovascular bundle. The motor unit is rotated on its pedicle and attached proximally to the coracoid process and distally to the biceps tendon (Fig 3–16). The lateral clavicular attachment of the pectoralis major is retained to preserve shoulder adduction.

Satisfactory results are obtained using this procedure. The motor unit has a work capacity of 16.4 m/kg, compared with 4.8 m/kg for the biceps in forearm supination. Three patients had excellent results, but 1 did not have sufficient power in the elbow and later underwent a Steindler flexor plasty. Transfer of the pectoralis minor along with the pectoralis major protects their common neurovascular bundle and provides strong elbow flexion to patients with loss of active flexion.

(3–32) J. Hand Surg. 8:186–190, March 1983.

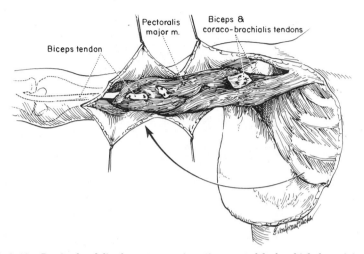

Biceps tendon
Pectoralis major m.
Biceps & coraco-brachialis tendons

Fig 3–16.—Proximal and distal anastomoses in patient treated for brachial plexus injury using both the pectoralis major and pectoralis minor muscles. (Courtesy of Tsai, T.-M., et al.: J. Hand Surg. 8:186–190, March 1983.)

3–33 **Development of the Fasciocutaneous Flap and Its Clinical Applications.** David E. Tolhurst, Barend Haeseker, and Rein Jac. Zeeman (Rotterdam, The Netherlands) encountered only one complication in 20 consecutive patients having fasciocutaneous flaps raised on the thigh and trunk. One of 11 such flaps on the lower leg had some necrosis. The flaps are useful in closing skin defects on the lower leg, especially when bone or bare tendon is exposed in the depths of a wound. Patients with postburn axillary contractures have been managed with flaps raised over the latissimus dorsi muscle. Even long, narrow flaps with a base-to-length ratio of 1:4 or greater survived. Fourteen flaps were used for axillary contractures and two for partial breast reconstruction; partial necrosis occurred in one of the latter flaps. Three flaps were raised successfully in previously grafted areas.

Flaps with large length-base ratios can be designed using the fasciocutaneous approach. These flaps can be used safely with a random-pattern design in most regions of the body where deep fascia is present. Their dissection is simple. The underlying muscle is left intact, and there is no question of functional impairment. The blood supply of the deep fascia is illustrated in Figure 3–17. Experimental studies in pigs support the hypothesis that the fascia has an important role in the blood supply of the overlying fat and skin.

The inclusion of deep fascia in flaps designed in various parts of the body appears to confer an element of safety, presumably because of

(3–33) Plast. Reconstr. Surg. 17:597–606, May 1983.

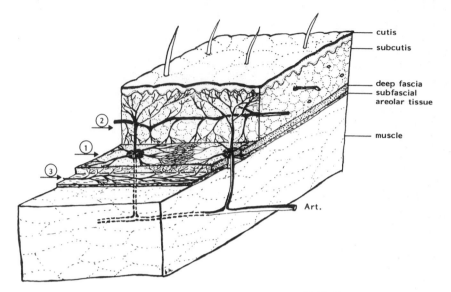

Arterial bloodsupply of the deep fascia ①②③

Fig 3–17.—Blood supply of the deep fascia. Indicated are the (1) perforating arteries, (2) subcutaneous arteries, and (3) subfascial arteries. (Courtesy of Tolhurst, D. E., et al.: Plast. Reconstr. Surg. 71:597–606, May 1983.)

the rich vascular plexuses associated with the deep fascia. The usual 1:1 base-length ratio need not be adhered to. This reliable, versatile flap is popular in Europe.

▶ [Another in this year's series of thoughtful papers on innovative ways of enhancing transferred tissue survival.—R.J.H.] ◀

3–34 **Repair of Cosmetic Defect of Lower Leg With Myocutaneous Free Flap.** Free flaps now are widely used in the repair of defects and restoration of function. A. Lamont, W. D. F. Malherbe, and J. Middelhoven (Univ. of Stellenbosch, Tygerberg, South Africa) report the successful outcome of free flap transfer for correction of a disfiguring tissue loss on the lower leg of a young woman. The defect was corrected in one stage with a full-thickness myocutaneous free flap.

Woman, 21, seen 2 years after an accident, had a substantial soft tissue defect of the posterior right calf in a skin-grafted area. The fibula was readily palpated through the skin. Arteriography showed normal vascular anatomy in the lower leg. A latissimus dorsi myocutaneous flap was dissected using a template of the area to be repaired. The full volume of the muscle was included. A microvascular team performed the arterial anastomosis first, using the posterior tibial artery, and then one venous anastomosis. A warming blanket was used during surgery, and local irrigation was done with heparinized saline. The length of ischemia was 55 minutes. Antibiotics were given

(3–34) S. Afr. Med. J. 62:642–644, Oct. 23, 1982.

for a brief time, and physiotherapy was begun immediately after surgery. There were no complications. The defect was overcorrected to compensate for expected atrophy of the transferred muscle. The patient was left with a restored contour of the calf and an acceptable scar within the brassiere line on her back.

▶ [Unfortunately, the authors have omitted a view of the scarring of the back (which must have been significant), allowing the reader to evaluate the trade-off.—F.J.M.] ◀

3–35 **Gluteal Thigh Flap in Reconstruction of Complex Pelvic Wounds.** Soft tissue perineal defects resulting from trauma, surgery, irradiation or inflammation can present a significant reconstructive surgical challenge; however, a new flap has been used that is ideally suited to this site. Bruce M. Achauer, Ivan M. Turpin, and David W. Furnas (Univ. of California, Irvine) used 9 flaps in 7 patients with difficult wounds, all of which healed successfully. The gluteal thigh flap is based on the inferior gluteal artery, which ends as a cutaneous vessel to the midposterior part of the thigh after supplying the distal half of the gluteus maximus (Fig 3–18). The point of rotation is 5 cm above the ischial tuberosity. The flap usually is no more than 12 cm wide, which allows primary closure of the donor defect, and can be extended to the popliteal fossa. Flap elevation is illustrated in Figure 3–19. The flap is most easily transferred as an island. Primary closure over suction drains is suggested.

This flap permits the resection of pelvic and perineal malignancies

Fig 3–18.—Landmarks of gluteal thigh flap. (Courtesy of Achauer, B. M., et al.: Arch. Surg. 118:18–22, January 1983.)

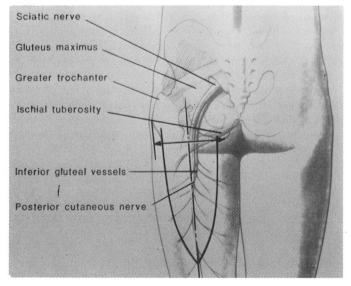

Sciatic nerve

Gluteus maximus

Greater trochanter

Ischial tuberosity

Inferior gluteal vessels

Posterior cutaneous nerve

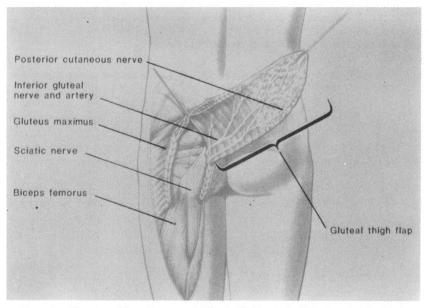

Fig 3–19.—Elevation of flap. (Courtesy of Achauer, B. M., et al.: Arch. Surg. 118:18–22, January 1983.)

previously considered unresectable, or whose complications, such as loss of the vagina, was unacceptable to patients. Three patients who required vaginal reconstruction after tumor resection, and 3 with radiation wounds, have been treated. No complications resulted from flap necrosis. The only persistent complication has been dysesthesia associated with sensory nerve transection. The flap is thick, does well as an island, and can safely be folded. The procedure can be combined with a primary ablative or debriding operation. The sensory innervation of the flap is an advantage in both vaginal reconstruction and the treatment of pressure sore.

▶ [The authors bring to our attention a flap on the posterior thigh that is based on the inferior gluteal artery and posterior gluteal nerve. It is a very neat flap that can be used for pelvic defects.—R.O.B.] ◀

3–36 **Reconstruction Following Amputation of the Penis in Children.** Edward S. Tank, Robert J. Demuth, and Stuart Rosenberg (Oregon Health Sciences Univ.) report two cases of traumatic penile amputation in boys in whom reconstruction was undertaken by mobilizing the residual erectile tissue.

CASE 1.—Boy, 6, had reconstruction in two stages, involving mobilization of the residual corporeal bodies and temporary scrotal implantation, followed by release in the second stage. Initial mobilization gained 3.5 to 4 cm of

(3–36) J. Urol. 128:386–388, August 1982.

length. A tunnel was created in the scrotum through which the corpora were passed to provide cover for the raw area created by the release. The second stage was done after 6 months. The boy has sensation in the penile skin and has had erections.

CASE 2.—Boy, 3, had a one-stage reconstruction by mobilization of the corporeal bodies to gain 3 to 4 cm of length. Split-thickness skin grafting was used to cover the new penile shaft. The patient voided with a good stream 6 months postoperatively and had erections.

The goals of reconstruction of the amputated penis include adequate phallic length with a urethral opening at the tip of the penis, a functional seminal conduit, cosmetically acceptable results, and preservation of sensation and erectile potential. Construction of a neourethra is unnecessary. The use of residual erectile tissue has provided an acceptable phallus and the potential for complete penile function.

▶ [The authors have outlined a very clever and what appears to be a very worthwhile maneuver. I have used this in situations where too much skin was excised for the urethral graft in the treatment of a hypospadias.—R.O.B.] ◀

3–37 **Burn Specific Health Scale.** The outcome of burn care is traditionally assessed in terms of mortality. Betsy Blades, Nick Mellis, and Andrew M. Munster (Baltimore) constructed a Burn-Specific Health Scale (BSHS) in an attempt to gain understanding of morbidity and other sequelae of burn injury. The 114 items of the scale were selected by professional and patient judges from among a large pool of items taken from the Sickness Impact Profile, Index of Activities of Daily Living, General Well-Being Schedule, and other items suggested by the burn center staff and burned patients. The scale is self-administered. Most items are rated on a 5-point basis.

Preliminary internal consistency and reliability testing of the BSHS gave satisfactory results. The scale was tested on a sample of 40 adult burn patients after discharge. All had flame burn injuries, with second- and third-degree involvement of at least 10% of body surface. Patients with burns of more than 40% of body surface had the most dysfunction, but the differences were significant only for the psychologic (affective) and body-image areas. Postburn recovery appeared to be dynamic, undergoing marked changes for at least a year after hospitalization. Greater dysfunction was observed in patients with face and hand burns, largely because of psychologic and body-image differences. No significant effects of sex or marital status were evident.

The BSHS appears useful for assessing both individual and group performance after burn injury. The findings to date indicate that postburn recovery is a dynamic process, and this must be taken into account when patients are evaluated for any purpose. The BSHS may prove most useful for indicating the need for changes in treatment. The psychosocial performance of patients with major burn injury lags

(3–37) J. Trauma 22:872–875, October 1982.

behind their performance in other areas, and alternative clinical strategies for supporting them must be examined. The BSHS can help determine the need for specialized centers for treating burn-injured patients.

▶ [The development and use of the BSHS is an effort to quantify problems and difficulties outside usual clinical aberrations. It will prove useful to the extent that it provides reliable physical, psychological, and body image data.—B.W.H.] ◀

3–38 **Identification of High-Risk Population for Serious Burn Injuries.** W. P. Glasheen, E. O. Attinger, A. Anne, B. W. Haynes, J. T. Hiebert, and R. F. Edlich examined the epidemiologic correlates of serious burn injuries occurring in the Commonwealth of Virginia in a 21-month period in 1978–1979. A total of 1,552 burn-injured patients required hospital treatment during this time, and 79 of them died. An estimated 2 or more Virginians per 10,000 population required inpatient treatment for burn injury during the review period.

Caucasian patients constituted 49% of the burned group and nonwhite male patients, 18%. Peak incidence was in young adults aged 20–29 years, followed by children aged 9 and younger. Injuries were least frequent in persons aged 80 and older. Flame and scald liquid burns accounted for 60% of all cases. Hot surface injuries were prominent in both infants and the elderly. After age 2, flame burns were the chief cause of serious burn injuries. More than 80% of fatal injuries were caused by flame burns. Major types of injury showed no significant seasonal variation. Injuries were most frequent on residential property. Among work-related injuries, craftspersons were most frequently affected. Use of alcohol was implicated in 5.4% of cases, child abuse in 2.2%, criminal assault in 1.6%, and smoking in 1.5%.

Age, race, and sex all were determinants of serious burn injury in this survey of the Virginia population. An inverse relationship between socioeconomic status and the incidence of serious burn injuries is evident. Targeted educational programs now are being instituted to inform citizens about how to prevent these unnecessary injuries. By making such information available to appropriate groups, the incidence of serious burn injuries may be substantially reduced.

▶ [This study targets a population which has an increased likelihood for burn injury and points out, in particular, the socioeconomic impact. Such studies point the way for effective prevention programs.—B.W.H.] ◀

3–39 **Thermoregulatory Responses of Patients With Extensive Healed Burns.** Since healed burn wounds are incapable of sweating, burned patients can be expected to be less tolerant than normal subjects to heat exposure. Yair Shapiro, Yoram Epstein, Chaim Ben-Simchon, and Haggai Tsur examined the thermoregulatory responses of 10 male patients who recovered from deep second- and third-degree burn injuries. Four patients had healed burned areas of 45% to 55%

(3–38) Burns 9:193–200, January 1983.
(3–39) J. Appl. Physiol. 53:1019–1022, October 1982.

of total skin surface, and 6 had 20% to 30% burned skin area. Ten healthy male subjects also were studied. Patients and control subjects were exposed for 1 hour a day over 5 days to a temperature of 40 C at a relative humidity of 50% while stepping on a bench 32 cm high at a rate of 12 steps per minute, for an oxygen uptake of about 1 L per minute. A 3-hour exposure on day 6 was used to test heat tolerance. The study was done at the end of winter to exclude natural acclimatization differences.

Patients with more extensive injuries had higher rectal temperatures, mean skin temperature, and heart rates than the other patients or control subjects. Maximal evaporative cooling capacity was 4.9 W/kg in this group, 7.2 W/kg in the patients with less extensive injuries, and 10.2 W/kg in the control group. The required evaporation capacity for thermoequilibrium was similar in all groups. Total sweat rate normalized to healthy skin area was highest in the patients with extensive injuries and lowest in control subjects. Sweating sensitivity normalized to healthy skin area was comparable in all groups.

It appears that in patients with extensive burn injuries that have healed thermoequilibrium is not maintained despite a high compensatory sweating rate in healthy skin. In patients with less extensive injuries, compensatory sweating from healthy skin is adequate for thermoequilibrium. Elevated rectal temperature appears to be the chief drive of sweat regulation. The sweating rate is a function of change in rectal temperature and healthy skin surface area.

▶ [In the extensively burned and grafted patient, one observes a lack of sweating over the graft and an excessive sweating over unburned areas. This study clarifies the problem one step further by demonstrating that, in very extensive burns, thermoequilibrium may not be maintained and sweating is controlled by core temperature and its effectiveness by healthy skin surface area.—B.W.H.] ◀

3–40 **Molten Metal Safety Boot Burns: Analysis and Treatment.** Metal refinery workers are vulnerable to molten metal splash that trickles past the boot top and can cause serious foot burns. Safety boots and shoes have failed to completely prevent these injuries. William K. Boss, Jr., and Marvin S. Arons (New Haven, Conn.) reviewed data on 20 male patients seen in 1967 to 1981 with deep dermal burns of the foot or ankle, or both, which were caused by molten aluminum and brass alloys that tend not to adhere to the skin, in contrast to molten zinc. In these 20 patients the metal burned through the pants, rolled along the leg past the boot top, and settled on the ankle or foot.

Up to three burns were present on each foot-ankle; size ranged from 2 × 2 cm to 8 × 11 cm. Although they appeared to be full-thickness burns, this was found not to be the case. The first 7 patients were given a 2-week period for primary healing, but all eventually required grafting. They did not have exposed tendon or deep structures after burn eschar was removed. Subsequent patients had early tangential excision and debridement of their wounds. Dermabrasion-debridement was a useful approach. Skin grafts were applied and affected extremities were elevated constantly for 10 days. Progressive ambulation was then instituted. Patients were able to return to work with elastic support stockings a month after operation. Graft take was essentially complete in all cases. No secondary procedures were necessary. No contractures, hypertrophic scars, or inclusion cysts developed.

Tangential excision and early wound closure seem to be indicated in these cases, although not all foot burns necessarily require early debridement and grafting. Present safety boots and shoes do not provide complete protection of the feet and ankles for metal refinery workers. Improvement in shoe design and boot top protection could reduce the occurrence of these injuries.

▶ [In this study, the problems of molten metal burns of the foot are highlighted, and since most are deep dermal, the authors recommend tangential excision. Given the circumstance of a very hot burn source and deep dermal injury, tangential excision and primary grafting should shorten healing time, decrease cost, and lessen time off of work.—B.W.S.] ◀

3–41   **Management of Full-Thickness Burns of Scalp and Skull.** Acute morbidity is frequent in cases of full-thickness burn injury of the scalp, and wound closure remains controversial. John Hunt, Gary Perdue, and Thomas Spicer (Univ. of Texas, Dallas) reviewed the cases of 17 men aged 6–58 years, who sustained full-thickness scalp burns with associated necrosis of part of the periosteum or calvarium. The average burn size was 19% of the total body surface area. Most injuries were caused by high-voltage electrical accidents. One fifth of patients had associated head and neck trauma. The outer table was visible at admission in 6 patients.

Initial wound excision or debridement was done a mean of 5 days after injury. Wound closure was most often by dermabrasion of or drilling of holes into the outer table, followed by immedate or delayed split-thickness autografting; or total excision of the outer table with partial or total excision of the inner table and delayed split-thickness autografting. An average of two further operative procedures was necessary to completely cover the wounds. Burn wound cellulitis led to delayed eschar excision in 3 cases. Half the patients having bony debridement had systemic or local septic complications, or both. Two CSF leaks resulted from dural tears during debridement of the inner table. One patient developed *Pseudomonas aeruginosa* meningitis after repair of a dural tear. The infection resolved after insertion of a spinal catheter and intrathecal aminoglycoside therapy.

Early eschar excision followed by immediate local flap coverage is

(3–41) Arch. Surg. 118:621–625, May 1983.

the recommended treatment for full-thickness burns of the scalp. With such treatments hospitalization is shortened, and the risk of sepsis is virtually eliminated. If the periosteum of the outer table is intact, the wound can be covered simply with split-thickness autograft. If the periosteum is burned and the calvarium nonviable, the simplest and safest procedure is dermabrasion with an electric burr followed by coverage with a rotation scalp flap. Immediate autografting is not uniformly successful. A local scalp flap sometimes can be used after removal of the full-thickness of the necrotic outer table. Otherwise the bone is left to granulate and skin is grafted later. Excision of necrotic inner table is a high-risk procedure.

▶ [This interesting paper emphasizes the use of local flap coverage for exposed skull after burn injury. This technique is useful when flap coverage is available and, as others have shown, produces healing by resorption of devascularized bone. I have found that a simple method is often useful. If bone damage is above the inner table, one can burr off the outer table to bleeding bone and apply split grafts directly. The method is useful for tibial injuries also. Good takes are usually possible, which become durable, effective, and permanent skin cover.—B.W.H.] ◀

3–42 **Clinical Trials of Amniotic Membranes in Burn Wound Care.** Human amniotic membrane has been suggested as a plentiful substitute for autografts and allografts in burn wound management. William C. Quinby, Jr., Herbert C. Hoover, Michael Scheflan, Philemon T. Walters, Sumner A. Slavin, and Conrado C. Bondoc assessed the healing of partial-thickness skin graft donor sites dressed with amniotic membrane or with 5% scarlet red ointment gauze dressing. The efficacy of amniotic membrane dressings in preventing infection in fresh, shallow, second-degree burn wounds was compared with that of 0.5% silver nitrate or 1% silver sulfadiazine dressing. Amniotic membranes and allograft dressings were compared in open contaminated wound areas of limited size. Membrane changes were made every 8–12 hours on contaminated granulating wounds.

Healing of donor sites covered with amniotic membrane was comparable to that of sites covered with standard dressings of scarlet red ointment gauze. Pain was greatly reduced with the use of membranes. Patients with clean shallow burns had much less pain when membranes were used, and healing was equivalent to that seen with topical agents or allografts. Freshly excised wounds did as well after secondary grafting when membranes were used initially as when allografts were used. Autografting was successful in most contaminated wounds initially managed with membrane dressing.

Amniotic membranes have provided benefit similar to that obtained with allograft coverage in various settings, including skin graft donor sites and both clean and contaminated burn wounds. Although the absence of vascularization makes amniotic membranes less versatile than allografts for temporary wound closure or as biologic dressings for granulating wounds, their availability and rela-

(3–42) Plast. Reconstr. Surg. 70:711–717, December 1982.

tively low cost are important advantages, as is the reduction in pain obtained.

▶ [This study demonstrates the effectiveness of the amniotic membrane in the prevention of infection in second-degree burns, donor site healing, excised burns, and contaminated burn wounds, pointing out that it compares favorably with allograft. In addition to wound effectiveness, it is readily available in most hospitals and is inexpensive. The amniotic membrane does not, however, have the quality of allograft, which may vascularize and heal, but is functionally much like autograft until rejection. The authors state that vascularization does not occur, using chorion side down. Robson disagrees, stating that amnion side down does not vascularize but chorion does. (Robson, M.C. and Krizek, T.J., *Conn. Med.* 38:449, 1974.)—B.W.H.] ◀

3–43 **Early Surgical Decompression in Management of Electrical Injuries.** Deep damage to muscle and other tissues occurs in electrical injuries. Much tissue destruction is a result of progressive ischemia in the burned extremity, and early surgical decompression may be critical in preserving limb function. C. James Holliman, Jeffrey R. Saffle, Melva Kravitz, and Glenn D. Warden (Univ. of Utah Med. Center, Salt Lake City) reviewed the management of 80 patients seen in 1976–1981 with electrical injuries in whom the passage of current through the body was documented or highly probable. The 75 men and 5 women had an average age of 28 years. High-voltage injuries occurred in 68 cases, house current injuries in 8, and lightning injuries in 4. The mean total body surface area of injury was 13%, and the mean full-thickness burn area was 7.8%. Eleven patients required cardiopulmonary resuscitation, 10 of whom were long-term survivors. Early treatment included fluid resuscitation and, where indicated for acidosis or marked myoglobinuria, administration of bicarbonate or mannitol, or both. Decompressive escharotomy or fasciotomy was carried out for a charred or "mummified" distal extremity; a reduced or absent distal limb pulse; loss of distal sensation or motor function; gross limb swelling; or an intramuscular compartment pressure of over 30 mm Hg by the wick catheter technique.

Far more fluid was needed in the first 24 hours after injury than was predicted by commonly used burn resuscitation formulas. The mean requirement was 12 cc/kg/percent of total body surface area burned. One inadequately hydrated patient developed renal failure. Sixty-five patients had a total of 509 surgical procedures. Fifty-eight amputations were done in 22 patients. Fifty-three patients had a total of 87 complications from their electrical burns. Half the complications were cardiac in nature. There were no clostridial infections. Five patients (6.25%) died. They had a mean burn size of 42%, and all had multiple surgical procedures. Two deaths were due to sepsis. The average period of hospitalization was 3 weeks.

Early surgical decompression with fasciotomy and sequential wound debridement result in a low amputation rate and conservation of limb length in patients with electrical injuries. Early fasciotomy

(3–43) Am. J. Surg. 144:733–739, December 1982.

may permit the return of adequate perfusion to damaged tissue before secondary tissue loss from ischemia occurs. Fasciotomy also permits assessment of the viability of deep tissues. Scanning with technetium Tc 99m-pyrophosphate is helpful in locating hidden areas of muscle damage.

▶ [This study summarizes much of the current thinking regarding treatment of electrical injuries. Although fasciotomy is valuable, the crucial approach is prompt and sequential debridement of devitalized muscle leading to early wound closure by graft. Estimation of viability of muscle is difficult, and contracture is the best test. Vascularity and color are less reliable. Technetium-99m pyrophosphate scanning may assist in locating hidden muscle damage.—B.W.H.] ◀

3–44 **Prophylactic Antibiotics as Adjunct for Skin Grafting in Clean Reconstructive Surgery Following Burn Injury** are discussed by J. Wesley Alexander, Bruce G. MacMillan, Edward J. Law, and Romaine Krummel (Shriners Burns Inst., Cincinnati). A randomized prospective double-blind trial was conducted to determine the effectiveness of cephalothin versus placebo given perioperatively for prevention of infections associated with skin grafting in clean reconstructive surgery done after burn injury. The incidence of infection associated with skin grafting is relatively low, but infections caused by gram-positive organisms are common and are often associated with marked graft loss when hemolytic *Streptococcus* is present.

The study included 249 patients, 127 of whom were given antibiotic treatment; 122 served as controls. Cephalothin (Keflin) was given in a dose of 15 mg/kg in 50 ml of 5% dextrose in water (D/W). An identical volume of 5% D/W was used for the placebo. The first dose of placebo or antibiotic was given with preoperative medication, the second dose at the beginning of the skin incision, and the third dose 4 hours after the skin incision was made, during the recovery phase. The antibiotic was effective in reducing infection (0.8% in treated patients, 5.7% in controls, $P < .03$), reducing graft loss ($P < .02$), and shortening the hospital stay. Graft take in infected patients was significantly less than in patients with noninfected grafts, and their hospitalization was 6.45 days longer.

Others also report that three doses of an antibiotic administered perioperatively are effective in preventing wound infections. Continued administration of antibiotics for more than the first postoperative day does not further reduce the infection rate. The only cause of significant graft loss in the control group was infection, and prevention of infection resulted in a 99.9% graft take. It is recommended that an antibiotic effective against gram-positive organisms be administered routinely during the perioperative period in patients under treatment for burn injuries.

▶ [This nice study demonstrates that cephalothin does decrease postgraft wound infection in clean reconstructive surgery. In spite of the fact that this drug has a short half-life and has not given good results in the past, the timing and dosage were the

---

(3–44) J. Trauma 22:687–690, August 1982.

likely reasons for its success. To achieve effective prophylaxis against postoperative wound infection, it is only necessary that an effective drug against the pathogens encountered perfuse the wound in high concentration during the operation. Antibiotics administered outside this time frame have little, if any, value.—B.W.H.] ◄

3-45 **Improved Survival With Aggressive Surgical Management of Noncandidal Fungal Infections of the Burn Wound.** Fungal infections of burn wounds, although infrequent are difficult to treat and are frequently fatal. Michael J. Spebar, Michael J. Walters, and Basil A. Pruitt, Jr. (Brooke Army Med. Center, Fort Sam Houston) reviewed experience since 1973 with patients who developed fungal infections of burn wounds. In 1978 an aggressive diagnostic and surgical approach was instituted, including biopsy of any new, darkening wound areas and culture for bacterial and fungal organisms. If fungal elements were found, wide excision down to muscle fascia was carried out with a peripheral margin of 3–5 cm. No topical antifungal agents were used. Intravenous amphotericin B was reserved for patients with multifocal, systemic, or muscle invasion by fungi.

Of 1,513 patients admitted during the review period, 118 (8.2%) developed fungal infections of burn wounds. *Candida* invasion accounted for 38.5% of cases. Most of the rest were due to *Fusarium, Aspergillus,* and the phycomycetes. Forty-eight percent of cases of *Candida* infections and 41% of cases of noncandidal infections were diagnosed before death in 1973–1977. In 1978, 64% of cases of *Candida* infections and 67% of cases of noncandidal infections were diagnosed before death and treated. Mortality for patients with noncandidal infections fell from 87% in 1973–1977 to 25% in 1978, but mortality was not decreased for those with *Candida* infections. No patient with noncandidal infection that invaded muscle or its fascia or who had infection in more than one body region survived.

Mortality from fungal infections of burn wounds can be markedly reduced if they are recognized and surgically excised. Frequent observation of wounds for darkening is important. Excision of infected wound areas before signs of deep or multicentric invasion develop can improve the survival of patients with noncandidal infections. The prognosis is poor for patients with *Candida* invasion of the burn wound.

► [A good case is made for excising invasive fungal infections, and it is supported by improved mortality. The Brooke unit has the largest experience in managing these unusual infections, and their report is authoritative.—B.W.H.] ◄

3-46 **Unexplained Fever in Burn Patients Due to Cytomegalovirus Infection.** Infection in burned patients most often is attributed to bacteria and fungi, but infections with cytomegalovirus (CMV), herpes simplex virus, and adenovirus are not infrequent. George S. Deepe, Jr., Bruce G. MacMillan, and Calvin C. Linnemann, Jr. (Univ. of Cincinnati) reviewed the data on 4 patients with unexplained fever

(3–45)   J. Trauma 22:867–868, October 1982.
(3–46)   JAMA 248:2299–2301, Nov. 12, 1982.

due to CMV infection, in whom the cause of fever was not readily appreciated because of the few physical signs and abnormal findings on laboratory tests. All 4 patients had fever that developed at least a month after hopitalization and lasted 1 to 4 weeks. The burn wounds were healing well and were not considered the focus of infection. Three patients received antibiotics empirically. Lymphocytosis was seen in 3 cases; 1 patient had marked leukopenia and neutropenia and was receiving two penicillins. One of the 3 patients studied had anicteric hepatitis. The fever was not associated with clinical deterioration.

Cytomegalovitus infection developed in 4 of 70 patients (5.5%) with burns of more than 40% of body surface area. The clinical presentation resembles that of CMV in immunocompromised hosts such as renal transplant recipients. The prolonged fever is associated with lymphocytosis without atypical lymphocytes, delayed onset of infection, and anicteric hepatitis. The pathogenesis of CMV infection in burn patients is unknown, but defective cellular immunity may have a role. Cytomegalovirus infection may be primary or may result from reactivation of latent infection. Reactivation usually is a result of immunosuppression. Identification of CMV as the cause of fever in burn patients may prevent unnecessary diagnostic tests and permit the discontinuance of inappropriate antibiotic therapy.

► [This unusual viral infection is to be suspected when unexplained fever occurs. The incidence in patients with severe burns seems to be about 5 percent, and recovery is promoted by discontinuing antibiotic therapy.—B.W.H.] ◄

3–47   **Control of Methicillin-Resistant *Staphylococcus Aureus* in a Burn Unit: Role of Nurse Staffing.** Methicillin-resistant *Staphylococcus aureus* has become an important hospital pathogen in the United States and has caused serious problems in burn centers. Paul M. Arnow, Patricia A. Allyn, E. Mark Nichols, Dianne L. Hill, Marie Pezzlo, and Robert H. Bartlett investigated the spread of this organism in a burn unit over an 8-month period in 1975. Methicillin-resistant *S. aureus* (MRS) colonization was identified by the recovery of more than 5 colonies of MRS from a burn unit patient. Infection was considered present if fever and purulence were present and MRS was the sole or predominant pathogen. Wound cultures were obtained from 102 patients, and 34% of cultures yielded a heavy growth of MRS. Cases were older, had more extensive burns, and were hospitalized longer than noncolonized controls. Seven patients who were infected with MRS were the oldest and had the most extensive burns. Antibiotic administration was no prominent risk factor. Spread appeared to occur chiefly by contact transmission involving personnel. Environmental sampling yielded few colonies of MRS.

Transmission continued despite barrier isolation and the treatment of colonized personnel with topical intranasal antibiotics. Cases

(3–47)   J. Trauma 22:954–959, November 1982.

ceased to occur after separate nursing personnel were assigned to work with culture-positive and culture-negative patients on each shift and these patients were placed in different areas of the burn unit. When separation of personnel into cohorts could not be maintained because of an increase in patients, further cases occurred. When separation into cohorts was resumed and the burn unit was cleaned with a phenolic disinfectant, no new cases occurred among 149 patients admitted in the next 6 months.

Nurse staffing may have been an important factor in the transmission of MRS in this burn unit. In view of the potential results of MRS infection in patients with burn injuries, isolation measures and surveillance measures should be promptly instituted when a case is detected. If further cases occur, a detailed epidemiologic study should be carried out to guide subsequent control measures.

▶ [This article is of special interest in relation to a study on the same subject (see abstract 3–48). Success in controlling of the methicillin-resistant *Staphylococcus* in a burn unit was achieved by separating nursing into cohorts, combined with effective disinfection.—B.W.H.] ◀

3–48 **Burn Units as a Source of Methicillin-Resistant *Staphylococcus Aureus* Infections.** Methicillin-resistant strains of *Staphylococcus aureus* were first reported in England in 1961, and their prevalence has increased substantially in recent years in hospitals in the United States. John M. Boyce, Rebecca L. White, William A. Causey, and William R. Lockwood (Univ. of Mississippi, Jackson) reviewed the cases of 245 patients at a university hospital who become colonized or infected with methicillin-resistant *S. aureus* over a 3½-year period in 1978–1981. In the first 18 months the incidence of colonization and infection was only 0.05% but, after a focal outbreak in the burn unit, the organism was acquired by significant numbers of patients on other wards. Patients without burns acquired the organism more often during periods when newly admitted burn patients acquired it. The rates of colonization and infection in the last 2 years of the review period were 0.16% and 0.28%, respectively. A total of 151 patients eventually were overtly infected by methicillin-resistant *S. aureus*. Acquisition of the organism by patients without burns on adult surgical and medical services declined significantly after the burn unit was closed. Less drastic measures failed to permanently reduce acquisition of the organism by hospital patients.

Of 146 hospitals with 300 or more beds surveyed, 88 had confirmed methicillin-resistant *S. aureus* infections. Outbreaks of 50 or more cases in 1975–1980 occurred more frequently in hospitals with burn units. The occurrence of large outbreaks was not associated with hospital size. It appears that the occurrence of methicillin-resistant *S. aureus* infections in burn units may lead to increased transmission of the organism to patients without burns, and that control of the infec-

(3–48) JAMA 249:2803–2807, May 27, 1983.

tion in burn units may reduce spread of the organism to patients without burns. Many hospitals have found it difficult to eradicate the organism without closing the burn unit, but some have eradicated the organism using varying combinations of measures such as isolating burn patients on wards with air locks, cohorting patients and personnel, in-service educational programs emphasizing handwashing, decreasing the use of prophylactic antibiotics, and administration of flucloxacillin to burn patients colonized with *S. aureus.*

▶ [Colonization of burn unit patients by methicillin-resistant *Staphylococcus* has become a serious problem. I have been fortunate in having only one case, and it was managed by strict isolation which prevented dissemination throughout the burn unit. The identification of the burn unit as a reservoir for widespread contamination of other patients indicates the urgency for tighter methods for control lest the care of the severely burned patient be jeopardized by burn unit closure.—B.W.H.] ◀

3–49 **Postburn Immunosuppression in an Animal Model: Monocyte Dysfunction Induced by Burned Tissue.** Many aspects of immunity are altered in severely burned patients. John F. Hansbrough, Verlyn Peterson, Eric Kortz, and Joseph Piacentine (Univ. of Colorado, Denver) examined cell-mediated immunity in burned mice by an assay involving the induction of contact sensitivity to dinitrofluorobenzene (DNFB). Painting the ears with DNFB and measuring swelling with calipers is a sensitive, quantifiable means of assessing cell-mediated immunity. A 25% to 30% body surface burn was produced by exposure of a dorsal area to steam. Escharectomy was performed, and control mice has a 30% skin area excised. Some mice received monocyte replacement using peritoneal exudate cells, or lymphocytes from mesenteric lymph nodes of donor mice.

Cell-mediated immunity was severely depressed for 2 weeks after burn injury. Removal of the eschar immediately after injury precluded the development of immunosuppression. Transfer of burned tissue subcutaneously to other mice led to severe immunosuppression. Cell-mediated immunity was restored by infusing peritoneal macrophages from unburned mice intravenously, but not by infusing lymphocytes. Infusion of macrophages from burned mice did not alter immunosuppression in burn-injured animals.

Cell-mediated immunity is greatly suppressed in burn-injured mice. The factors responsible appear to arise from or in response to the burn wound eschar. Further studies are needed to characterize the inhibitory material or materials. This model of postburn immunosuppression may prove useful in examining the widespread effects of burn injury on host defenses. It is expected that methods for avoiding host defense suppression in burn patients will have great clinical application in the near future.

▶ [This study relates depressed cell-mediated immunity to burned tissue and its restoration by transfusion of peritoneal macrophages from unburned animals. The substances in burned tissue need further identification and characterization.—B.W.H.] ◀

(3–49) Surgery 93:415–423, March 1983.

3–50 **Cold Treatment of Burns.** Cryotherapy for burn injuries provides a reduction or elimination of pain and inhibits postburn tissue destruction in the zone of action of the thermal agent. N. S. Pushkar and B. P. Sandorminsky (Kharkov, USSR) established parameters of therapeutic cooling of burn injuries using thermography and histologic study of tissue preparations from zones of thermal applications to rats.

Anesthetized rats were subjected to back burns, and cryoapplications were carried out at varying temperatures and times. Mean hot applicator temperature was 98 C, and mean cryoprobe temperature during contact with skin was − 110 C. Evans blue and sodium fluorescein were used to assess capillary permeability, and an India ink-gelatin mixture was used to examine the cutaneous microcirculation. Rats subjected to deep dorsal flame burns of 10%–15% of the body surface area had cryotherapy with a vapor-liquid nitrogen spray jet, which lowered the subcutaneous temperature to − 6 C to + 13 C. Toxicity was assessed by using full-thickness skin flaps material and a chicken embryo model.

Thirty-seven burn-injured patients, including 14 with deep burns, received cryotherapy up to 24 hours after injury, but 68 control patients did not. A vapor-liquid nitrogen spray was used at a distance of 10–15 cm for 20–30 seconds. Cooling in the range of − 6 C to +12 C yielded maximal therapeutic effects within the first 3 hours after burn injury. Destructive changes in burned skin were reduced by cryotherapy, local circulation of vascular tissue was improved, and toxicity was decreased. No adverse effects of cooling were evident. Patients had marked reduction in pain after cold treatment, without undesired side effects. The time of epithelialization of superficial burns was decreased, and the clearing of deep thermal injuries was accelerated. Two patients with symmetric limb injuries had necrosis only in the control extremity.

Cryotherapy appears to be an effective means of reducing postburn tissue destruction. Cooling lessens impairment of local circulation, decreases destruction and toxicity of injured skin, and stimulates healing.

▶ [It is a well-established fact that cold relieves the pain of burn injury. It is less well-established that cold diminishes depth of injury, even though there is considerable data, including this paper, which suggest that this is the case. Cold may also diminish fluid losses, but this, too, lacks definition.—B.W.H.] ◀

3–51 **Effects of Thermal Injury on Rat Skeletal Muscle Micro-circulation.** Mark K. Ferguson, Frank C. Seifert, and Robert L. Replogle (Univ. of Chicago) undertook an intravital microscopic study of the rat skeletal muscle microvasculature to evaluate blood flow changes occurring at a distance from thermal injury. Burns of 15% and 30% of the body surface were produced by immersion through a

(3–50) Burns 9:101–110, November 1982.
(3–51) J. Trauma 22:880–883, October 1982.

rubber template into water maintained at 97 C for 15 seconds. Saline and albumin were used for resuscitation. Dissection of the extensor hallucis proprius muscle was carried out after stabilization for 1 hour. Observations were continued for 4 hours after thermal injury. All animals maintained a mean arterial pressure above 100 mm Hg during the observation period.

Fluids were comparable in the two groups of rats with burns. Hematocrit values remained greater in the group with large burns. All of the arterioles examined showed spontaneous vasomotor activity, and there was no evidence of red blood cell sludging of leukocyte-endothelial interaction. Mean internal vessel diameters were similar in all groups. Mean red blood cell velocity was significantly greater in the large-burn group than in the small-burn and control groups. Disparity in blood flow values was more marked. Mean flow value in vessels of the large-burn group was 22.7×10^{-6} ml per minute, compared with 11.9×10^{-6} ml per minute in the small-burn group and 9.4×10^{-6} ml per minute in the control group.

Increased red blood cell velocity and blood flow were observed in the groups with large burn injuries compared with the group having minor burn injuries and the control groups. Major thermal injury is associated with increased arteriolar blood flow in skeletal muscle from the site of injury. Other studies have found selective increases in blood flow to the heart, brain, and liver after burn injury. The cause of the increase in arteriolar blood flow in skeletal muscle is unclear but it may represent a response to the release of unidentified vasoactive substances by the burn wound.

▶ [In demonstrating increased skeletal muscle arteriolar blood flow at a distance from the site of injury, the authors offer data to confirm several studies showing the characteristic hyperdynamic state in the patient with severe burns. Cardiac output of 15 L/min is not unusual 2 weeks post burn, with a return toward a normal value after wound healing.—B.W.H.] ◀

3–52 **Role of Granulation Tissue in Formation of Hypertrophic Scarring in Burn Lesions.** S. Teich-Alasia and G. C. Angela (Turin, Italy) analyzed the evolution of granulation tissue in burn lesions, with emphasis on the structural changes in hypertrophic scar formation. In first degree and superficial second degree burns, only the epithelial cells or, at most, the underlying dermis, become necrotic. The hair follicles and the epithelial cells that line the sebaceous and sweat glands are usually undamaged. With intense proliferation of these epithelial cells, rapid repair and complete reconstruction of the skin occur.

In deep second and third degree, or full-thickness, burns, the epithelial cells and hair follicles are destroyed and repair becomes complicated. Capillaries regain their normal permeability, thus ensuring partial reabsorption of the edema. Proliferation of capillaries and

(3–52) Ann. Plast. Surg. 9:132–138, August 1982.

small vessels ensues, with gradual progression of the process toward the superficial areas. Leukocyte infiltration is massive, and associated proliferation of macrophages and histiocytes occurs in the connective tissues of the skin; fibroblasts in the adventitia of the newly formed capillaries also increase in number. Many giant cells are seen. A morphologicofunctional characteristic of the granulation tissue is given by the intense laying down of collagen and mucopolysaccharide acids by the fibroblasts. The structural behavior of the granulation tissue conditions the successive structure of the repair. Histopathologic studies show that granulation tissue often has extremely irregular structure containing bands and tortuous arches, whorllike structures, nodules of vessels, and coarse bundles of collagen. This architecture could lead to the genesis of a hypertrophic scar. The intense formation of new blood vessels encourages the proliferation of fibroblasts. Histologic studies demonstrate how important it is that, after tangential excision, the remaining raw surfaces be covered immediately with skin grafts.

Early excision of damaged tissues and immediate coverage of raw areas with autoplastic which prevents the formation of granulation tissue, may be of fundamental importance in averting hypertrophic scarring, thus preventing serious esthetic and functional results.

▶ [The authors make a case for a direct relationship between granulation tissue and scar hypertrophy on the basis of extensive wound biopsy studies. It is clear that fibroblast proliferation occurs in granulation tissue, and that scar hypertrophy occurs most commonly in healing partial thickness wounds rather than in full thickness wounds grafted adjacently over granulating beds. The question is how the graft controls scar hypertrophy where reepithelization may not. It would not appear logical to incriminate granulation tissue, per se.—B.W.H.] ◀

3–53 **Burn Encephalopathy in Children.** Nearly 200 cases of neurologic sequelae of burn injury in children have been reported. Dhanpat Mohnot, O. Carter Snead III, and John W. Benton, Jr. (Univ. of Alabama, Birmingham) reviewed data on 287 children treated for burn injury in a 2-year period and found 13 (5%) with encephalopathy (acute onset of sensorial change, seizures, or abnormal neurologic signs after burn injury). The 11 boys and 2 girls had a mean age of 3 years. Seven had fire and flame injuries and 6 had scald injuries. Mean body surface area injured was 30%. Neurologic abnormalities appeared a mean of 16½ days after injury. Eight patients had seizures, which were generalized in 5 instances and focal in 3. Most patients had multiple metabolic abnormalities. Acidosis, hyponatremia, hypocalcemia, and wound infection were more frequent than hypoxia or hyperglycemia. The EEG findings were abnormal in 4 of the 6 patients studied. Three patients had recurrent encephalopathic symptoms after initially improving. Eleven patients recovered completely, 1 patient died of sepsis, and 1 had delayed speech development.

Earlier reports on burn encephalopathy indicated a stormy course

(3–53) Ann. Neurol. 12:42–47, July 1982.

including seizures, obtundation and, often, respiratory arrest, all apparently due to cerebral herniation. Better fluid management and abandonment of topical agents with neurotoxic effects, such as hexachlorophene, may help explain the apparent reduction in the severity of symptoms involving the CNS in burn-injured patients. Seizures were prominent in 9 of the present children. One patient had communicating hydrocephalus, which resolved. Children may be especially vulnerable to the effects on the CNS of metabolic and hemodynamic changes produced by burn injury because of the smaller surface area, higher initial metabolic rate, and developing brain. Laboratory studies and an EEG should be obtained in suspected cases. The cerebrospinal fluid may have to be examined if sepsis is present.

▶ [It is my impression also that this distressing complication of severe burn injury is diminishing. The etiology is complex. More effective monitoring, leading to more precise therapy, is probably responsible for the decline in its occurrence.—B.W.H.] ◀

3–54 **Body Image Development in the Burned Child** is discussed by Frederick J. Stoddard (Harvard). Body image development may be impaired by burn injury, as is evident from experience with patients aged 2–19 years with burn injuries of up to 90% of the body surface area. Because infants have a differentiating body image that is largely dependent on the mother for its stability, only inferences can be made about this group. Such children are vulnerable to severe regression at subsequent hospitalization because of memories of the original trauma. Body image disorders in this group are partially related to memories of separation anxiety. Injury in school-age children involves some degree of grief over the loss of the former image and some degree of adaptation to a disfigured body image. The retained memory of a "normal" body may either damage or enhance a patient's self-esteem. Previously stable but flexible defenses and supportive parents help children with burns face the ridicule of peers. Pubertal and adolescent patients exhibit anxiety, sadness, anger, and guilt in response to disfigurement. These reactions are integrated with the aggressive and sexual conflicts experienced at or before the time of the injury.

Many children with burn injuries adapt well and do not manifest serious emotional disorders. Disrupted body image integration from trauma can lead to hostility and anxiety. Night terrors and waking delusions of body fragmentation are also noted. A realistic body image may be absent, or anxiety states may cause distortion of the boundaries between the self and others. Misperceptions of others as mutilating or mutilated may serve to defend against anxiety. In children burned when young, reconstructive surgery early in life may reduce or prevent body image disorder. Personality disorders need not result from burn injuries that have caused disfigurement. When an emotional disorder is associated with failure to adapt to the real body,

---

(3–54)   J. Am. Acad. Child Psychiatry 21:502–507, September 1982.

psychotherapy is indicated. Mental health professionals may require education to help them set realizable psychotherapeutic goals.

▶ [This descriptive study of body image in children with burns provides insight into an important problem area. The author points out that with proper support, no personality disorders need follow these severe injuries.—B.W.H.] ◀

3–55 **Isolation of Immunosuppressive Serum Components Following Thermal Injury.** Immunologic problems are prevalent in patients with burns, and a significant number of severely burned patients are profoundly immunosuppressed. John L. Ninnemann, J. Thomas Condie, Stanley E. Davis, and Rebecca A. Crockett (Univ. of Utah, Salt Lake City) examined the role of specific burn serum-borne substances in lymphocyte suppression by separating suppressive sera into fractions with column chromatography and testing the fractions in mixed lymphocyte culture (MLC). Where possible, suppressors were confirmed by radioimmunoassay, virus plaque assay for interferon, or limulus reactivity for endotoxin. In addition, various immunologically active compounds were tested for suppressive activity in MLC and their elution behavior on column chromatography was examined.

Plasma was obtained from 10 burned patients, aged 3–37 years, whose estimated change of survival was less than 50%. Reduced lymphocyte responsiveness appeared to be mediated by the generation of nonspecific suppressor T cells, the activity of which was mitomycin-resistant. Serum immunosuppressive activity appeared very soon after injury, often within 24 hours. The suppressive material was not found in normal serum. It acted through a specific subpopulation of lymphocytes. Suppression was not confined to a single molecular weight species. Significant suppression of MLC was observed with E prostaglandins, especially PGE_2. Serum interferon levels were sufficient to produce immunologic effects. Four of the five endotoxins tested produced significant suppression in MLC.

The question of whether a discrete "burn toxin" participates in the immunologic changes following burn injury remains unresolved, but the present findings suggest that a combination of immunologically active materials present in early post-burn serum makes an important contribution. Prostaglandins, interferon, endotoxin, and the "burn toxin" complex may all participate in the immune depression that often accompanies thermal injury.

▶ [This is further discussion of postburn immunosuppression, adding further data to explain the etiology (see abstract 3–56).—B.W.H.] ◀

3–56 **Anergy, Immunosuppressive Serum, and Impaired Lymphocyte Blastogenesis in Burn Patients.** John H. N. Wolfe, Andrew V. O. Wu, Nicholas E. O'Connor, Inna Saporoschetz, and John A. Mannick (Harvard Med. School) performed skin testing with four recall

---

(3–55) J. Trauma 22:837–844, October 1982.
(3–56) Arch. Surg. 117:1266–1271, October 1982.

antigens serially in 21 patients with major thermal burn injuries in an attempt to correlate anergy, immunosuppressive serum, and impaired lymphocyte responsiveness to phytohemagglutinin (PHA). Serum or plasma levels of cortisol, endotoxin, and prostaglandin E_2 were also measured. Serum immunosuppression was tested by the ability to inhibit the PHA-induced proliferation of normal allogeneic peripheral blood lymphocytes. The patients, with a mean age of 40 years, were treated with human plasma protein fraction and Ringer's lactate for 48 hours. All received penicillin prophylactically. Topical therapy was with silver sulfadiazine.

Four of 6 patients estimated to have less than a 35% chance of surviving became persistently anergic, and 3 of them died. Two of 6 patients with a 35% to 70% chance of surviving became persistently anergic, but all patients in this group survived. All 5 with anergia of some degree had staphylococcal or *Pseudomonas* septicemia. Two of the 9 patients with a 70% or greater chance of surviving were anergic, and 1 of them developed sepsis. Anergy was not closely related to either the severity of burn injury or the predicted outcome, but it was related to the actual outcome. All 4 deaths occurred in persistently anergic patients. More anergic patients became septicemic, but the relationship was not a significant one. Anergy was related to coexisting serum immunosuppression exceeding 50%. Impairment of peripheral lymphocyte responsiveness to PHA was associated with anergy or relative anergy. Serum immunosuppressive activity could not be related to the levels of endotoxin, cortisol, or PGE_2.

Although the initial steps in the immunodeficiency that follows severe trauma are unknown, anergy to skin-test antigens can be attributed to a failure of the cellular immune response that seems to involve a serum suppressor factor and impaired lymphocyte function. Circulating suppressor cells may be the cause of impaired lymphocyte function in this setting. Skin testing with recall antigens is useful in identifying patients with impaired resistance to sepsis.

▶ [This article supports the relationship between anergy and mortality from burn injury, offering correlations with immunosuppressive serum and lymphocyte response to mitogens. Others have found anergy less specific and less directly related to the severity of the injury. Perhaps it is fair to say that anergy is not always a clear indication of prognosis.—B.W.H.] ◀

3–57 **Depressed Immune Response in Burn Patients: Use of Monoclonal Antibodies and Functional Assays to Define the Role of Suppressor Cells.** Circulating suppressor leukocytes may be important in mediating the immune suppression associated with trauma and burn injury, but functional assays of suppressor cells have been insensitive and cumbersome. Andrew J. McIrvine, John B. O'Mahony, Inna Saporoschetz, and John A. Mannick (Harvard Med. School) investigated the role of suppressor cells, using monoclonal antibodies to

---

(3–57) Ann. Surg. 196:297–304, September 1982.

identify T-lymphocyte subsets with suppressor/cytotoxic (OKT8) and helper/inducer (OKT4) function, in 22 patients with burns of more than 30% of the body surface, and in 14 normal subjects of similar age. The patients were resuscitated with Ringer's lactate in the first 24 hours and then Plasmanate as needed. Twelve patients had excision within 5 days after admission; the mean number of grafts was 3.

The ratio of suppressor to helper subsets was 0.55:1 in normal subjects and 1.4:1 in the patient group. The ratio in patients peaked in 5–7 days, followed by a return to normal by 2 weeks after injury. Reduced lymphocyte responsiveness to phytohemagglutinin coincided with the elevated suppressor-to-helper-cell ratio. Functional assays showed circulating suppressor cells in 9 patients during the same period. These changes were not predictive of the outcome, but subsequently, systemic sepsis in 8 patients was associated with the return of an increased suppressor-to-helper-cell ratio and a decreased mitogen responsiveness. Six patients had circulating suppressor cells on functional assay at this time. Five of these 6 patients died of sepsis.

Severe burn injury regularly appears to induce an early, transient increase in circulating suppressor cells and depressed lymphocyte activation. A later rise in suppressor cells to levels detectable by functional assays correlates with death from sepsis. It has been suggested that immunosuppression may be a defense against autoimmunity that otherwise might result from intense tissue antigenic bombardment after injury.

▶ [This study discusses, in detail, the depressed immune response postburn injury, emphasizing suppressed cellular immunity. This response seems counterproductive. The speculation is that it is a defense against major autoimmune responses which result from massive tissue destruction.—B.W.H.] ◀

3–58 **Treatment of Gram-Negative Bacteremia and Shock With Human Antiserum to a Mutant *Escherichia coli*.** Mortality from gram-negative bacteremia continues to be high despite the use of potent antibiotics and aggressive support. Endotoxin would appear to be an important factor in mortality. Studies with the J5 mutant of *Escherichia coli* O111:B_4, a mutant unable to incorporate exogenous galactose into its lipopolysaccharide, indicate that lipopolysaccharide core determinants are the cross-protective antigens in bacteremia. Elizabeth J. Ziegler, J. Allen McCutchan, Joshua Fierer, Michel P. Glauser, Jerald C. Sadoff, Herndon Douglas, and Abraham I. Braude treated bacteremic patients with a human antiserum to endotoxin core, prepared by vaccinating healthy men with heat-killed *E. coli* J5. The lack of lipopolysaccharide oligosaccharide side chains in the mutant exposes the core for antibody formation.

Antiserum was given to 103 of 212 patients with gram-negative bacteremia or gram-negative bacteria isolated from infected foci in the presence of antibiotic therapy. The most common isolates were *E.*

(3–58) N. Engl. J. Med. 307:1225–1230, Nov. 11, 1982.

coli and *Pseudomonas aeruginosa*. The groups were comparable with respect to severity of illness and antibiotic use. Deaths from gram-negative bacteremia were less frequent in patients given J5 antiserum than in those given nonimmune serum. Mortality in the former group was about half that in controls. Antiserum was especially effective in hypotensive patients. Antibody titers were correlated with survival among patients in profound shock. The antiserum was safe and easy to administer. A possible adverse reaction occurred only twice in over 300 cases.

Human J5 antiserum substantially lowers mortality from gram-negative bacteremia and septic shock. Protective immunoglobulin in a form suitable for intravenous use could become an important part of the management of gram-negative bacteremia. Preliminary experiments suggest that the IgM antibody is more potent against infection than the IgG antibody, possibly because its size permits more efficient blocking of the lipopolysaccharide core on bacterial surfaces.

▶ [This fascinating paper presents convincing evidence that mortality from gram-negative bacteremia can be decreased by a human antiserum to endotoxin core that has been exposed for increased antibody formation by loss of its lipopolysaccharide side chains. This vaccination technique seems to offer more protection through IgM production and by its ability to block endotoxin core on the bacterial wall.—B.W.H.] ◀

3–59 **Regulation of Granulopoiesis Following Severe Thermal Injury.** Overwhelming bacterial infection is the chief cause of death after thermal injury. The neutropenia often associated with septicemia in these patients suggests a defect in regulation of granulopoiesis. Verlyn Peterson, John Hansbrough, Charles Buerk, Christine Rundus, Stephen Wallner, Hunter Smith, and William A. Robinson (Denver) correlated serially measured serum colony stimulating factor (CSF) levels with cell counts in 22 patients with burns of more than 30% of the body surface. Cases of chemical and electrical burns were excluded. Six patients with a mean burn of 58% developed gram-negative septicemia and died, while 16 with a mean burn of 38% had no fatal septicemias. A CSF assay was performed on marrow cells obtained from the posterior iliac crest of normal subjects.

Patients who died had initially low CSF levels and had persistent monocytopenia. Survivors had prompt increases in CSF and developed monocytosis. The rise in serum CSF in surviving patients peaked on day 3 after injury. In nonsurvivors, serum CSF rose slowly and did not peak until day 5. Serum CSF levels subsequently drifted downward in nonsurvivors, although 5 of the 6 had serious infections during this period. Mean granulocyte counts were comparable in the two groups despite episodes of fulminant sepsis in the nonsurvivors. The nonsurvivors had significant monocytopenia compared with the surviving patients. In nonsurvivors, monocyte counts fell even further during periods of sepsis.

(3–59) J. Trauma 23:19–24, January 1983.

While sepsis is uncommon in less severely burned patients, and survival is the rule, patients who fail to survive burn injury have delayed peak serum CSF levels and have significant monocytopenia. These patients apparently have an aberration in granulocyte regulatory function shortly after burn injury, which may have a role in the development of fatal septicemia in patients with severe burns.

▶ [This study finds a cause for neutropenia in burns, that is, diminished CSF levels, and the authors postulate diminished host defense on this basis. The production of CSF is dependent upon monocyte-lymphocyte interrelationships, and alteration of this dependency may be at fault. It is encouraging to see progressive studies such as this one approach the keys to controlling granulocytes and their functions.—B.W.H.] ◀

3–60 **Heterotopic Para-articular Ossification of the Elbow With Soft Tissue Contracture in Burns.** A flexion contracture at the elbow after burn injury may rarely be combined with new bone formation in the para-articular tissues. Dugald A. Dias (Bombay, India) encountered 12 cases of ossification in the triceps, with or without involvement of other periarticular tissues, along with soft tissue contracture anteriorly. The incidence of para-articular ossification at the elbow was 0.3% among 3,683 patients seen in 1971–1974 with burn injuries. Two patients had bilateral bone blocks. All patients were women; most were aged 18–30 years. Six patients had no movement at all; fixation was at 90–100 degrees of flexion. Three other patients had movement of only 5 degrees. Six patients were operated on 4–6 months after burn injury, and the other 3 evaluable patients were treated after an interval of 2–3 years.

In all these cases a 10-cm linear posterior incision was used. A subperiosteal dissection was done posteriorly and anteriorly when necessary, taking care to preserve the triceps tendon. After bone was removed, the raw surfaces were covered with fascia lata. The extensor tendon was sutured back in place to preserve extension. The soft tissue contracture anteriorly then was corrected and skin-grafted. The extremity was suspended in full extension, and physiotherapy was begun after 1 week. The bone block was mainly in the triceps tendon in all cases. Physiotherapy is continued for at least 6 months after operation. Seven patients recovered full motion, but 2 lost 5–10 degrees of motion. No recurrence of new bone formation was observed on follow-up for at least 2 years.

Considerable care may be needed to safely remove new bone from around the ulnar nerve in cases of heterotopic para-articular ossification of the elbow. The new bone formation is related to immobility and progressive bone atrophy. The operative results cannot be assessed until after 3–6 months. New bone formation does not recur after removal and early physiotherapy.

▶ [Heterotopic bone formation around the elbow is an unusual but important postburn complication. Any prolonged burn recovery with decreased elbow range should be suspect. An x-ray is diagnostic, and removal of the triceps block is useful.—B.W.H.] ◄

3–61 **V-W Plasty.** Although contracting scars often can be corrected by single or multiple Z-plasties if the surrounding skin is not right, it is preferable to remove the scarred area as widely as possible at the time the contracture is released. Hisao Koyama and Ryosuke Fujimori (Kyoto, Japan) have found a Y-V advancement to be useful for this purpose. If, however, the angle of the triangular flap becomes too wide, flap transfer will be very difficult. A new "V-W plasty" technique combines the use of two juxtaposed Y-V plasties, which when advanced, create a W-shaped sutured wound that can be used to correct bridle-burn scar deformities.

This technique has been used to release contractures and improve the appearance of scars in the neck, axilla, elbow, knee, and other regions. Its application in one case is illustrated in Figure 3–20. No flap necrosis has resulted, and the contractures have been successfully corrected. The extending length is greater than in the Y-V advancement, and contracted scars can be more readily extended in the V-W plasty because of the many release incisions. The cosmetic results are better than those obtained with traditional or modified Z-plasty in cases of contracted scar that are unsuitable for Y-V ad-

Fig 3–20.—**A,** design of V-W plasty for patient with contracting scar after burn on right elbow region. **B,** incisions are finished; flaps will now be advanced. (Courtesy of Koyama, H., and Fujimori, R.: Ann. Plast. Surg. 9:216–219, September 1982.)

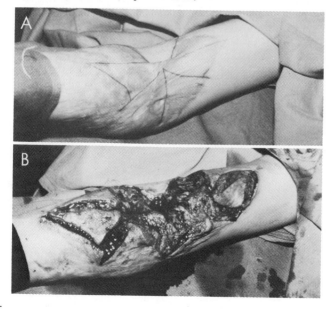

vancement. The Y-V advancement, where inadequate, can easily be altered to a V-W plasty.

▶ [This is an interesting example of the use of the V-W plasty in providing some scar removal in addition to the release of a wound contracture.—B.W.H.] ◀

3–62 **Complications of Surgery for Radiotherapy Skin Damage.** Ross Rudolph (Univ. of California, San Diego) reviewed data on 28 patients who were operated on for skin damage from therapeutic irradiation between 1976 and 1981. Twenty-two pateints had skin ulcers. One had excision of damaged tissue because of severe pain. Five patients had myocutaneous flap reconstruction of an absent breast in an irradiated area. All the patients were adults, irradiated an average of 9 years previously. Two had been treated for benign conditions. The average radiation dose in recent cases was 6,522 rad. Most ulcers were on the trunk. Ten patients had multiple operations. Nine skin grafts, 11 skin flaps, 19 myocutaneous flaps, and 3 omental flaps were carried out.

Split-thickness skin grafting for ulcers produced significant problems including partial graft loss, especially when grafts were placed on acute wounds after ulcer excision rather than on chronic granulating wounds. Both nondelayed and delayed local flaps had high rates of complications. Only 1 nondelayed flap survived without complication. The myocutaneous flap procedures for breast reconstruction were uncomplicated, but those used in the treatment of ulcers were frequently complicated by the flap pulling away from the radiation-damaged tissue. The flaps were placed over Marlex mesh and used to cover full-thickness chest wall excisions. Most of the radiation wounds ultimately closed. Only 5 ulcers were not totally healed, and pain was relieved in 3 of these patients. All nonulcerated lesions healed, with multiple operations where necessary.

The only uncomplicated procedures in this series were omental flap operations for ulcers and myocutaneous flap operations for breast reconstruction. Myocutaneous flaps may be useful in treatment of ulcers, especially if the radiation damage can be fully excised. If possible, the effects of gravity should be avoided by careful myocutaneous flap design. The deeper penetration of modern radiotherapy makes skin grafts and local flaps less useful.

▶ [These two papers add to our knowledge and capacity to deal with the difficult irradiated wound. The ability to cover irradiated wounds with skin grafts will relate not only to the type of radiation, but also to the dose and the degree of premorbid vascularity of the anatomical area involved, i.e., face vs. trunk. The ability to determine the healing capacity of a wound, and to favorably modify this capacity chemically or mechanically, may aid us in the future. Precise definition of the severely damaged tissue, its removal, and its replacement, remain the keystones of success.—S.H.M.] ◀

3–63 **Ultrastructure and Etiology of Chronic Radiotherapy Damage in Human Skin.** Ross Rudolph, Thomas Arganese, and Marilyn

---

(3–62) Plast. Reconstr. Surg. 70:179–183, August 1982.
(3–63) Ann. Plast. Surg. 9:282–292, October 1982.

Woodward (Univ. of California, San Diego) undertook an electron microscopic study of surgical specimens of ulcerated and nonulcerated skin from 5 patients with chronic radiation skin damage. Four ulcerated and four nonulcerated skin specimens were examined. Notable fibroblast disorganization was evident, with swollen and degenerating mitochondria, vacuoles, and dilated, irregular rough endoplasmic reticulum. Unusual crystalline inclusions were present in some fibroblasts. Engulfment of necrotic cells by other cells, probably macrophages, was observed in nonulcerated skin. In the ulcer specimens, stromal collagen was dense and elastosis was seen. Contractile fibroblasts were seen in two of the four specimens. The microvasculature showed occasional luminal occlusion and vacuolation of endothelial cells, but no consistent abnormalities. The changes in vessels were sporadic throughout the irradiated tissues.

These findings suggest that permanent damage to fibroblasts or fibroblast stem cells may have an important role in chronic radiation-induced skin ulceration. Myofibroblasts may be reduced in quality or quantity in radiation-induced skin ulcers, which explains why spontaneous contraction and wound closure do not occur. A reduction in myofibroblasts are probably due to fibroblast stem cell damage.

3–64 **Myocardial Infarction After Electric Injury.** Muscle damage is a well-known sequel of electric injury. Arrhythmias, ischemic myocardial changes, and direct myocardial injury have been described, but myocardial infarction secondary to coronary occlusion is an uncommon complication. Thomas J. Kinney (Akron, Ohio) reports a case of myocardial infarction occurring immediately after a high-tension electric injury.

Man, 57, with no history of chronic disease or heart disease, was standing behind a crane holding a welding torch that may have touched the crane body when it contacted a high-tension line rated at 23,000 volts. He reportedly was thrown 6 to 8 feet into the air, and he admitted having felt an electric shock. He may have lost consciousness for a few seconds. Immediately, severe pain was noted in the left anterior area of the chest. All extremities were burned. An ECG showed ST elevations in leads II and III and AVR with reciprocal changes in the other leads. Frequent premature ventricular beats were abolished by a lidocaine drip. Total creatine phosphokinase 12 hours after injury was 3,850 and the CPK-MB was 500. An echocardiogram showed poor inferior wall motion. Chest pain resolved within 2 days, but a cardiac friction rub developed for 2 days. The extremity burns were managed by debridement and local treatment.

Mild congestive heart failure developed toward the end of the patient's hospital stay. Studies 2 months later showed subtotal obstruction of the left circumflex coronary artery beyond a 30% to 40% obstruction at its origin. Exertional chest pain and controlled congestive heart failure persisted. A recent ECG showed an old inferior wall myocardial infarction.

Only a few reports of myocardial infarction that complicated elec-

(3–64) Ann. Emerg. Med. 11:622–625, November 1982.

tric injury have appeared in the English literature. The infarction in the present patient probably was secondary to coronary insufficiency or spasm. The electric injury may have caused a massive CNS and hormonal sympathetic discharge, overstressing a borderline coronary supply. A temporary arrhythmia also could have been responsible.

▶ [An unusual presentation of myocardial damage from coronary occlusion rather than direct injury.—B.W.H.] ◀

3–65 **Mechanisms of Burn Shock Protection After Severe Scald Injury by Cold Water Treatment.** Previous studies have suggested that histamine is released from moderately severe scald burn wounds, causing local and distant increases in vascular permeability and formation of edema, and that cold water treatment (CWT) reduces histamine release and can prevent formation of edema. Joseph V. Boykin, Jr., and Stephen L. Crute (Med. College of Virginia, Richmond) examined the cardiovascular response to CWT of a severe scald injury in adult guinea pigs subjected to a 3-second subxiphoid immersion in water at 100 C. Treated animals were immersed in water at 15 C for 15 minutes immediately after the scald injury. Cardiovascular responses and serum histamine and lactate levels were monitored for up to 24 hours after injury.

The serum histamine and lactate levels were significantly reduced by CWT for up to 8 and 24 hours, respectively, after injury, compared with levels in untreated animals. Hematocrit values were significantly lower in the first 8 hours after injury in animals given CWT. Blood pressures were higher in these animals for the first 8 hours. Peripheral resistance rose progressively in both groups, but was significantly lower in treated animals 24 hours after injury. Cardiac output remained depressed in untreated animals 24 hours after injury but was significantly improved in animals given CWT.

Severely burned animals given CWT appear to do better hemodynamically than untreated animals. The present findings confirm that cold inhibits release of tissue histamine from burn wounds after severe scald injury. Improved cardiovascular function after CWT may be correlated with decreased serum histamine and lactate levels. Decreased scar formation also has been described with early cooling or CWT. Cold water treatment can also inhibit acidosis. Effective pharmacologic antagonists of burn hypovolemia could substantially reduce the need for massive fluid resuscitation, eliminate complications of volume replacement, and improve early recovery from severe thermal injury.

▶ [This study summarizes the beneficial effect of cold after burn injury, as it inhibits histamine release thereby causing less edema formation. It is also possible to diminish burn edema pharmacologically using histamine inhibitors. Such agents (e.g., cimetidine) act most effectively if given before burn injury, and lose their effectiveness with time. The potential for controlling edema exists, however.—B.W.H.] ◀

(3–65) J. Trauma 22:859–866, October 1982.

-66 **Fluid of Choice for Resuscitation of Severe Shock.** J. A. R. Smith (Royal Hallamshire Hosp., Sheffield, England) and J. N. Norman (Univ. of Aberdeen, Scotland) compared various resuscitative solutions in a standardized canine shock model in which refractory shock is induced in adult mongrel dogs by bleeding to a mean aortic pressure of 40 mm Hg for 2 hours, after which the remaining shed blood is reinfused and the central venous pressure is maintained at 0–2 mm Hg by fluid infusion for 2 hours before killing. Fifty-five animals were treated with Ringer's lactate, dextran 70, hydroxyethyl starch, Haemaccel (polygeline), or a standard crystalloid-colloid perfusate. The standard perfusate contained dextrans 40 and 70, electrolytes, and normal saline, in a ratio of crystalloid to colloid of 2:1. Colloidal solutions were preferable to crystalloid solutions alone in terms of oxygen debt, volumes required, and evidence of pulmonary overload. Very similar results were obtained with dextran 70, hydroxyethyl starch, and Haemaccel. Total peripheral resistance was lowest after administration of dextran 70. Use of the standard perfusate gave better results than either crystalloid or colloid alone. Oxygen consumption was greater with the standard perfusate than with dextran 70 solution. The cumulative oxygen debt was significantly greater with dextran 70 than with the standard perfusate. Mean arterial lactate was lower with the perfusate, but not significantly so.

Better results were obtained using a mixture of crystalloid and colloid than with either crystalloid or colloid alone in this canine shock model. Much of the controversy over whether crystalloid or colloid is preferable is artificial. A mixture of the substances is needed to properly resuscitate severely shocked patients, both to effectively restore blood volume and improve regional flow.

▶ [The authors step into the crystalloid vs. colloid controversy regarding resuscitation from shock, and quite rightly conclude that a combination is better than either one alone. In my opinion, the same conclusion would apply to burn patient resuscitation.—B.W.H.] ◀

3–67 **Fluid Resuscitation in the Burned Child: A Reappraisal.** Recent studies have suggested that adults with burn injuries may be resuscitated with half the amount of Ringer's lactate recommended by the Parkland formula (4 ml/kg/percent burn). James A. O'Neill, Jr. (Univ. of Pennsylvania, Philadelphia) examined fluid requirements in 40 children with a mean burn size of 45%. The mean age was 5.8 years. Twenty-eight patients had injuries of over 30% of the body surface. Five had associated inhalation injuries.

The patients were initially thought to require 3 ml/kg/percent burn by the modified Brooke formula. All had apparently adequate urine flow in the first 48 hours, but this often required administration of excessive fluids in the first 24 hours after injury. All patients had an adequate cardiac output at 48 hours. The initial estimate of fluid re-

(3–66) Br. J. Surg. 69:702–705, December 1982.
(3–67) J. Pediatr. Surg. 17:604–607, October 1982.

quirements was adequate for patients with 20% to 30% burns, but those with 35% and greater burn injuries required 4 ml/kg/percent burn and sometimes more. The total amount of fluids given these patients in the first 48 hours averaged 20% more than the Brooke estimate. Twenty-six of the 40 patients required more, and 9 less, than the Brooke estimate. The patients with inhalation injury all required more than 4 ml/kg/percent burn, as did the 5 with extensive, particularly deep full-thickness burns. Maximum weight gain paralleled the amount of fluid administered. Serum electrolytes and osmolality remained within acceptable ranges in the first 72 hours after injury in all patients. Half the patients became hyperglycemic, but this generally resolved as a satisfactory clinical response was achieved. Three patients required insulin.

The apparent increase in fluid needs for burned children compared with adults probably results from a greater metabolic rate and insensible water loss. Children with small burns will respond well to 3 ml/kg/percent burn of Ringer's lactate in the first 24 hours, while those with more extensive injuries require about 4 ml/kg/percent burn. While inordinate edema should be avoided, administration of inadequate fluid is a more frequent cause of early mortality than is administration of excessive fluid volumes.

▶ [In our experience, the Parkland formula closely predicts the fluid requirements of the severely burned child, and, therefore, is in agreement with the author. In contrast, most adults require less for good resuscitation, especially if some colloid is used.— B.W.H.] ◀

3–68 **Parkland Formula in Patients With Burns and Inhalation Injury.** James J. Scheulen and Andrew M. Munster (Baltimore) reviewed data on 101 consecutive adults with 20%–60% body surface burns who were resuscitated according to the Parkland formula, 4 ml/kg/percent burn. All patients were intubated, most of them within 4–6 hours after burn injury. Many patients had signs of upper airway injury that were directly visualized, and several also had findings consistent with lower airway injury. In most cases fluid therapy was instituted in the field within 2 hours of injury. The other patients were treated within 4 hours after injury. An attempt was made to maintain a urine output of 30–70 ml per hour. Initial topical therapy was with silver sulfadiazine.

Mean volumes of urine output were very close to the upper desired limit of 70 ml per hour, and median volumes were close to 30–50 ml per hour. Patients with inhalation injury clearly required fluids well in excess of the calculated Parkland prediction, and they received an average of 37% above the calculated amount, representing nearly 4 liters of additional Ringer's lactate in the first 24 hours. Patients without inhalation injury required an average of 5.6% of additional fluid, or about 520 ml in the first 24 hours. Patients with inhalation

(3–68) J. Trauma 22:869–871, October 1982.

injury required 31% more fluid than the other to maintain identical urine volumes. The additional fluid was delivered not solely as fluid challenges, but also through a general increase in the rate of infusion over the calculated rate.

Fluid administration should be minimized in patients with inhalation injury in order to prevent pulmonary edema and respiratory distress syndrome. No one formula has proved superior to others in resuscitating patients with such injury. Urine volumes in the range of 20–35 ml per hour are acceptable if other monitored parameters remain normal in these patients. The wider use of invasive monitoring procedures such as use of a Swan-Ganz catheter may be warranted.

▶ [In evaluating the Parkland formula in patients with respiratory injury, the authors concluded that unnecessarily large fluid loads may have been given. They observed no adverse pulmonary function, and also concluded that all formulas might be equally effective.

I would conclude that the formula that calls for the least amount of fluid to support the circulation and renal function (urine output 25–50 cc/hr) and maintain normal electrolytes, is the best.—B.W.H.] ◀

3–69 **Characterization of Acute Renal Failure in the Burned Patient.** Acute renal failure has been reported in from 1% to 30% of burn-injured patients. Mercé Planas, Thomas Wachtel, Hugh Frank, and Lee W. Henderson (San Diego) reviewed data on 35 patients with second- and third-degree burn injuries of 30% or more of body surface area. Acute renal failure, defined as a serum creatinine level of 1.5 mg/dl or above in the absence of shock and persisting in the face of aggressive vascular volume expansion, developed in 11 of the 29 patients surviving more than 48 hours after admission. Patients received modified Ringer's solution, 3 ml/kg of body weight per percent of second- and third-degree burns, in the first 24 hours. In the next 24 hours, plasma and 5% dextrose in water were given to maintain a urine volume of at least 0.5 ml/kg of body weight per hour. Topical therapy was with silver sulfadiazine.

The 11 patients with renal failure were older than the others but had comparable burn injuries. Mortality for these patients was 73%, compared with 17% for patients without renal failure. The fractional excretion of urinary sodium remained low, and the urine-plasma osmolality ratio commonly was above unity, suggesting reduced glomerular filtration with a proximal tubular defect that produced a "downstream" osmotic diuresis. The onset of acute renal failure in these patients was relatively late.

Acute renal failure in burn-injured patients is associated with increased mortality. Renal failure in patients surviving more than 48 hours after injury is predominantly of the polyuric type. All but 1 of the present patients had "normal" to high 24-hour urine volumes. The cause of this form of renal failure is not clear, but a primary

(3–69) Arch. Intern. Med. 142:2087–2091, November 1982.

reduction in glomerular filtration rate may be responsible, along with proximal tubular dysfunction. The osmotic architecture of the concentrating mechanism may be impaired, but not destroyed. The reduced glomerular filtration rate may be due to burn-related dysfunction of afferent and efferent resistances, with reduced filtration pressure and normal renal blood flow resulting.

▶ [This study demonstrates that renal failure in patients surviving over 48 hours is often polyuric, and the authors postulate a reduction in the glomerular filtration rate (GFR). In a series of severely burned patients who did not have renal failure, the GFR was observed to be elevated, renal plasma flow was normal, with increased filtration fraction (Haynes, et al.: *Ann. Surg.* 134:617, 1951). Since shock was not a factor in renal failure in this study, alteration of GFR by glomerular resistances may be the correct explanation.—B.W.H.] ◀

3–70 **Correction of Serum Opsonic Defects After Burn and Sepsis by Opsonic Fibronectin Administration.** Both depression of the reticuloendothelial system (RES) and depletion of opsonic fibronectin have been observed in patients with burn injuries. Marc E. Lanser (Royal Victoria Hosp., Montreal) and Thomas M. Saba (Albany Med. Coll., Albany, N.Y.) examined the effects of thermal injury and sepsis on circulating opsonic fibronectin levels in rats, and the results of administering purified opsonic fibronectin. Rats were subjected to a 26% to 28% full-thickness immersion burn of the dorsum and, after resuscitation with saline, had *Staphylococcus aureus* injected intraperitoneally. Purified rat opsonic fibronectin was administered intravenously 45 minutes after burn injury. In vivo RES function was assessed using a colloid clearance technique.

Burn injury led to acute depletion of fibronectin, which resolved within 6 hours. Severe "hyperopsonemia" was present at 12 and 24 hours. Administration of purified opsonic fibronectin reversed the acute depletion in both nonseptic and septic rats given low doses of bacteria, but not in animals given a high-dose bacterial challenge. Burn injury caused a sharp fall in serum opsonic activity, measured in vitro using a liver slice bioassay. Fibronectin administration partially restored opsonic activity. Burn injury also affected RES function adversely, and this effect was not significantly influenced by administration of opsonic fibronectin.

Opsonic fibronectin deficiency may be a significant factor in RES dysfunction following burn injury and sepsis. Administration of opsonic fibronectin corrected the opsonic fibronectin deficiency and improved RES function in the present rat model. Preservation of RES function after burn injury may depend on the appropriate manipulation of many factors, one of which is opsonic fibronectin.

▶ [Saba's studies of reticuloendothelial opsonization by fibronectin have characterized one aspect of host defense against bacterial challenge. The present study points out that fibronectin deficiencies in severe burns may be aided by repletion therapy.— B.W.H.] ◀

(3–70) Arch. Surg. 118:338–342, March 1983.

3–71 **Fibronectin and Phagocytic Host Defense: Relationship to Nutritional Support** is discussed by Thomas M. Saba, Bruce C. Dillon, and Marc E. Lanser (Albany Med. Coll. of Union Univ., Albany, N.Y.). Fibronectin is a glycoprotein found in blood and tissue fluid and in association with basement membranes, connective tissue, and the extracellular matrix of many cells. It has binding sites for collagen, fibrin, fibrinogen, actin, heparin, and *Staphylococcus aureus*. It appears to bind to receptors to monocytes, leukocytes, and alveolar and peritoneal macrophages. Tissue fibronectin may function as an adhesive or structural glycoprotein, while plasma fibronectin behaves as an opsonic glycoprotein. Exchange between the two pools may occur. Plasma fibronectin appears to be involved in phagocytic function.

Multiple organ failure in septic trauma or surgical patients may be related in part to Kupffer cell dysfunction mediated by plasma opsonic fibronectin deficiency. Deficiency of plasma opsonic fibronectin in septic trauma patients can be reversed by infusing fibronectin-rich fresh plasma cryoprecipitate. Particle clearance by the reticuloendothelial system may influence circulating particulates and aggregates of activated leukocytes, and an imbalance might lead to lung microembolization. Disordered fibronectin function might alter microcirculatory responses to severe septicemia and intraperitoneal infection. Nutritional failure is common in septic surgical and trauma patients. Fibronectin deficiency develops rapidly with fasting, and is reversed by feeding.

The results of fibronectin deficiency induced by total food deprivation or protein-calorie malnutrition, in terms of host defense against bacteremia, remain to be defined. Cryoprecipitate therapy to reverse fibronectin deficiency in septic trauma patients remains experimental. Injection of pure fibronectin or fibronectin-rich cryoprecipitate without knowledge of the fibronectin concentration may be undesirable, since the potential negative effects of excessive plasma fibronectin levels are unknown.

▶ [The authors summarize the data which suggests that poor nutrition decreases opsonic fibronectin and thus the effectiveness of phagocytosis. The article is a review and worth reading.—B.W.H.] ◀

3–72 **Anergy in High-Risk Surgical Patients: Role of Parenteral Nutrition.** Abnormal delayed hypersensitivity responses have been associated with infectious complications and mortality, and some studies have indicated that nutritional support can convert anergy to responsiveness and improve the outcome. David A. Simonowitz, E. Patchen Dellinger, Michael R. Oreskovich, Joseph C. Stothert, and William A. Edwards (Univ. of Washington, Seattle) performed weekly skin tests with four antigens on 98 high-risk patients referred to Har-

(3–71) JPEN 7:62–68, January/February 1983.
(3–72) West J. Med. 137:181–185, September 1982.

borview Medical Center for nutritional support. The 64 men and 34 women had an average age of 56 years.

Thirty-eight patients had trauma that required surgery, 22 had elective surgery, and 38 had acute problems such as myocardial infarction and pancreatitis. Mean hospital stay was 39 days. Sixty-seven patients received total parenteral nutrition (TPN) for a mean of 19 days. All patients received an average of 35 kcal/kg and 1.2 gm/kg of amino acids daily, as well as fats and trace elements. Testing was with purified protein derivative, streptokinase-streptodornase, mumps antigen, and Dermatophitin.

Twenty patients were initially reactive on skin testing and remained so through follow-up. Six were anergic initially and became reactive. A total of 70 patients were anergic and remained so, but 2 initially reactive patients became anergic during follow-up. The reactive and anergic patients did not differ clinically or demographically. Most patients in both groups received parenteral nutrition. No patients who were reactive died. Incidence of sepsis and infectious complications combined was 23%. Mortality in the anergic group was 33%. Sepsis and infectious complications occurred in 68% of these cases. The results of nitrogen balance studies and skin testing were not correlated. Most conversions of skin test findings resulted from appropriate surgical treatment rather than nutritional support.

Although these high-risk patients require nutritional support, anergy on delayed hypersensitivity testing should not be the sole indication for giving such assistance or for delaying surgery. Skin test responsiveness correlates with the outcome, but in most instances the outcome is chiefly influenced by conventional medical and surgical treatment. Parenteral nutrition may reduce postoperative complications only in very high-risk patients.

▶ [The data in this article show that no patients died who were reactive, and that mortality in the anergic group was 33% with a high incidence of complications. While there was correlation of skin test to outcome, parenteral nutrition seemed to reduce complications only in the high-risk group. While the role of parenteral nutrition is still evolving, my clinical impression is that it is influencing the clinical course of burn patients significantly, and possibly mortality as well.—B.W.H.] ◀

3–73 **Plasma Thromboxane Concentrations Are Raised in Patients Dying With Septic Shock.** Endotoxic shock in animals is associated with increased metabolism of arachidonic acid to prostaglandins and thromboxane A_2, a proaggregatory/vasoconstrictor substance. Inhibition of thromboxane synthesis has improved survival and reduced both lysosome labilization and the severity of coagulopathy. H. D. Reines, P. V. Halushka, J. A. Cook, W. C. Wise, and W. Rambo (Med. Univ. of South Carolina, Charleston) measured central venous plasma levels of thromboxane B_2 (TXB$_2$), the stable metabolite of thromboxane A_2, in 12 patients in septic shock, most of whom had intra-abdominal sepsis related to surgery. Eight of the 12 patients died. Six samples from controls also were analyzed.

All the study patients had systolic hypotension at the outset. Intrapulmonary shunting was significantly more severe in nonsurviving patients. The prothrombin and partial thromboplastin times were significantly prolonged in nonsurvivors, and platelet counts and fibrinogen levels were lowest in these patients. Central venous TXB_2 levels were similar in surviving patients and controls, but were raised about 10-fold in nonsurviving patients. Steroid therapy did not have any apparent effect on plasma TXB_2 levels.

Metabolism of arachidonic acid to thromboxane A_2 appears to be increased in patients dying of septic shock, but not in patients who survive septic shock. The highest TXB_2 values in patients dying of neurologic trauma without evidence of sepsis of pulmonary disorder are lower than those in any patients dying of septic shock. The possibility that the severity of disseminated intravascular coagulation and respiratory distress is associated with increased TXA_2 formation deserves investigation. Treatment with cyclo-oxygenase inhibitors or thromboxane synthetase inhibitors may prove useful in the management of patients in septic shock.

▶ [The demonstration that thromboxane B_2 (TXB_2) is markedly elevated in septic shock in man opens up to speculation whether a relationship exists between this abnormality, observed coagulation deficits, and abnormal pulmonary oxygen transport. There is much to be learned about the arachidonic acid chain of thromboxanes, which are specific and critical in their relationship to clotting and wound healing.— B.W.H.] ◀

3–74 **Mechanisms of Insulin Resistance Following Injury** are discussed by Preston R. Black, David C. Brooks, Palmer Q. Bessey, Robert R. Wolfe, and Douglas W. Wilmore (Boston). To assess the mechanisms of insulin resistance developing after injury, the relationship between insulin levels and glucose disposal in 9 nonseptic, multiple trauma patients were examined 5–14 days post injury. Average age was 32 years, and the Injury Severity Score (ISS) was 22. All patients were hemodynamically stable and had normal values for electrolytes, pH, blood volume, and urinary output at the time of study. Seventeen age-matched normal persons severed as controls.

By means of a modified euglycemic insulin clamp technique, insulin was infused in 35 two-hour studies using at least one of four infusion rates (0.5, 1.0, 2.0, or 5.0 mU/kg/minute). Basal glucose levels were maintained by a variable infusion of 20% dextrose using bedside glucose monitoring and a servo-control algorithm. The amount of glucose infused reflected glucose disposal. Glucosuria did not develop, and no urinary correction was necessary. Tracer doses of $(6,6,{}^2D_2)$ glucose were administered in selected patients to determine endogenous glucose production. At plasma insulin concentrations of less than 100 μU/ml, responses in patients and controls were similar. However,

(3–74) Ann. Surg. 196:420–435, October 1982.

maximal glucose disposal rates were significantly less in the patients (9.17 mg/kg/minute vs. 14.3, $P < .01$). Insulin clearance rates in the patients were almost twice those observed in controls. To further characterize this decrease in insulin responsiveness, 6 additional patients and 12 controls were studied after acute elevation of the glucose level to 125 mg/dl above basal (hyperglycemic clamp). Despite exaggerated endogenous insulin production in the patients (80–200 μU/ml vs. 30–70 μU in controls), glucose disposal was significantly lower (6.23 vs. 9.46, $P < .02$).

The findings demonstrated that the maximal rate of glucose disposal is reduced in trauma patients, that the metabolic clearance of insulin in injured patients is almost twice normal, and that insulin resistance developing after injury appears to occur in peripheral tissues, probably skeletal muscle, and is consistent with a postreceptor defect.

▶ [This study, including the discussions which follow the article, is highly recommended in its entirety. It clarifies the effects of injury on glucose metabolism by demonstrating that glucose disposal is reduced, while insulin clearance is greatly increased. It is likely that insulin resistance occurs in peripheral tissues, possibly skeletal muscle.—B.W.H.] ◀

3–75 **Beneficial Effect of Early Excision on Clinical Response and Thymic Activity After Burn Injury** is discussed by C. E. Echinard, E. Sajdel-Sulkowska, P. A. Burke, and J. F. Burke. Severe burns produce immunodepression, cause of frequent septic complications. Late rejection of allograft and an increased ability for tumor growth after severe burns have also been described. Theories proposed to explain immunodepression include increased cortisol levels, acting especially on thymus and lymphoid organs, or an immunosuppressive factor released into blood after burn trauma.

Catabolic response and immunodepression were studied in guinea pigs with scald burns that were excised on day 1 post burn and in those whose scald burns were unexcised. Weight gain returned to normal by day 6 in the excised group, but remained depressed in burned animals whose wounds were not excised or whose nonexcised wounds were treated by application of topical silver sulfadiazine. Animals with unexcised burns had wound infection after 5 days, whereas those with excised burns had no infection. Thymic deoxyribonucleic acid (DNA) synthesis returned to normal by day 6 in those with burn excision, but remained depressed in the untreated animals. Plasma and thymic-free cortisol values returned to nearly normal by day 8 in the excised group, but remained markedly elevated in those with unexcised wounds. The choice of anesthetic was determined by comparing the effect of sodium pentobarbital and halothane. Synthesis of DNA seems to be a little less decreased by pentobarbital. Halothane is immunosuppressive, but this is noticeable only after exposure and disappears after 3 days. The fact that sodium pentobarbital required

(3–75)   J. Trauma 22:560–565, July 1982.

very high doses made halothane the agent of choice. The methods of closing the wound were compared in animals treated with homografts, autografts, or silastic sheet, as well as primary suture. The latter was chosen to close the skin defect. The differences in clinical and immunologic behavior in the two groups of animals probably resulted from the retained burn eschar and development of sepsis in unexcised burns.

These studies indicate that early excision and early wound closure reduce catabolic response and immunodepression in guinea pigs after burn injury.

▶ [Removal of burn injury by excision, and healing by graft, minimizes a large series of events designed to promote host survival. This may be ideal, but in larger burn injuries, survival, even with staged excision, is dependent on the quality of host response, including humoral and cellular immunity, wound healing, optimum nutrition, and other responses. The veritable explosion of studies and data in these areas is reassuring.—B.W.H.] ◀

3–76   **Determinants of Pulmonary Interstitial Fluid Accumulation After Trauma.** The cause of respiratory failure following shock and trauma is not completely understood. Robert F. Tranbaugh, Virgil B. Elings, Janet Christensen, and Frank R. Lewis (Univ. of California, San Francisco) used the thermal-green dye double indicator dilution method of measuring extravascular lung water (EVLW) to make sequential measurements in 16 severely injured patients presenting in shock over a 2-year period. The 15 men and 1 woman had an average age of 32 years. All had surgery for penetrating or blunt trauma. Five patients died, 3 of sepsis. Initial resuscitation was with crystalloid only.

The EVLW remained normal in 10 patients, 9 of whom survived, and 1 of whom died a neurologic death. These patients had an average initial blood pressure of 40 mm Hg and received an average of 18 L of crystalloid in the first 2 hospital days, as well as 1 L of colloid and 12.7 L of blood. Six patients had elevations of EVLW, and 4 of them died, 3 of sepsis and 1 of cardiovascular collapse. They had the same degree of shock and similar resuscitation as the former patients. The 4 patients with severe lung contusion had an initial moderate rise in EVLW followed by a rapid return to normal. The EVLW increased greatly in association with sepsis 4–7 days after injury.

Severe hemorrhagic shock and massive transfusion do not lead to accumulation of EVLW. Accumulation does not follow massive crystalloid resuscitation with resultant hemodilution of the plasma colloid oncotic pressure. Posttraumatic elevations of EVLW are associated with severe pulmonary contusion, sepsis, and heart failure. The chief determinants of interstitial fluid accumulation after trauma appear to be elevated capillary hydrostatic pressure and changes in capillary permeability due to lung contusion or sepsis.

▶ [Pulmonary edema (EVLW) is, for the most part, related to sepsis, and it is likely that the cause is primarily a change in capillary permeability. It is important to rec-

(3–76) J. Trauma 22:820–826, October 1982.

ognize that increased EVLW is not caused by large crystalloid fluid loads (e.g., burn patient resuscitation), shock per se, or multiple transfusions.—B.W.H.] ◄

3–77 **Adrenal Response to Repeated Hemorrhage: Implications for Studies of Trauma.** Although most serious traumatic injuries involve at least two major insults, most studies on endocrine responses have focused on either acute injuries or elective surgical intervention. Michael P. Lilly, William C. Engeland, and Donald S. Gann (Brown Univ., Providence, R.I.) attempted to determine whether moderate stimuli evoke similar responses when repeated, using a hemorrhage of 7.5 ml/kg as the stimulus to adrenocortical and medullary responses. Splenectomized dogs anesthetized with pentobarbital were bled 2 days after adrenal vein cannulation, and secretion rates of cortisol and catecholamines were determined in timed adrenal blood samples. The bled volume was reinfused after 1 hour, and the procedure was repeated the following day.

A significant cortisol response was observed following hemorrhage on each study day; the response on day 2 was 40% greater. Secretion rates of catecholamines did not change significantly after initial bleeding, but both epinephrine and norepinephrine responded dramatically on day 2, increasing to 14 times baseline levels. No significant cardiovascular changes in heart rate, arterial pressure, central venous pressure, or cardiac index were noted following bleeding on either day.

Severe potentiation of both adrenal cortical secretion and adrenal medullary secretion was observed in response to moderate hemorrhage when the stimulus is repeated after 24 hours. The physiologic role of the increased secretion of adrenal hormones on the second day is unclear, but differences in distribution, metabolism, or excretion of the hormones on the second day might require increased secretion rates to maintain constant circulating hormone concentrations. Models using two suitably timed or graded stimuli might be useful in examining responses to traumatic injury followed by surgery.

► [This paper emphasizes potentiation of adrenal response to repeated hemorrhage, and points out the relationship to trauma and surgery as repeated hemorrhages. These data recall a common clinical impression, in vogue some years ago, that secondary operations often succeeded where primary ones failed, and wound dehiscence being one example.—B.W.H.] ◄

3–78 **Treatment of Keloids and Hypertrophic Scars With Adhesive Zinc Tape.** Keloids and hypertrophic scars are benign proliferative connective tissue formations characterized by excessive collagen deposition, which are cosmetically unsightly and can produce discomfort. It has been reported that fewer keloids form when adhesive tape containing zinc oxide is used on wounds.

Thor Söderberg, Göran Hallmans, and Lennart Bartholdson (Univ. of Umeå, Umeå, Sweden) undertook a prospective study of the effects

(3–77) J. Trauma 22:809–814, October 1982.
(3–78) Scand. J. Plast. Reconstr. Surg. 16:261–266, 1982.

of zinc tape application on keloids and hypertrophic scars in 41 patients. These keloids had formed after surgery, trauma, burns, acne, and vaccinations, most commonly on the shoulder, sternal region, and arms. Two patients had failed to benefit from attempted surgical excision. Age of the 41 ranged from 2 to 67 years. The keloids had been present for up to 30 years. Ordinary adhesive tape that had zinc oxide included with the gum-resin adhesive was applied directly to the scar surface without tension and was kept on day and night.

The scar was reduced to the level of the surrounding skin in 23 cases, in 11 of which keloids had been present for a year or longer. Most patients with unresponsive keloids were treated with zinc tape for more than a year. More keloids in the sternal and shoulder regions failed to respond to zinc tape therapy. Itching was reduced in all affected patients, and often was eliminated. The only complication was an allergic reaction that cleared up when a tape coated with a polyacrylate-zinc oxide substance was used in place of the ordinary zinc tape.

The precise cause of abnormality in keloids and hypertrophic scars remains unknown. Zinc tape treatment obviously has an effect on the volume of these lesions, although spontaneous regression may explain some of the results. The mechanism underlying the beneficial effect of zinc tape in some instances is unclear, but both the synthesis and degradation of collagen may be involved in keloid formation and may be influenced by exposure to zinc. The effect of zinc tape should be compared with that of a tape not containing zinc.

▶ [Is it the mechanical effect of the tape or the chemical benefit of the zinc? The study should be repeated with tape containing no zinc, and a demonstration should be done illustrating whether zinc, or any other substance, will pass through the scar epithelium in sufficient concentration to affect wound healing. The genesis of all keloids and hypertrophic scars is undoubtedly multifactorial and several factors may need to be modified to prevent or treat them.—S.H.M.] ◀

3–79 **Acceleration of Wound Healing by Topical Application of Honey: An Animal Model.** The use of honey as an adjuvant in wound healing is a widely accepted folk remedy. Topical honey reportedly is helpful in the treatment of infected wounds, decubitus ulcers, and burn injury. Arieh Bergman, Joseph Yanai, Jerry Weiss, David Bell, and Menachem P. David examined the usefulness of honey in mice having an area of tissue 10 × 10 mm in size removed from the nape of the neck to the depth of muscle. Study animals had a thin layer of pure, unboiled commercial honey applied before dressing.

The distance of epithelization from the periphery of the wound was greater in honey-treated animals than in saline-treated control animals up to 9 days after wounding. Granulation tissue was thicker in the study animals. The area of the wound remained smaller in honey-treated animals than in controls. No wounds were clinically infected.

Wound healing appeared to occur much more rapidly in rats in this study with honey-treated wounds than in control animals. Honey

---

(3–79) Am. J. Surg. 145:374–376, March 1983.

may accelerate wound healing through its energy-producing and bacteriocidal properties and its hygroscopic effect.

▶ [Another testimonial that shows that folk medicine contains much intuitive wisdom—but it is a little hard to swallow without more objective data.—R.J.H.] ◀

3–80 **New Method of Dosimetry: Study of Comparative Laser-Induced Tissue Damage.** Dan Castro, Alan Stuart, David Benvenuti, Richard M. Dwyer, and Malcolm A. Lesavoy (Univ. of California at Los Angeles) undertook studies of laser-induced damage of pig skin in a carefully controlled setting using an argon laser, a yttrium/aluminum/garnet: neodymium (YAG:Nd) laser, and a broad-band infrared light source. A beam scan technique was used for accurate measurement of the laser intensity incident on the tissues and to standardize dosage measurements. The depth of penetration, vascular coagulation, damage to adnexal structures, and scar formation were quantitated. Comparable histologic changes were reproduced with the different energy sources used in the study. Tissue damage produced with the argon laser at 1,130–7,550 joules/sq cm was obtained with the YAG:Nd laser at 170–990 joules/sq cm, and with the infrared light source at 23–184 joules/sq cm. The argon laser did not penetrate past the mid-dermis. The blue-green argon laser showed great affinity for vascular coagulation. With the other energy sources, both vascular coagulation and adnexal damage were consistently dose related. Scar formation was less marked with the argon laser than with the YAG:Nd laser and the infrared light source. With the latter devices, scar formation was related to dosage and time.

This appears to be an accurate means of quantifying laser-induced tissue damage. Work is in progress to elucidate the biochemical effects of laser energy sources in order to better control various therapeutic modalities.

▶ [This study is an important one to all who use lasers, or who are about to use them. It provides a better understanding of the physiology of laser-induced damage to the skin and its underlying structures.—R.J.H.] ◀

3–81 **Wound Healing Accelerated by *Staphylococcus Aureus*.** Stanley M. Levenson, Dorinne Kan-Gruber, Charles Gruber, John Molnar, and Eli Seifter (Albert Einstein College of Medicine) found, while studying wound healing in rats with incisions made by a heated scalpel and a cold scalpel, that inoculation of the incisions with a strain of *Staphylococcus aureus* dramatically accelerated the gain in wound strength. Incisions then were purposely contaminated with several species of bacteria. Paramedian incisions 7 cm long were made in the back skin of rats and closed with interrupted fine monofilament steel sutures. Incisions made with the heated scalpel and those made with the cold surgical scalpel healed similarly over 6 weeks postoperatively.

The accelerating effect of *S. aureus* on wound healing was evident

(3–80) Ann. Plast. Surg. 9:221–227, September 1982.
(3–81) Arch. Surg. 118:310–320, March 1983.

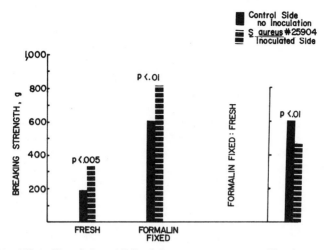

Fig 3–21.—Effect of inoculation with *Staphylococcus aureus* on wound breaking strength in 1 or 2 dorsal skin incisions in rats (7-day wounds). (Courtesy of Levenson, S. M., et al.: Arch. Surg. 118:310–320, March 1983; copyright 1983, American Medical Association.)

4 days postoperatively, which was the initial time of testing, and persisted for 28 days postoperatively. The effect was most marked 6–7 days postoperatively, but remained highly significant on day 18. Seven strains of *S. aureus* exhibited the effect, but it was not observed with *Staphylococcus epidermidis, Staphylococcus hominis,* or *Pseudomonas aeruginosa.* Accelerated wound healing was also noted with *S. aureus* in germ-free rats. As few as 10^2 organisms significantly accelerated the gain in breaking strength. Heat-killed organisms were ineffective, as was a filtrate of the medium in which the staphylococci had grown. The results are shown in Figure 3–21. Intravenous injection of *S. aureus* just after wounding led to a significant but modest acceleration in healing.

Contamination of skin incisions with *S. aureus* accelerates wound healing in rats. The effect probably is the result in part of incitement of an "optimal" inflammatory reaction to wounding. Purposeful contamination of clinical incisions is not recommended, because clinical wound sepsis is too great a risk. If, however, chemical components of *S. aureus* or compounds produced in the wound as a result of interaction with the organism are active factors, introduction of the appropriate chemical agent would be a possibility.

▶ [The conclusion of this article would be a serendipitious finding should further study achieve identification and isolation of the long sought after safe accelerator of wound healing.—R.J.H.] ◀

3–82 **Effect of Epidermal Growth Factor on Wound Healing in Mice.** Communal licking and grooming are common observations in

(3–82) J. Surg. Res. 33:164–169, August 1982.

mammals, particularly after injury. Margaret Niall, Graeme B. Ryan, and Bernard McC. O'Brien (Melbourne) have obtained evidence that delivery of saliva to an injured area may represent a physiologic response to injury mediated by epidermal growth factor (EGF). This growth factor is synthesized in high concentration in the submaxillary gland of the male mouse and is present in high concentration in saliva, where its release is under α-adrenergic control. Synthesis of EGF is stimulated by testosterone in both sexes. The effects of topical application of EGF on wound healing were examined in control and sialectomized mice of both sexes. Sialectomized mice received EGF intraperitoneally at a rate of 10 μg daily for 8 days.

Epidermal growth factor had a highly significant stimulatory effect on wound closure in both control and sialectomized male mice. A dose of 1 μg was used to simulate that applied by communal licking. Topical EGF therapy abolished the difference in wound closure noted between control and sialectomized animals. Castrated male mice responded like those with intact gonads. Topical EGF was much less effective in both control and sialectomized female mice, but female mice given testosterone responded to EGF like male mice. Topical application of arachidonic acid appeared to promote wound closure in sialectomized animals. Administration of indomethacin with EGF inhibited the effect of EGF in accelerating wound closure in control and sialectomized animals. Dexamethasone had a similar inhibitory effect whether it was given alone or with EGF.

Possible evolutionary advantages of communal licking can be explained in part by the presence of EGF in saliva. The testosterone dependence of EGF synthesis makes teleologic sense in the context of an acute response to injury caused by fighting. Prostaglandins in injured tissue may modulate the acute effects of EGF. Epidermal growth factor is a potent mitogen for murine fibroblast and epithelial cell lines, and it may also participate in longer term effects integral to wound healing.

3–83 **Behavior of Synthetic Absorbable Sutures With and Without Synergistic Enteric Infection.** Synthetic absorbable sutures are being used increasingly in intestinal anastomosis and abdominal wound closure because of their slow dissolution compared with that of catgut. C. R. Kapadia, J. B. Mann, D. McGeehan, J. E. Jose Biglin, B. P. Waxman, and H. A. F. Dudley (London) examined the behavior of polyglycolic acid (PGA) and polydioxanone (PDS) sutures in a guinea pig model using synergistic enteric bacteria. Dorsal pouches 2 cm long were made down to the deep fascia; suture loops were placed in the pouches before they were inoculated with a saline suspension of an organism, either *Escherichia coli* or *Bacteroides fragilis*. More than 600 wounds were made in about 100 animals.

Braided PDS produced an increased incidence of infection of 42%.

(3–83) Eur. Surg. Res. 15:67–72, Mar.–Apr. 1983.

The infection rate of 36% with monofilament PDS did not differ significantly from the control rate of 30%. The PGA sutures were associated with an infection rate of 26%, not significantly below the control rate. No significant reduction in breaking strength was noted with infection when monofilament PDS suture material was tested, but PGA sutures showed an accelerated rate of breakdown in the presence of infection, as did braided PDS sutures.

Braided PDS suture material was associated with an increased rate of infection in this guinea pig model, and its dissolution was enhanced by the presence of infection. Polyglycolic acid sutures appear to be indifferent to, or marginally inhibitory of, infection, and their dissolution seems to be unaffected by the presence of sepsis. There would seem to be no contraindications to using PGA or monofilament PDS when enteric infection is a possibility. Studies of the effects of these materials on wound healing in the gut are needed.

▶ [Reassuring is the word for this article, but other studies, in the presence of different bacterial wound infections, are needed.—R.J.H.] ◀

3–84   **Development of New Miniature Method for Study of Wound Healing in Human Subjects.** William H. Goodson III, and Thomas K. Hunt (Univ. of California at San Francisco) describe a method for studying wound healing in human beings that is minimally invasive and is well accepted by patients. A small subcutaneous wound is made in the lower lateral part of the upper arm, and a tube of expanded polytetrafluoroethylene (PTFE) 1 mm in diameter and 7 cm long is placed in the wound as shown in Figure 3–22 About 1 cm of tubing is left outside the skin and secured with a loop of nylon suture through the tubing and skin. Studies in mice indicated that reproducible amounts of hydroxyproline accumulated in connective tissue in the PTFE tubing, and that the course of accumulation followed that of wound healing.

Initial studies showed that the method is safe in human beings. Catheters then were placed in 30 patients expected to heal normally and in 13 undergoing comparable surgical procedures in whom poor wound healing was a possibility for various reasons. Tubing having a nominal pore size of 90 μm was placed for up to 7 days. Rapid accumulation of hydroxyproline in the tubing was observed, as in the animal studies. Significantly less accumulation was noted in the patients at risk. The difference was not attributable to age or sex. Histologic studies on days 5–7 indicated that increased hydroxyproline accumulation at this stage correlated with an increase in visible tissue.

This appears to be a useful means of assessing wound healing in the clinical setting. Using local anesthesia, the tubing can be placed in outpatients, making the method applicable to systematic studies in

(3–84)   J. Surg. Res. 33:394–401, November 1982.

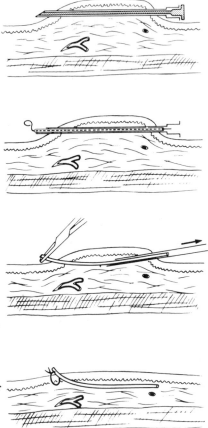

Fig. 3–22.—Insertion of PTFE tubing in wound. Needle and trochar are placed through subcutaneous tissue; the trochar is removed, and PTFE tubing (over stylette) is placed in the needle; the tube is held and the needle removed in the opposite direction; the tube is then secured in the subcutaneous position with sutures. (Courtesy of Goodson, W. H., III, and Hunt, T. K.: J. Surg. Res. 33:394–401, November 1982.)

populations, as well as to the observation of patients requiring surgery.

▶ [This is an exciting and ingenious paper because it is written by seasoned students of wound healing physiology who describe a minimally invasive technique for analyzing products and events in the healing cycle. For the first time, general populations can be studied accurately in human beings as well as animals.—R.J.H.] ◀

3–85 **Op-Site Skin Closure: Comparison With Subcuticular and Interrupted Sutures.** Op-Site skin closure involves a polyurethane membrane coated with a firm adhesive, having a central line of fenestrations lying across the incision. There is theoretically a lesser risk of wound contamination by staphylococci carried on a needle or suture. G. M. Watson, C. J. Anders, and J. R. Glover (Chertsey, England) compared Op-Site skin closure with both interrupted silk sutures and subcuticular nylon sutures in a series of 209 consecutive

---

(3–85) Ann. R. Coll. Surg. Engl. 65:83–84, March 1983.

abdominal operations and inguinal herniorraphies done by a single surgeon. All wounds were closed primarily. There were 120 "clean" procedures, 62 operations with an "intermediate" risk of wound infection, and 27 "contaminated" procedures. Five patients later were moved from the intermediate into contaminated group because of positive results of peritoneal swab culture.

Op-Site skin closure was associated with less frequent erythema and tenderness than were the other methods, but at the expense of some loss of precision of wound edge alignment. Similar trends were noted at all levels of wound contamination, although subcuticular sutures were not used in the contaminated groups. Three patients with silk sutures and 3 with subcuticular sutures required formal incision of a wound abscess. All four Op-Site-treated wounds that discharged pus drained freely, and in three instances there was no tenderness or reddening.

Although Op-Site skin closure permits freer drainage of secretions from the surgical wound and is associated with less tenderness and erythema than are silk or subcuticular nylon sutures, there is a tendency for the wound edges to slip out of alignment or invert. The method should not be used in patients who are likely to become confused postoperatively, or when early, copious discharge of fluid through the wound is expected. Op-Site skin closure may prove to be especially useful when a wound is contaminated.

3–86 **Current Concepts in Soft Connective Tissue Wound Healing** are reviewed by L. Forrest (Manchester, England). Most experimental studies of wound repair have involved skin wounds, but the general applicability of concepts derived from such studies remains to be established. The strength and integrity of soft tissues are related to the forces existing between collagen fibrils, and these in turn are dependent on collagen fibril size, density, and architecture. Fibril size is influenced by the genetic type of collagen, enzymatic changes in the collagen monomer, and the proteoglycan environment. Tissue continuity is restored and tissue strength regained after wounding through the formation of a myofibroblast-reticulin network, which later disappears as the healing wound ages. The extent of the network determines the area in which repair tissue will be laid down. Connective tissue synthesis is regulated through monitoring of the local physicochemical environment.

An initial change in the tension or compression state of the tissues may be communicated to the local connective tissue cells via changes in the charge distribution on the collagen molecules and the egress of intravascular components to the extracellular wound space, leading to induction of the clotting, complement, and kinin systems. Contact of platelets with collagen leads to the release of granule contents and induces platelet synthetic activity involving the release of products of

(3–86) Br. J. Surg. 70:133–140, March 1983.

the prostaglandin synthetase pathway, some of which are central to the inflammatory process. Fibroblasts derived from local tissue cells and new capillaries appear in the wound 24–48 hours later than do white blood cells.

Current studies are focusing on the operation of the fibroblast capillary system in the locally hypoxic, acidotic conditions of the wound space. An understanding of connective tissue biology is basic to the knowledge of all healing processes and to virtually all aspects of human pathology.

▶ [This is an erudite update on current concepts in the physiologic sequence of events in wound healing in human beings. It is concise, highly readable, and based upon an encyclopedic bibliography.—R.J.H.] ◀

3–87 **Factors Influencing Wound Complications: A Clinical and Experimental Study** is reported by Timothy E. Bucknall (Westminster Med. School, London). Burst abdomen, incisional herniation, and sinus formation remain major wound healing problems after laparotomy. A prospective study of 1,129 major laparotomy wounds in patients operated on from 1975 to 1980 revealed burst abdomen in 1.7%, incisional hernia in 7.4%, and sinus formation in 6.7%. All of these complications were significantly associated with wound infections. The occurrence of dehiscence lessened substantially when mass wound closure was adopted.

A study in rats using different microorganisms confirmed that infection reduces wound strength because of reductions in fibroblast concentration and activity. A monofilament nonabsorbable suture was the most suitable type for use in closing infected abdominal wounds. Both monofilament and braided nylon sutures retained their strength during the study in rats previously infected by injection of *Staphylococcus aureus*. Ultrastructural study showed that bacteria lodged in the interstices of infected multifilamentous materials, especially silk and nylon. A vigorous polymorph reaction was associated with the presence of trapped organisms. A clinical trial comparing polyglycolic acid and monofilament nylon sutures in the closure of abdominal wounds confirmed the experimental findings. The wound failure rate was significantly higher with polyglycolic acid sutures, and sinus formation was not reduced.

It is recommended that a mass closure technique using monofilament nylon sutures be used for laparotomy closure. This material provides no place for cells and bacteria to be trapped. In addition, sinus formation is impeded. Suture strength should suffice to hold the abdominal fascia together even if healing is delayed by infection. Efforts must continue to reduce wound sepsis.

3–88 **Efficacy of Triamcinolone Acetonide Following Neurorrhaphy: Electroneuromyographic Evaluation.** A major obstacle to

(3–87) Ann. R. Coll. Surg. Engl. 65:71–77, March 1983.
(3–88) Ann. Plast. Surg. 9:230–237, September 1982.

successful functional reinnervation appears to be development of excessive scar at the level of nerve repair. Previous studies indicated that less scar forms around injured nerves when triamcinolone is used in conjunction with neurorrhaphy. William P. Graham, III, Thomas S. Davis, Stephen H. Miller, and Irena Rusenas examined the effects of locally instilled triamcinolone acetonide on functional reinnervation after neurorrhaphy in stump-tail monkeys, as assessed by electroneuromyography. The median nerve was transected proximal to the wrist, and perineural repair with 10–0 nylon was carried out under magnification. Either 2.5 mg of triamcinolone or its vehicle alone was instilled into the repair site after closure of the incision, and the nerves were evaluated from 1 to 14 months after operation.

Evoked responses were first obtained from the thenar muscle at 3 months. The configuration of the response in corticosteroid-treated monkeys more closely approached animals that were not operated on. The trend at 8 months was toward delayed latency, slightly reduced amplitude, and a prolonged time course in responses evoked from vehicle treated nerves. Triamcinolone-treated nerves showed only a persistently reduced amplitude. At 14 months the difference in spread of the evoked response differed significantly between corticosteroid and vehicle groups. Fewer axons were present in vehicle-treated nerve fascicles. Large myelinated axons were abundant in corticosteroid-treated monkeys, besides many small axons. The number of large diameter axons correlated inversely with the duration of the evoked response.

It appears that triamcinolone acetonide, instilled locally just after a neurorrhaphy, benefits regeneration of motor nerves in a primate model. The improved reinnervation is most likely due to the anti-inflammatory action of the corticosteroid.

▶ [The authors present a well-documented study of the beneficial effects of triamcinolone on nerve anastomosis and regeneration. They postulate that since treated nerves maintain an intact perineurium longer, axons are directed into the distal segment with more frequency. Another factor is decreased scar formation at the neurorrhaphy site. The authors provide logical explanations for their good results.— F.J.M.] ◀

3–89 **Nerve Regeneration Across Extended Gap: Neurobiologic View of Nerve Repair and Possible Involvement of Neuronotrophic Factors.** Recognition of agents such as nerve growth factor that support the growth of neurons, and of trophic factors that may influence the orientation of elongating axons, forms the basis for new approaches to nerve repair. Göran Lundborg, Lars-Bertil Dahlin, Nils Danielsen, Hans-Arne Hansson, Ann Johannesson, Frank M. Longo, and Silvio Varon evaluated an experimental system in which a transected nerve regenerates directly through a cylindrical chamber formed from autologous mesothelial tissue and into the distal nerve segment. The results obtained in rats having sciatic resections were

(3–89) J. Hand Surg. 7:580–587, November 1982.

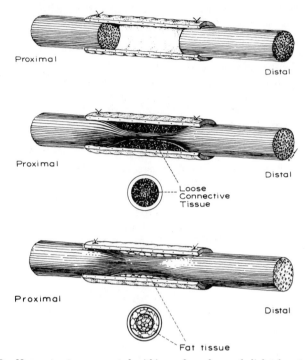

Fig 3–23.—Nerve structure generated within preformed mesothelial tube at various times. **Top,** after resection of a sciatic nerve segment, the nerve stumps are introduced into the openings of the mesothelial chamber, leaving a gap of 10 mm. **Center,** after a month, a thin nerve structure is generated through the chamber, bridging the gap between the nerve stumps. The remaining space inside the chamber is occupied by loose connective tissue. **Bottom,** after 3 months, the newly formed nerve structure has a larger diameter. The remaining space is filled with fat tissue. (Courtesy of Lundborg, G., et al.: J. Hand Surg. 7:580–587, November 1982.)

compared with those in animals having autologous nerve grafting. In both cases a 10-mm gap was created. The mesothelial tube method is illustrated in Figure 3–23.

A solid cord of tissue containing well-myelinated axons arranged in small bundles was present after 1 month in the mesothelial chamber group. A well-defined regenerated nerve was present after 3 months, consisting of a multifascicular trunk containing myelinated and non-myelinated axons, Schwann cells, vascular elements, perineurium, and an epineurium. There was abundant invasion of axons into the distal nerve segment. Significant action potentials were recorded from the intrinsic foot muscles. Similar findings were obtained in the nerve graft group in terms of axonal density and distribution of axonal diameters; mean conduction velocities across the gaps also were comparable in the two groups. When the gap was left empty, however, little or no regeneration was observed.

These findings indicate that, if the regrowing proximal nerve stump is in an appropriate environment, a well-organized, well-oriented nerve trunk can develop. The loose cellular stroma and interstitial fluid, which contains trophic activity, may make the mesothelial chamber technique useful clinically. Restoration of the proper microenvironment appears to be necessary for optimal nerve regeneration.

3–90 **Nerve Anastomosis by a Fibrinogen Tissue Adhesive.** The problems encountered in various nerve suture techniques may be overcome by using artificial or biologic glues. D. Boedts (Univ. of Antwerp) evaluated a fibrinogen tissue adhesive consisting of a human plasma cryoprecipitate solution having a fibrinogen content of about 80% and a bovine thrombin solution of high concentration. The cryoprecipitate solution was applied to the sciatic fascicle ends after section of the nerve in guinea pigs and clotted with the second component. Aprotinin and factor XIII were added to the thrombin solution. A piece of aluminum foil was placed beneath the nerve stumps to facilitate the procedure and prevent adhesion.

The fibrin structure was absorbed within 3 days and transformed into connective tissue, which lay longitudinally along the anastomosis. Axonal regeneration through the site of section began after 3 weeks when apposition was optimal. The longitudinal arrangement was less compact than in normal fascicles. Early axonal myelination was evident 10 weeks later. Stricture formation resulted from connective tissue proliferation when apposition was suboptimal or poor. In 1 case, total disruption of the nerve stumps and neuroma formation were observed.

This sealing method that uses blood clotting substances, simulates normal wound healing. Little or no tension should be present at the line of coaptation. If this approach cannot entirely replace surgical suturing, it at least provides a useful tool for nerve anastomosis and nerve grafting. Nerve grafting or rerouting is indicated if end-to-end anastomosis is not possible without tension and exact coaptation is not feasible.

3–91 **Role of Platelets and Fibrin in Healing Sequence: In Vivo Study of Angiogenesis and Collagen Synthesis.** The factors that initiate the healing response are largely unknown, but it is reasonable to think that products of coagulation have a role in the cellular response to wounding because activation of platelets and the clotting cascade are among the first reactions to injury. David R. Knighton, Thomas K. Hunt, K. K. Thakral, and William H. Goodson, III (Univ. of California at San Francisco) performed studies on rabbit cornea to determine whether the products of activated platelets produce neovascularization and collagen synthesis, and to assess the role of fibrin in eliciting macrophage migration and subsequent angiogenesis in

(3–90)   J. Head Neck Pathol. 3:86–89, 1982.
(3–91)   Ann. Surg. 196:379–388, October 1982.

vivo. Autologous platelets and platelet-free fibrin were isolated from rabbit blood. Released and control platelets and autologous and commercial fibrin were implanted in rabbit corneas.

Thrombin-released platelets produced both angiogenesis and opacification, with fibroplasia, corneal thickening, and neovascularization. Control platelet preparations produced no angiogenesis or histologic changes. Collagen synthesis was elevated to twice baseline in thrombin-activated platelet preparations. Fibrin injections elicited cellular exudation from the limbal vessels, followed by angiogenesis and corneal opacification. A mononuclear infiltrate was associated with neovascularization and fibroplasia. Injections of rabbit skin collagen and fibroblasts produced no such response.

Thrombin-activated platelets can stimulate angiogenesis and increase collagen synthesis in the in vivo rabbit corneal assay. Fibrin, fibrinopeptides, or fibrin degradation products cause leukocyte migration into the cornea and subsequent neovascularization. It would seem that fibrin acts as an activator of the production by leukocytes of growth and angiogenic factors. The findings suggest that impaired wound healing in patients with thrombocytopenia, leukopenia, or clotting disorders might be related to the absence of chemoattractant and mitogenic factors necessary for normal wound repair. The deficit might be corrected by administering platelets, leukocytes, or frozen plasma.

▶ [As evidenced in the discussion following this elegantly devised study (*Ann. Surg.* 196:388, October 1982), the nature and causes of angiogenesis and angioneogenesis are fundamental to a variety of processes. These include normal processes such as wound healing and pathologic processes such as arthritis, psoriasis, tumor growth, etc. With an exact understanding of which factors stimulate and which factors inhibit angiogenesis, will come better clinical management and control of these processes.—R.J.H.] ◀

3–92 **Flexor Tendon Healing and Restoration of Gliding Surface: Ultrastructural Study in Dogs.** Immediate protected mobilization of healing tendons was proposed in order to minimize adhesion formation. Richard H. Gelberman, Jerry S. Vande Berg, Goran N. Lundborg, and Wayne H. Akeson (Univ. of California at San Diego) undertook a microscopic study of healing tendons to compare the effect of immediate mobilization with that of continuous immobilization. Dogs had longitudinal incision of the synovial sheaths of the flexor tendons in the forelimb and transverse incision of the flexor digitorum profundus tendons at the level of the proximal interphalangeal joint. The tendons were repaired with 4-0 braided Dacron suture under magnification, using a 6-0 nylon epitenon suture to invaginate the free tendon ends. The digital sheaths were not repaired. The animals managed by either total immobilization or early controlled passive mobilization to the limits of the dorsal extension block.

The immobilized tendons healed by ingrowth of connective tissue from the digital sheath and cellular proliferation of the endotenon.

(3–92) J. Bone Joint Surg. [Am.] 65–A:70–80, January 1983.

The epitenon response was overwhelmed by an ingrowth of reparative tissue from the digital sheath. Collagen resorption was prominent, whereas protein synthesis was limited. The mobilized tendons, in contrast, healed by proliferation and migration of cells from the epitenon. Ingrowth of reparative tissue from the sheath was relatively sparse. The epitenon cells showed greater activity and more collagen production at all intervals up to 42 days after repair, compared with findings in the immobilized repairs. Fibroblasts within the area of repair of the mobilized tendons exhibited active protein synthesis. No adhesions or surface irregularities were seen protruding from the inner lining of the flexor tendon sheath.

Cells involved in repair in mobilized tendons are chiefly from the surface layer (Fig 3–24). The early epitenon response is much more marked than is the delayed proliferative response of the endotenon seen in immobilized tendons (Fig 3–25). It would appear that the gliding surface of a tendon may be induced from an early stage by

Fig 3–24 (top).—Healing mobilized tendon with epitenon cellular ingrowth.
Fig 3–25 (bottom).—Immobilized tendon healing by adhesion and endotenon cellular ingrowth. (Courtesy of Gelberman, R. H., et al.: J. Bone Joint Surg. [Am.] 65–A:70–80, January 1983.)

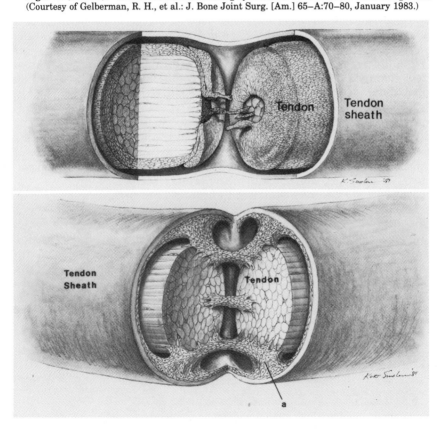

limited motion, with a mechanically stronger and functionally superior repair resulting.

▶ [This is a neat and histologically well-documented study from orthopedic colleagues. It reemphasizes the importance of controlled passive motion at an early stage in stimulating an intrinsic healing response in tendons.—R.J.H.] ◀

3–93 **Healing of Split Flexor Tendon Graft: Experimental Study in Chickens.** Restoration of strength and function in a partially lacerated flexor tendon without operation has been described. Alfred W. Farmer, Leslie G. Farkas, and Morley A. Herbert (Toronto) found the half-thickness flexor tendon graft to be an adequate replacement in experimental tendon defect repair in chickens. Leghorn chickens, aged 6 months, had a split tendon graft about 42 mm long taken from the deep flexor of the third toe. The sublimis flexor was excised in the other foot, and a defect was created in the deep flexor by removing a 37-mm segment and was bridged by split tendon graft by side-to-side anastomosis with 5-0 silk sutures. After the toe was immobilized for 4 weeks in plaster, some animals were kept caged with perching rods for 9 weeks more and others spent 10 weeks in a free-ranging, natural environment.

The caged birds regained 59% of normal flexion, compared with 75% for the free-ranging animals. The strength of the healing tendons averaged 42% of normal. The donor flexors regained an average of 90%, and the grafted part of the recipient flexors, 85%, of their original diameter. Free-ranging birds exhibited greater restoration of tendon diameter and greater strength and return of active flexion than did those that remained caged. Histologic study showed near restoration of the fascicular architecture in the damaged area in free-ranging birds. Healing of the split tendon graft in the recipient deep flexor was advanced. The epitenon formed in the previously defective area appeared normal. In caged birds the defective side of the donor tendon was filled with connective tissue resembling young tendon tissue. The epitenon was thicker in the area of the defect.

The raw surface of a split tendon injury that is surrounded by its sheath can heal without the formation of permanent firm adhesions. The split tendon graft may be used in emergency situations when multiple tendon injuries of the hand are present and other tendon replacement methods are not applicable. In certain experimental animals, healing may be better in the natural environment rather than in standard cages.

▶ [A thoroughly controlled and documented study by seasoned investigators using a proven experimental model. Their findings suggest a useful clinical application of split tendon grafts for repair of multiple tendon defects in man when donor material may be scarce.—R.J.H.] ◀

3–94 **Treatment of Therapeutically Resistant Nonunions With Bone Grafts and Pulsing Electromagnetic Fields.** Electrothera-

(3–93) Ann. Plast. Surg. 10:284–289, April 1983.
(3–94) J. Bone Joint Surg. [Am.] 64–A:1214–1220, October 1982.

peutic methods offer a possible alternative to bone grafting in the management of ununited fractures. C. A. L. Bassett, S. N. Mitchell, and M. M. Schink (New York) used both bone grafting and pulsed electromagnetic fields to achieve union in 83 adults with ununited fractures. Of these, 38 had combined treatment at the outset, after a total of 100 unsuccessful surgical attempts at repair, 33 of which involved bone grafting; 45 other patients had combined treatment after there was no response to pulsed electromagnetic field therapy alone. Nearly a third of all patients had a history of infection. Fresh autogenous cortical-cancellous or cancellous iliac bone grafts were used in all patients but 1, who received a preserver allogeneic cortical graft. Electromagnetic field therapy was self-administered for 10 hours a day at home, usually at night. Strict nonweight-bearing was observed postoperatively by patients with an unstable nonunion in the lower extremity.

The rate of successful healing in patients having combined treatment from the outset was 87%. In the patients initially treated unsuccessfully with electromagnetic field therapy alone, 93% of fractures healed after combined treatment. The failure rate after 2 attempts at treatment, 1 of which was operative, was 1.5%. The median time to union in the overall group was 4 months. No complications resulted from either bone grafting or the use of pulsed electromagnetic fields.

A marked reduction in the failure rate was achieved with this approach (Fig 3–26), An example is shown in Figure 3–27. There is clinical and laboratory evidence to suggest that a synergistic effect occurs between bone grafts and pulsed electromagnetic fields. The latter technique should be strongly considered for use as an adjunct to any extremity bone graft, whether in a primary or a salvage situation. It does not lead to an increase in cortical diameter; however,

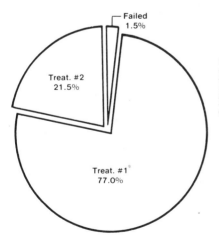

Fig 3–26.—Comparison of results of the first attempt to produce union with pulsing electromagnetic fields, incorporating data from the second attempt. Overall failure rate was 1.5%. (Courtesy of Bassett, C. A. L., et al.: J. Bone Joint Surg. [Am.] 64–A:1214–1220, October 1982.)

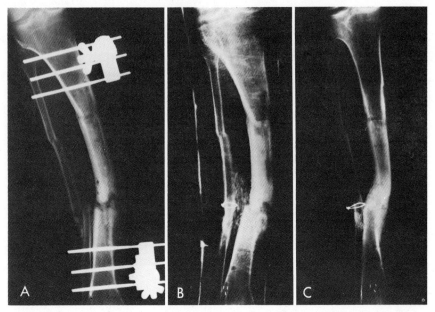

Fig 3–27.—Anteroposterior radiographs of patient with open fracture of the right tibia and fibula occurring in 1978. Four attempts were made to repair the fracture operatively and the wound was actively draining. **A,** after 12–13 months, coils and external fixation were applied. **B,** the fracture healed within 6 months, but the leg was refractured in October 1980; at this time the patient had a bone graft and the limb was immobilized in plaster. **C,** By February 1981, the fracture was healed and drainage ceased. (Courtesy of Bassett, C. A. L., et al.: J. Bone Joint Surg. [Am.] 64–A:1214–1220, October 1982.)

after bone grafting of a major stress-concentrating defect, pulsed electromagnetic field therapy helps ensure early union and return of function.

▶ [This is a most impressive and prodigious study, which uses carefully selected patients treated clinically over many years by the senior author and his associates. The long debate about the efficacy of pulsing electromagnetic fields in healing established bone nonunions seems to come to an end with this presentation of the amazing success rates of these conservative and dedicated workers.—R.J.H.] ◀

3–95 **Fibrin Adhesive System (FAS) Influence on Bone Healing Rate: Microradiographic Evaluation Using Bone Growth Chamber.** Push/pullout methods of quantifying bone ingrowth adjacent to hard tissue implants do not permit histologic analysis of the interface. T. Albrektsson, A. Bach, S. Edshage, and A. Jönsson used an experimental model, the bone growth chamber, to examine the effects of the fibrin adhesive system (FAS) on bone growth in the rabbit. A titanium implant containing two canals (Fig 3–28) was inserted into the tibial metaphyses of adult rabbits. On one side the implants were pretreated with FAS and on the other side they were bathed in autol-

(3–95) Acta Orthop. Scand. 53:757–763, October 1982.

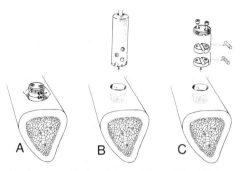

Fig 3–28.—A, titanium bone growth chamber consisting of 3 separate parts held in place by 2 screws. One proximal and 1 distal canal penetrate the implant at the level of the junctions between the titanium sections. The chamber was inserted in the rabbit tibia, after which bone began to grow into the canals *(arrows).* **B,** after 4–5 weeks, the chamber with a surrounding bone collar was removed with a trephine. **C,** the implant was taken apart for microradiographic and histologic examination of the tissue that had grown into the proximal and distal canals. (Courtesy of Albrektsson, T., et al.: Acta Orthop. Scand. 53:757–763, October 1982.)

ogous blood and marrow. Either implant was placed so that the top canal was at the level of cortical bone and the lower one was in the marrow space, or the top canal was in the marrow space close to the proximal cortex and the distal canal was deep in the marrow space. The implants were removed after 4–5 weeks.

Microradiographic and microdensitometric studies showed that FAS-treated implants tended to contain less bone than did the medullary cell-treated implants. Implants with the top canal at the level of cortical bone consistently contained more bone than the others did. Histologic study showed normal bone tissue with osteoblastic activity in control implants. Test bone exhibited a tendency toward inflammation and, in two instances, inflammation was very evident.

The dividable titanium implant permits estimates of early bone ingrowth rates under varying conditions. In the present study in rabbits, bone tissue did not grow more rapidly into FAS-treated implants than into those treated with autologous blood and medullary cells. More evidence is needed before FAS treatment can be recommended to accelerate bone regeneration in cases of bone injury.

3–96 **Osteogenic Properties of Reimplanted Decalcified and Undecalcified Autologous Bone in Rabbit Radius.** Whereas undecalcified devitalized bone is not generally thought to produce new bone when implanted into muscle, decalcified cortical bone has such a capacity. J. Wittbjer, B. Palmer, and K.-G. Thorngren examined the differences in osteogenic capacity between decalcified and undecalcified autologous bone reimplanted in an operative resectional defect in the rabbit radius. Bone removed from a 12-mm segment of radius was

(3–96) Scand. J. Plast. Reconstr. Surg. 16:239–244, 1982.

either decalcified in 0.6 N HCl for 24 hours and stored for 2 days in cold saline, or stored without being decalcified; the bone was replaced 3 days later. The animals were followed roentgenographically for 4 weeks postoperatively.

Thin radiopaque bands were sometimes seen at 2 weeks in sites of implanted decalcified bone matrix. Further mineralization was evident at 3 weeks in these specimens, but there were large individual differences in the degree of radiopacity. Specimen radiography confirmed substantial mineralization in defects implanted with decalcified bone, but no new bone formation in undecalcified implants. Histologic study showed immature woven bone with many osteocytes throughout the decalcified implants. Small islands of newly formed bone were present in limited areas of the periphery of undecalcified implants. Fluorescence microscopy showed more extensive fluorescence in decalcified specimens in all instances but one.

When bone is retransplanted to a defect in the rabbit radius, decalcification appears to accelerate osteogenesis in comparison with undecalcified bone implants. The osteogenic process is impaired by infection.

3–97 **Lymphedema Following Ilioinguinal Lymph Node Dissection.** Ilioinguinal lymph node dissection is thought to lead frequently to poor wound healing and postoperative edema. J. H. James (Århus, Denmark) reviewed the results of ilioinguinal node dissection in 90 consecutive patients, 37 of whom were living at the time of review. A standard procedure was used in all cases, the goal being to remove disease radically with a minimum of complications. A skin strip 3–5 cm long is included in the excised tissue overlying any palpable nodes. All tissue superficial to the muscles and femoral vessels and nerve are excised en bloc in a subfascial plane of dissection before performing a suprainguinal or iliac dissection. If necessary, the wound is closed with a sartorius muscle flap or an abdominal transposition flap to cover the femoral vessels.

Healing was complicated in 54.5% of the patients, but usually the complications were minor. Three patients required drainage of a lymph collection. Fifty patients experienced postoperative edema. In the 33 patients examined, edema developed in 8 of 19 who had no healing complications and in 11 of 14 who did have complications. Leg edema usually was noted soon after discharge from hospital and was most severe in the first 6 months after operation. Edema lasted for more than a year in about two thirds of the patients. Elastic support was helpful occasionally, but bed rest and diuretics were not. Also, 25% of the patients reported impaired mobility resulting from leg edema. Severe edema was observed in 30% of the patients, some edema in 50%, and no edema in 20%. Measurements of leg circumfer-

(3–97) Scand. J. Plast. Reconstr. Surg. 16:167–171, 1982.

ence correlated well with measurements of leg volume by the water displacement method.

Ilioinguinal node dissection may result in postoperative edema, and this may be associated with healing complications. However, the possibility that these complications might develop is not a contraindication to the operation.

4. Esthetic Surgery

SKIN, SUBCUTANEOUS, AND HAIR

4-1 **Serious Complication Following Medical-Grade Silicone Injection of the Face.** Serious complications of silicone injections into the breast region are well documented, and some investigators have observed chronic inflammatory reactions to facial injections. Bruce M. Achauer (Univ. of California, Irvine) describes a patient who developed severe chronic inflammatory changes after facial injections of silicone and required en block excision of the injection area and flap reconstruction.

Woman, 53, had developed painful inflammatory subcutaneous nodules in the buttocks, arms, and right side of the face at age 34, which resolved, leaving areas of atrophy that failed to respond to corticosteroid and antibiotic therapy. Atypical mycobacteria were found in the facial lesions, and isoniazid and para-aminosalicylic acid were given for several months. Liquid silicone injections were administered by an FDA-approved investigator. About 12 cc was administered in 0.5- to 2-cc increments over 4 years. Inflammation in the injection area began 11 years after the initial injections and occurred with increasing frequency. The reaction became progressively less responsive to antibiotics and local corticosteroid treatment, and the involved tissue was finally excised. A free latissimus dorsi flap was used to reconstruct the region. Facial nerve function was preserved. Examination of the excised specimen showed lipid material, chronic inflammation, and necrosis.

This patient appears to have had Weber-Christian disease, a condition of relapsing, nodular, nonsuppurative panniculitis. The lipodystrophy that follows the acute stage is characterized by symmetric losses of subcutaneous fat from the face. This patient had a severe inflammatory reactions some time after the start of liquid silicone injections to augment a deficient facial area. She also had rheumatoid arthritis. Caution is indicated when liquid silicone injections are used in patients with Weber-Christian disease or autoimmune states. It is not entirely clear whether this patient had a reaction to silicone or a reactivation of the panniculitis, although the former is more likely.

▶ [The authors have brought to our attention a tragic case. This is the first reported complication from the injection of silicone by an FDA-approved investigator. Based on the experience with this patient, it would appear that any patient with Weber-Christian disease is not a candidate for such a procedure.—R.O.B.] ◀

4-2 **Clinical Utilization of Injectable Collagen** is outlined by Ernest

---

(4–1) Plast. Reconstr. Surg. 71:251–253, February 1983.
(4–2) Ann. Plast. Surg. 10:437–451, June 1983.

N. Kaplan, Edward Falces, and Hale Tolleth (Stanford Univ.). Injectable collagen is a highly purified, reconstituted, fibrous dispersion isolated from cowhide. Shortly after implantation the carrier saline is resorbed, leaving collagen fibers that condense into a soft implant, a latticework of collagen fibers into which host fibroblasts and capillaries grow. The vascularized implant is subsequently incorporated by host tissues. A test site is monitored for 4 weeks before definitive treatment is carried out. The overall rate of untoward responses has been about 3%. Soft, distensible lesions with relatively smooth margins are best corrected with injectable collagen. Several deposits of material may be helpful in indurated lesions. The best correction is obtained when the material is placed within the dermis. Appreciable correction is obtained only when a lesion can be overcorrected to 1.5 to 2 times its initial depth.

Over 400 patients have been treated to date, and fewer than 2% have had problems. In patients with acne, saucer-shaped depressions, especially those due to corticosteroid injections, have been successfully treated. Crater-shaped lesions are also well-treated with injectable collagen, but acne scars that are sharply marginated and deep do not respond. Injectable collagen has been used to augment some age-related rhytids, especially skin furrows and creases resulting from movement of underlying muscles. The treatment is less effective in such age-related defects as drooping skin and "cobblestone" skin. Injectable collagen has been useful in the treatment of some herpes zoster lesions, especially diffuse, superficial pockmarks. Soft, atrophic scars and linear, depressed scars have been substantially corrected with injectable collagen. Keloids and hypertrophic scars are not treated in this way. Soft, shallow skin grafts with an inadequate volume of underlying tissue, and broad areas of atrophy less than 5 mm deep that chiefly involve the dermis, may respond well to injectable collagen therapy.

▶ [Injectable collagen is indicated in the types of problems presented by these authors.—R.O.B.] ◀

▶ ↓ The authors of the following two articles have introduced the use of a fascial or mersilene tape passed under the platysma after its fixation to the sternocleidomastoid muscle. I would suppose this is to control downward pressure of the deeper neck structures against the platysma and skin for the most beneficial effect. The second paper is also devoted to providing deep support. Plication is appealing because of its safety.—R.O.B. ◀

4–3 **Rhytidectomy in Male Patients.** James W. Smith, Robert Nelson, and Karl Weaver (New York) performed face-lift operations on 27 males in 1979 and 1980. Eyelid operation was the most commonly requested procedure, followed by facial operation. Males constituted 4% of all patients operated on by the authors in this period, and most were in the sixth decade. Most wished to improve the appearance of the neck or midfacial region. Most patients were actors, designers of clothing for young people, or successful businessmen devoted to pro-

(4–3) Aesthetic Plast. Surg. 7:41–45, 1983.

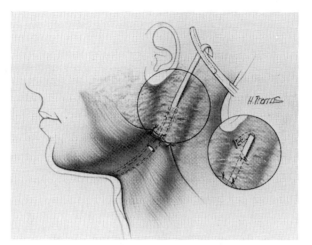

Fig 4–1.—Once band is in place and is seen to have no kinks in it and to lie perfectly flat in neck, and when it can be observed that skin is stretched out properly over chin and upper and lower parts of neck, because of exactness of its location, then small stab wound is made in fascia overlying platysma, and clamp is inserted and passed to stab site in platysma where tape can be identified and pulled through. The tape is then turned back on itself and reintroduced through original incision where surgical stapler is used to hold it in place. (Courtesy of Smith, J. W., et al.: Aesthetic Plast. Surg. 7:41–45, 1983; Berlin-Heidelberg-New York: Springer.)

moting youth-oriented enterprises. Patients were prepared with vitamins C and K for a week before operation. Markings were made just before operation. The patients received Nembutal, morphine, and Compazine as premedication and Valium intraoperatively. The local anesthetic usually was 0.5% Xylocaine with 1:200,000 epinephrine.

The incisions are placed in nearly the same sites in men and women. Significant problems with scars and sideburns have not occurred. In the neck, the dissection is carried across the midline from one side to the other. The subcutaneous dissection is wide enough to permit lateral plication of the platysma. A strip of bovine fascia lata or Mersilene tape is placed after plication of the lateral platysma borders on each side. The sling acts as a retaining ligament. The fascia or Mersilene is passed behind the platysma, starting about one fingerbreadth below the mandibular angle. The Mersilene tape is passed through the fascia overlying the sternocleidomastoid and back on itself as shown in Figure 4–1. A surgical staple is inserted to make a loop on each side and hold it in place under the desired tension. Where indicated, a malar plication is also carried out at the level of the lower border of the zygomatic arch, where the superficial musculoaponeurotic system is tightened with several 3-0 Dexon sutures.

4–4 **Multiple-Tiered Deep Support of Cheeks in Meloplasty and Rhytidectomy.** It may be difficult to obtain effective long-term re-

(4–4) Aesthetic Plast. Surg. 7:21–25, 1983.

sults from cosmetic procedures on the aging face. More permanent results can be obtained by adding deep support to superficial skin support. John R. Lewis, Jr. (Inst. of Aesthetic Plastic Surgery, Atlanta) has long used deep support of the cheek fascia in meloplasty and rhytidectomy. The undermining and support of the facial fascia (SMAS) in the posterior part of the cheek has become popular recently, but plication of the fascia in the cheeks is at least equally as effective and safe.

The undermining procedure is illustrated in Figure 4–2. It seldom extends to the nasolabial fold or the external orbital margin. In the neck, undermining usually is not carried completely across the midline in the submental region. The cheek fascia is anchored to the zygomatic fascia in the upper preauricular area, and a second tier of four to six sutures is placed more anteriorly in the cheek. The superior tier of sutures prevents the lower tier from pulling the superior tissues downward. The goal is support of all tissues upward and backward. A third tier of sutures may be placed farther forward in the

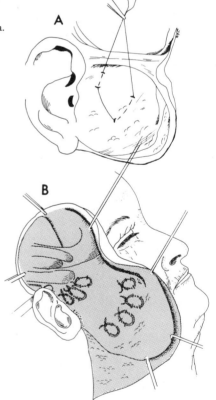

Fig 4–2.—Undermining and support of fascia. **A,** anchoring of fascia of cheek to zygomatic fascia. **B,** position of sutures. (Courtesy of Lewis, J. R., Jr.: Aesthetic Plast. Surg. 7:21–25, 1983; Berlin-Heidelberg-New York: Springer.)

cheek in cases of marked ptosis with prominent nasolabial folds and heavy jowls. In a patient with a prominent zygomatic arch and deeply hollowed cheeks, plication may be done in the hollowed area only. Braided white nylon has given satisfactory results. The neck is generally supported by carrying the cheek incision into the postauricular area and occipital part of the scalp. The platysma is most often supported by partial severence with sling support.

There appears to be no advantage in undermining the facial fascia for support of the cheek in meloplasty. Plication of the fascia in multiple tiers seems to be more effective. It is less time consuming and less hazardous than undermining, and the procedure adds to support of the platysma in the neck.

4–5 **Seagull Incision in Posterior Cervical Lift: Indications, Limitations, and Surgical Technique.** The posterior cervical lift described by Gonzalez-Ulloa creates an obvious vertical scar and a deformity of hairline contour in the nape area. José Guerrerosantos, Sharadkumar Dicksheet, and Mario Sandoval (Zapopan, Mexico) have used a one-stage procedure involving anterior and posterior neck lift, with a modified horizontal incision in the form

Fig 4–3.—Seagull incision in posterior cervical lift. **A,** outline of seagull incision 3 to 4 cm above hairline. **B,** seagull incision joining retroauricular incision on either side. **C,** skin from entire posterior part of neck is undermined. **D,** to estimate correct amount of tissue to be excised, vertical cuts in distal portion of inferior flap are made, pilot sutures are placed, and excess skin is then excised. **E,** final suturing is done in 2 layers. (Courtesy of Guerrerosantos, J., et al.: Plast. Reconstr. Surg. 70:388–396, September 1982.)

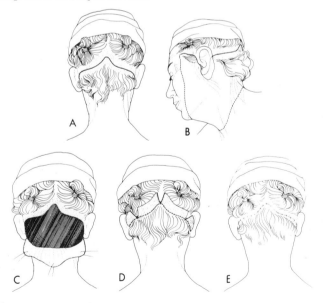

of a seagull on the occipital part of the scalp, over a 15-year period.

TECHNIQUE.—An extensive cervicofacial procedure is carried out with basal narcosis supplemented by local infiltration and nasal intubation. After the anterior neck and cheek lifts, the patient is turned prone, the anterior aspect of the neck is bandaged to prevent hematoma formation, and a seagull incision is marked above the occipital hairline in the posterior part of the scalp (Fig 4–3). It joins the retroauricular incision on either side. The entire posterior cervical flap is elevated by dissection in the deep subcutaneous fat just above the muscular fascia. Thorough hemostasis is essential. Excess skin is resected by a small flap at a time, with the knife blade beveled parallel to the hair follicles. Final suturing is done in two layers.

Four of 28 patients with flaccidity in both the upper and the lower anterior neck regions underwent a neck lift with skin undermining all around, and they still had flaccidity in the upper part of the neck 2 to 3 years later. The other 24 patients had a rhytidoplasty including anterior and posterior neck lift, with wide cervical skin undermining all around, cervical lipectomy, plastysma and submandibular gland uplifting, and pulling of the cheek flap up and posteriorly. Follow-up 3 years later showed great improvement in both the anterior upper and anterior lower neck regions.

Posterior cervical lift improves the lower anterior neck flaccidity that sometimes accompanies upper anterior neck flaccidity. It is readily added through a seagull incision, but it must be accompanied by an entire anterior cervicofacioplasty with correction of all underlying structures. The procedure is not indicated in all cases of rhytidoplasty.

▶ [This procedure is not without danger to the blood supply to the scalp. Particular attention should be paid to protecting the superficial temporal vessels. The operation has merit in those patients with marked laxity of the lateral and posterior neck. Correct positioning of the patient to perform this procedure is not all that easy.— R.O.B.] ◀

4–6 **Midforehead Lift** is described by Calvin M. Johnson, Jr., and S. Randolph Waldman (Tulane Univ.). The upper third of the face should be included in rejuvenation operations. The ideal procedure eliminates furrows, corrects tissue ptosis, and weakens any hyperdynamic action of the underlying musculature without creating further deformity. The upper limb of the excision should be placed in a midforehead crease. The vertical dimension of the excision depends on the elevation desired; it may vary in width if some areas are to be elevated more than others. The deformity is overcorrected by 0.5 to 1 cm since the brows will descend postoperatively. Upper blepharoplasty should follow the midforehead lift. The forehead skin excision should not contain frontalis muscle. The inferior flap is developed down to the supraorbital rims and root of the nose in a subcutaneous plane, and a subgaleal-frontalis muscle flap is then developed in the middle third of the forehead, staying medial to the supraorbital nerve

(4–6) Arch. Otolaryngol. 109:155–159, March 1983.

trunks. The skin is approximated in two layers. Six months are allowed for complete maturation of the scar.

The midforehead lift may be effective in patients with an aging face and brow-glabellar ptosis who are not candidates for the coronal forehead lift. They include most males as well as selected females. Careful operative technique and good esthetic judgment should yield rewarding results.

▶ [Many patients will not accept the scar from the midforehead lift recommended by these authors, however, it will give a greater correction of eyebrow ptosis than can be achieved through coronal incision.—R.O.B.] ◀

4–7 **Reduction Mentoplasty.** A hypertrophic chin tends to masculinize the face, but chin reduction has received less attention than chin augmentation. Peter McKinney (Northwestern Univ.) and Pamela B. Rosen (Mount Sinai Med. Center, New York) reviewed the results of reduction mentoplasty in 8 patients treated in a 15-year period. The 7 females and 1 male had an average age of 28 years. Four patients had had previous orthodontia. Six had rhinoplasty at reduction mentoplasty. Operation was performed with local anesthesia in 6 cases.

TECHNIQUE.—The periosteum and soft tissue are elevated from the mandible and "degloved" over the rim through a labial sulcus incision. The area to be resected, usually the triangular section of bone forming the mental prominence (Fig 4–4), is marked with dye and removed en block with a mechanical saw, and the edges are softened before the lip is closed. Excision of the mentalis muscle is not recommended.

An average decrease in bony projection of 4 mm was obtained. Over-resection is suggested, since elevation of the soft tissues alone ac-

Fig 4–4.—Silver tape indicates area of mandible usually resected. Note relation to foramina from which nerves emerge. (Courtesy of McKinney, P., and Rosen, P. B.: Plast. Reconstr. Surg. 70:147–152, August 1982.)

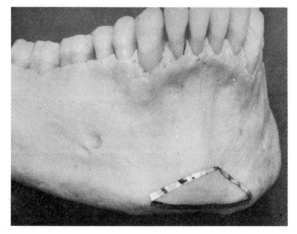

counts for a 1- to 2-mm increase in projection. No infections occurred. Transient numbness of the lip was frequent. No patient had muscle weakness.

Reduction mentoplasty can balance the profile, especially after a rhinoplasty. Dental and facial bone relations must first be carefully assessed. The operation should remove at least 2.5 to 3 mm of bone; it can be done with local anesthesia.

▶ [In discussing this article, Dr. Henry Kawamoto (*Plast. Reconstr. Surg.* 70:142–152, August 1982) points out the danger of the soft tissues slipping down under the reduced chin when the patient smiles. An effort should be made to fix the soft tissues to the bone during the early postoperative healing phase.—R.O.B.] ◀

4–8 **Alternative Flap in the Treatment of Baldness.** Punch grafts of hair often can be detected easily at conversational distance, and the Juri flap procedure is rather hazardous. William D. Walker (Hamilton, Australia) designed a large single flap based on a large pedicle on one side of the scalp. The flap should provide a good frontal hairline with the hair pointing forward to disguise the transition zone. The donor area is the back of the occipital region on one side. A deep U-shaped flap is prepared, as shown in Figure 4–5, and raised without delay at the level of the periosteum. Dissection is continued down into the neck at the deep fascial level. The flap base can safely be narrowed about 1 cm, providing a 2-cm increase in flap length. About a 3-cm-wide piece of frontal skin is removed and used to cover the flap defect as several split-skin autografts. Homografts from a previous operation or from stored skin also may be necessary as a biologic dressing. The flap is cut off after 2 weeks and the bridge segment returned, removing the homografts and some autografts. The donor area may be closed after about a month. Local flaps may be swung in to break up the graft into less conspicuous areas.

Six of these operations have been performed. One had a significant

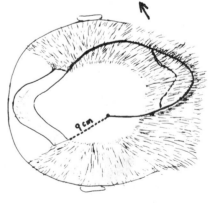

Fig 4–5.—Posterovertical view of flap with base of approximately 8 or 9 cm. (Courtesy of Walker, W. D.: Aesth. Plast. Surg. 6:75–79, 1982.)

(4–8) Aesth. Plast. Surg. 6:75–79, 1982.

complication, a small area of residual alopecia near the front. Two patients had temporary alopecia. Hematoma formation was not an important problem. The flap looks best when raised on the right side with the hair combed to the right. If desired, a single delay may be done to improve the blood supply and avoid any alopecia. The operation is major, and does nothing to cover the bald vertex. Presently, a combination of a second flap and partial excision of the bald areas is being used.

▶ [The authors have described a rather ingenious procedure using a large flap. Areas are taken from the occipital area and inset into a denuded area in the frontal region, creating a new hairline. I think this procedure is worth trying.—R.O.B.] ◀

4–9 **Tattoo Removal: Comparative Study of Six Methods in the Pig.** Removal of unwanted tattoos has always been a challenge, and several different methods of removal have been developed. C. Rolando Arellano, Donald A. Leopold, and Bruce B. Shafiroff (State Univ. of New York, Syracuse) compared the results of 6 popular methods of

Fig 4–6.—*(Top)* Tattoo after treatment with tangential excision and dextranomer dressing 1 month after third and final monthly treatment; *(center, left)* tattoo after dermabrasion and dextranomer 1 month after completion of 3 treatments; *(center)* tattoo 1 month after third treatment with dermabrasion alone; *(center, right)* tattoo after dermabrasion and rubbing with salt 1 month after third salabrasion treatment; *(bottom, left)* tattoo 1 month after third and final treatment with tannic acid overtattooing; *(bottom, center)* laser-treated tattoo showing different mode and power settings 1 month after final treatment; *(bottom, right)* tattoo treated with CO_2 laser 1 month after 3 monthly treatments. (Courtesy of Arellano, C. R., et al.: Plast. Reconstr. Surg. 70:699–703, December 1982.)

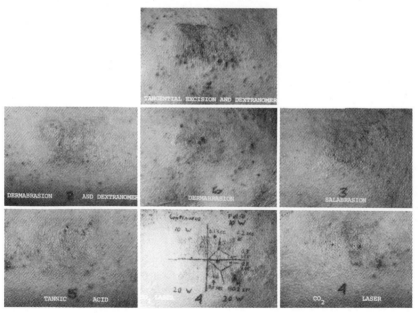

tattoo removal in a white pig with a rose design tattooed on the flank using reciprocating vibrator-driven needles. Black, red, yellow, and green pigments were used, all mixed with titanium dioxide. Removal was attempted after 1 month by split-thickness tangential excision and dextranomer (Debrisan) dressings; superficial dermabrasion and dextranomer dressings; salabrasion; CO_2 laser ablation; tannic acid solution overtattooing; and simple superficial dermabrasion. Split-thickness tangenital excisions were done progressively at 0.008, 0.012, and 0.014 inches.

The results are shown in Figure 4–6. Moderate residual pigment remained after split-thickness tangential excision. Superficial dermabrasion with and without dextranomer dressings and salabrasion all left minimal residual pigment. Tannic acid solution overtattooing left no residual pigment and acceptable scarring. Complete removal of pigment was achieved in two CO_2 laser treatments at a continuous 20-W power setting. Dextanomer was of some use in removing residual pigment after early changes in dressing. Biopsy findings showed that most pigment was in the dermis at an average depth of 0.5 mm in skin that was 2-mm in average thickness. Regenerated epidermis had an average thickness of 0.07 mm, which was its approximate thickness before tattoo ablation. Minimal fibrosis occurred in areas with no residual pigment.

Tannic acid solution overtattooing and the CO_2 laser were the most effective methods of removing tattoo pigment in this study. Both methods left acceptable scars. The overall appearance of the laser-treated areas was the most esthetically acceptable.

▶ [An interesting study in the pig model. Are the authors using one of these methods, tannic acid or CO_2 laser, in their patients? If so, what type of healing has occurred, especially in the deltoid region?—S.H.M.] ◀

EYE

4-10 **Recognition of Acquired Ptosis in Patients Considered for Upper Eyelid Blepharoplasty.** Robert B. Wilkins and Michael Patipa (Univ. of Texas, Houston) point out that surgeons performing upper eyelid blepharoplasties must be aware that simultaneous ptosis might be present. Levator dehiscence is the most common cause of involutional ptosis and often occurs with dermatochalasis of the upper eyelids. Careful preoperative evaluation of affected patients will help avoid unsatisfactory surgical results.

Woman, 25, had a history of allergies with significant recurrent lid swelling at age 17 years, and her eyelids had drooped progressively since that time (Fig 4–7). Review of old photographs showed bilateral ptosis that had gradually worsened. The palpebral fissures measured 6 mm bilaterally. Excellent levator function was demonstrated. There were moderate dermatochalasis and hyperpigmentation of all lids. The patient had high lid creases bilater-

(4–10) Plast. Reconstr. Surg. 70:431–436, October 1982.

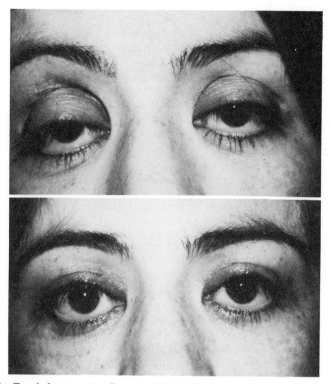

Fig 4–7.—**Top,** before operation. Presence of bilateral ptosis and high upper lid creases indicate levator aponeurosis dehiscence or disinsertion. **Bottom,** after bilateral reattachment of levator aponeurosis onto tarsus and lower lid blepharoplasty. (Courtesy of Wilkins, R. B., and Patipa, M.: Plast. Reconstr. Surg. 70:431–436, October 1982.)

ally. The upper lid tissues were so thin that iris pigment could be seen through them. Levator dehiscence was repaired in both upper eyelids. The dehisced distal edge of each levator aponeurosis was found high above the tarsus beneath the fat pads. The aponeurosis was reattached to the anterior part of the tarsus. An ellipse of upper lid skin was removed, and a lower lid blepharoplasty was done. The patient had symmetric lid heights postoperatively.

Patients being evaluated for blepharoplasty should be asked about lid trauma, recurrent lid edema or inflammation, previous operations, and congenital ptosis. Both lid fissures should be carefully measured in primary gaze. A levator aponeurosis dehiscence or disinsertion is corrected by locating the distal margin of the aponeurosis through a lid crease incision and reattaching it to the tarsus. A levator tuck operation has been effective where no disinsertion has been found. In patients with ptosis after upper lid blepharoplasties, Neo-Synephrine may help raise the eyelid by stimulating contraction of Müller's muscle, previewing the efficacy of a Fasanella-Servat procedure before it is carried out. Critical evaluation of the operation is necessary if no ptosis was present before it.

▶ [The authors have brought to our attention the fact that we must be careful to evaluate the upper eyelids for levator dehiscence with a minor ptosis as this will need to be corrected at the time of the blepharoplasty.—R.O.B.] ◀

4–11 **Lateral Fat Compartment of the Lower Eyelid.** Herniated orbital fat from the lateral compartment of the lower lid may impair an otherwise excellent result from blepharoplasty. Salvador Castañares (Los Angeles) has removed the fat adequately by varying the direction of incision of the orbicularis muscle and opening the encapsulated fat compartment.

TECHNIQUE.—The muscle incision descends laterally from a point close to the inner canthus to the area of the central compartment and then ascends at a nearly 45-degree angle laterally and superiorly, directed to a point below and just lateral to the lateral canthus. This modification can preclude the need for another complete lower lid blepharoplasty or other complex operation. The capsule of the fat compartment is nicked and the fat gently pulled out. The base is then transected and the fat excised with scissors. Point cauterization is used. Closure is with three fine nylon sutures or a small subcuticular suture.

Compromise of the results of blepharoplasty by failure to remove fat from the lateral compartment of the lower lid can be easily prevented by modifying the orbicularis incision so as directly to remove the fat.

4–12 **Radical Correction of Senile Entropion and Ectropion.** The chief mechanism of senile entropion is ill defined. Most patients appear to be cured by the many methods devised to correct this condition, but the persistence of the cures is uncertain. Jacques C. van der Meulen (Rotterdam) developed a new approach to correcting senile entropion and ectropion. The operation for entropion combines the advantages of vertical and horizontal lid reduction (Fig 4–8). Transposition or imbrication of orbicularis muscle can be added if indicated. The rim is first incised in the lateral border of the demarcated segment and then cautiously in the median border to remove a triangular segment of eyelid. After excision a half-moon-shaped segment of conjunctiva in the deeper part of the inferior fornix, the lid is reattached to the lateral canthus, and the orbicularis is shortened or imbricated if necessary. The skin of the lower lid is closed after the excess skin is removed. No complications have resulted from this procedure, and gratifying results have been consistently obtained.

Generalized laxity may also be present in patients with senile ectropion, but the tension balance favors increased tension in the lower part of the eyelid. Only the method of Kuhnt and Szymanovski has proved to be useful over time. The lid is not presently split in the margin but is incised just below the ciliary border. Excess skin can

(4–11)   Aesthetic. Plast. Surg. 7:27–30, 1983.
(4–12)   Plast. Reconstr. Surg. 71:318–325, March 1983.

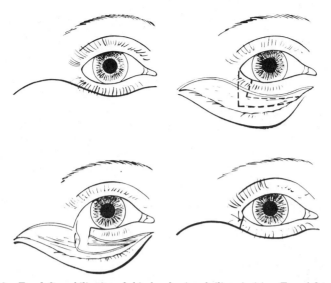

Fig 4–8.—Top left, mobilization of skin by classic subciliary incision. **Top right,** removal of triangular full-thickness wedge in most lateral part of eyelid and of half-moon-shaped segment of conjunctiva in deeper part of fornix, leaving eyelid attached to medial pedicle and orbicularis muscle intact. **Bottom left,** pedicled eyelid rim is reattached to lateral canthus with a few interrupted sutures. **Bottom right,** after reduction of skin surplus and, if necessary, shortening of orbicularis, incision is closed. (Courtesy of van der Meulen, J. C.: Plast. Reconstr. Surg. 71:318–325, March 1983.)

Fig 4–9.—Top left, mobilization of skin by classic subciliary incision. **Top right,** removal of triangular full-thickness wedge in most lateral part of eyelid and of inflamed conjunctiva and tarsus in upper part of fornix. **Bottom left,** pedicled eyelid rim is reattached to lateral canthus. **Bottom right,** skin incision is closed after reduction of its surplus. (Courtesy of van der Meulen, J. C.: Plast. Reconstr. Surg. 71:318–325, March 1983.)

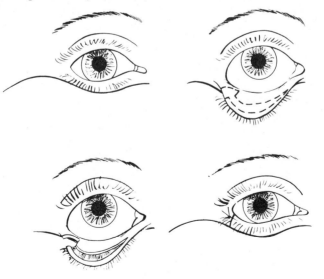

be effectively reduced through excision of a tarsoconjunctival wedge either in the center of the lid or in its most lateral portion. The vertical height of the eyelid is not reduced, leaving untreated one of the factors predisposing to ectropion. Where exposure of the lower lid margin has led to keratoconjunctivitis, the author has found it best to excise the inflamed conjunctiva in combination with resection of the tarsoconjunctival wedge in the lateral part of the lid rim, resulting in a reduction in vertical height and the correction of both horizontal and vertical laxity (Fig 4–9). The few patients followed after this procedure have indicated that it is highly effective. Only once has it been necessary to resuture the lid margin after dehiscence.

NOSE

4–13   **Onlay Graft For Nasal Tip Projection** is discussed by George C. Peck (Clifton, N.J.). Nasal tip projection is necessary for good esthetic results after rhinoplasty. Sheen's triangular nasal tip graft was an important breakthrough in technique to increase nasal tip projection; however, it has several shortcomings, including appreciable loss of the tip projection in some cases. The onlay graft for nasal tip projection is based on obtaining autogenous conchal cartilage and shaping grafts to represent the combined domes of the lower lateral cartilages. Resorption is not a concern. Segments of removed lower lateral cartilages can be used in some primary rhinoplasties, although this cartilage is usually too thin or weak. The operation is indicated for short nasal tip projection both in primary cases and after rhinoplasty.

Nasal tip projection can be augmented by 2–6 mm using this technique. If necessary, the onlay can be combined with a strut placed between the medial crura, which creates an umbrella-type reconstruction. The pocket is made just large enough to accommodate and hold the cartilage graft in the desired position. The average size of the conchal cartilage graft is 4 × 9 mm. Generally, the rim incision can be closed with one suture. A double-layered cartilage graft sometimes is necessary, which may be sutured together before insertion.

The onlay cartilage graft technique has been used without complication in 152 patients over 5 years. Esthetically good anatomic results have been obtained.

▶ [Onlay graft for nasal tip projection as presented by the author certainly has merit. Because of its location it is less apt to slip out of position. However, the key to these grafts is to create the least possible pocket.—R.O.B.] ◀

(4–13) Plast. Reconstr. Surg. 71:27–39, January 1983.

4–14 **Controlled Tip Sculpturing With the Morselizer** is described by Frank F. Rubin (Brookline, Mass., Hosp.). Modification of the nasal tip is the most difficult aspect of rhinoplasty. Various iatrogenic deformities are frequently produced with all methods. The author has used the morselizer to advantage in sculpting the nasal tip and avoiding deformities, in both thick-skinned and thin-skinned patients.

TECHNIQUE.—Both sides of the external surface of the lobule are marked, and a rimometer is used to transfer the markings to the undersurface of the lobule. The incision is extended through the cartilage to the columella and laterally for about half the distance from the tip to the base of the nose. The cephalic segment is freed from the overlying skin and actively morselized on its anterior surface. Both cephalic and caudal segments are approximated with an absorbable suture placed through the vestibular skin about one third of the distance from the tip to the base (Fig 4–10).

The morselized cephalic segment of lower lateral cartilage increases in length and serves as a lateral strut to help maintain tip projection, eliminating both the tendency toward retrodisplacement of the tip and uncontrolled rotation. This technique has been used in 40% of author's patients, with excellent results. The caudal cuff of the lower lateral cartilage may also be reshaped by freeing the skin retrograde and morsel-

Fig 4–10.—Drawing demonstrating cephalic segment delivered and morselized by placing teeth of morselizer directly on cartilage and smooth surface on vestibular skin. (Courtesy of Rubin, F. F.: Arch. Otolaryngol. 109:160–163, March 1983; copyright 1983, American Medical Association.)

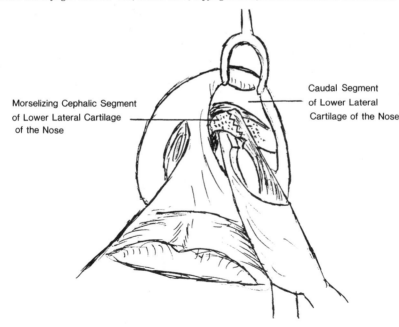

Morselizing Cephalic Segment of Lower Lateral Cartilage of the Nose

Caudal Segment of Lower Lateral Cartilage of the Nose

(4–14) Arch. Otolaryngol. 109:160–163, March 1983.

izing it. In patients with a marked bulbous tip or asymmetry of the lower lateral cartilages, the cephalic section of the lower lateral cartilage is severed at the most medial aspect of the incision and delivered as a chondral flap, and cartilage is trimmed from both edges and from the medial end of the chondral flap, which is morselized and replaced adjacent to the dome. If the tip is unduly wide or box shaped, the caudal cuff of cartilage is also freed and morselized retrograde.

Less than 10% of the lower lateral cartilage is excised with all these methods. By developing a new morselized fulcrum along the lower lateral cartilage, the tip is readily rotated and maintained in the new position, and the tendency for a secondary parrot-beak deformity to develop is reduced.

▶ [Too much weakening of the cartilage in the crus area results in tip distortion whether it be from the morselizer or from excising too much lower lateral cartilage. Abstract 4–15 presents a transcolumellar incision for surgery on the difficult nasal tip. There is no question that the open scar approach is helpful for some of the more difficult cases.—R.O.B.] ◀

4–15 **Tip Rhinoplastic Operations Using a Transverse Columellar Incision.** Trudy Vogt (Zurich) reviewed experience with the transverse columellar incision in over 300 cases of esthetic and corrective rhinoplasty. The goal is better exposure of the nasal tip region. No unsightly scarring has resulted from this extramucosal approach, and scar retraction of the incisions has not occurred. The open approach

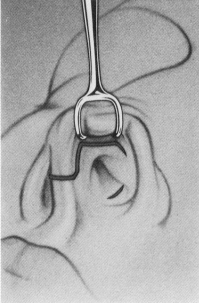

Fig 4–11.—Directions of incision. (Courtesy of Vogt, T.: Aesthetic Plast. Surg. 7:13–19, 1983; Berlin-Heidelberg-New York: Springer.)

(4–15) Aesthetic Plast. Surg. 7:13–19, 1983.

reveals the true anatomical conditions in cases of revision rhinoplasty.

TECHNIQUE.—An initial horizontal columellar incision is made very superficially at the level of the inferior to middle third of the columella. The cut turns at a right angle about 2 mm inside the vestibulum, extending up parallel to the columellar border into the area just caudal to the dome (Fig 4–11). It ends in a rim incision along the caudal reflection of the lower lateral cartilage. Short Ragnell scissors are used to dissect the columellar skin from the medial crura of the alar cartilages; dissection is kept close to the crural cartilages. All visible bleeders are coagulated. Caudal and lateral traction on the dome cartilages, after removal of the fibrous tissues extending from the depressor nasi to the skin of the tip, permits wide exposure of all the alar and crural cartilages. Any oversized tip cartilage structures then can be excised and missing cartilage added. At least 3 mm of width of the lateral alar cartilages is generally preserved. The columellar incision is closed with interrupted 6-0 nylon sutures. Packing is placed for tissue approximation, and splinting is by a transfixion sling suture. A plaster cast is left in place for 10 days.

Swelling has been minimal with this procedure, and no supratip deformities have resulted. No hypertrophic scars have developed. The scars soon become nearly invisible. The author believes that this open approach to rhinoplastic procedures offers many advantages.

4–16 **Columella Implants: Reconstruction of the Anterior Septum.** Carolina Gutierrez and Poul Stoksted (Odense Univ. Hosp., Denmark) followed up patients who had implants to replace the anterior septal cartilage of the nose. Implants included the cartilaginous septum, parts of the bony septum when cartilaginous septum could not be used, and bank cartilage when autograft material was insufficient. A total of 100 patients operated on in 1977–1979 were followed up for a year after columella implant surgery. Implants were made about the same size as the defects, and preferably slightly larger in the area of the inferior columella to increase its projection. A pocket was made in the columella between the mesial crura via the hemitransfixion incision. Holes were drilled in the inferior and superior edges of the implant, and traction sutures were placed. The implant was fixed with one or two mattress sutures.

Forty-four patients had had previous septal or rhinoplastic surgery. Twenty others had a crooked nose. The most common findings were septal dislocation and instability. Lines of fracture were found during surgery in 52% of cases. Satisfactory results were obtained in 66% of cases of bone implantation, 69.5% of cases of cartilage implantation, and 50% of the cases of bank cartilage implantation; the differences were not significant. The most difficult problem was in judging the proper implant size. Too small an implant resulted in instability, reduction in the nasolabial angle, and retraction of the columella. Poor results were more frequent in the patients who were operated on previously.

Two thirds of all patients in this series had completely satisfactory

(4–16)   Arch. Otolaryngol. 108:243–246, April 1982.

results from columella implant surgery. Adequate material is usually present for reconstruction of the anterior septum even after previous surgery on the nose. This technique is useful when the cartilaginous septum cannot be straightened because of multiple abnormalities that would cause postoperative deviation and possible obstruction if not corrected. Other indications for its use are a lack of support for the cartilaginous part of the nose, absence of a part of the septum, and the esthetic complex consisting of a drooping tip, sagging of the upper lateral cartilages, and columellar retraction.

4–17 **Cerebrospinal Fluid Rhinorrhea Following Rhinoplasty.** Cerebrospinal fluid rhinorrhea after rhinoplasty alone has not previously been reported. Geoffrey G. Hallock and William C. Trier (Univ. of North Carolina) report a case in which this potentially life-threatening complication occurred.

Woman, 26, underwent elective rhinoplasty for correction of a traumatic nasal deformity. The dorsal hump reportedly was removed through an intranasal, intercartilaginous incision made with a double-guarded osteotome. The caudal septum was shortened through a transfixion incision, and nasal tip correction was carried out. Infracture of the nasal bones was performed after lateral osteotomies with the use of a button-guarded osteotome introduced through piriform recess incisions. A clear nasal discharge was noted from both nostrils about 10 days postoperatively. After 2 months, the patient still exhibited a slow leak of clear fluid, greater on the right side. A glucose-oxidase strip test was grossly positive. Overpressure isotope cisternography with ^{99m}Tc-diethylenetriamine pentaacetic acid and intranasal pledgets confirmed CSF rhinorrhea. The tract was localized to a defect in the cribriform plate area, but scintigraphy showed no leak. Anterior fossa exploration revealed no source of leakage, although the dura was more firmly adherent in the right cribriform plate area, suggesting resolution of inflammation at this site. The olfactory tracts were divided, and the cribriform plate area was patched with a temporalis fascia graft. Rhinorrhea ceased postoperatively.

Most cases of CSF rhinorrhea are traumatic in origin. Whatever its cause, CSF rhinorrhea is a life-threatening problem. The diagnosis should be suspected in the presence of a profuse, watery discharge from the nose; the discharge need not be unilateral. Precise localization of the fistulous tract between the endocranium and the paranasal or nasal cavities is necessary. Overpressure cisternography is necessary in cases of intermittent leakage. Prophylactic antibiotic therapy is not of value. Use of the operating microscope has facilitated the identification of leaks. No single operative approach is uniformly effective. Failure of extracranial repair can always be followed by intracranial repair.

▶ [I thought this was worth bringing to our attention. Fortunately it is a very uncommon situation. The cribriform plate was probably exceptionally low.—R.O.B.] ◀

4–18 **A Compendium of Intranasal Flaps.** Marc S. Karlan, Robert H.

(4–17) Plast. Reconstr. Surg. 71:109–113, January 1983.
(4–18) Laryngoscope 92:774–782, July 1982.

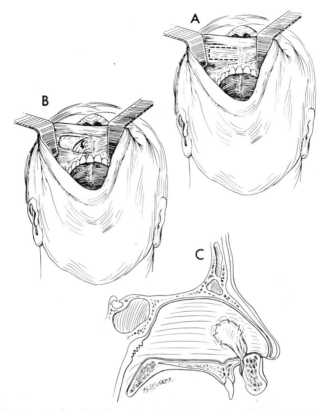

Fig 4–12.—Buccal sulcus flap of mucosa and submucosa with sufficient length for anterior lesions *(A)* passing through separate stab incision into nose *(B)*. Base of flap is compressed as it passes through stab incision *(C)*. (Courtesy of Karlan, M. S., et al.: Laryngoscope 92:774–782, July 1982.)

Fig 4–13.—*A*, nasolabial island pedicle flap *(outlines)* and intranasal rotation *(arrows)* half of Z-plasty for vestibular stenosis; *B*, rotations and advancements are complete. (Courtesy of Karlan, M. S., et al.: Laryngoscope 92:774–782, July 1982.)

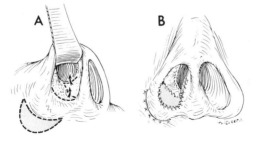

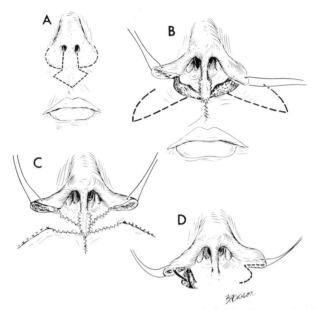

Fig 4–14.—*A,* preoperative scarred nasal tip with stenosis showing first stage incisions outlined for lengthening of columella, opening nasal vestibular stenosis and allowing access for nasolabial flaps; *B,* columellar fork flap folded on itself showing outline of nasolabial flaps; *C,* flaps all rotated; *D,* incision of alar edge and roll made from nasolabial flaps for reconstruction of nasal sill. (Courtesy of Karlan, M. S., et al.: Laryngoscope 92:774–782, July 1982.)

Ossoff, and George A. Sisson (Northwestern Univ. School of Medicine) describe a series of intranasal flaps used in intranasal reconstruction of tissue deficiencies. Intranasal exposure by speculum alone is fairly limited. Lateral alotomy is one of the easiest methods of increasing anterior exposure without esthetic sequelae. Open rhinoplasty methods require a columellar incision, but provide excellent exposure of the dorsal and anterior areas of the septum and vestibule with minimal external scarring. Transoral premaxillary approaches can provide nearly as good exposure without external esthetic sequelae. Lateral rhinotomy may be necessary for wide exposure of the entire nasal passage. Transethmoid approaches are necessary only for problems in the upper posterior area. The airway must be physically and physiologically maintained. Where possible, movement of intranasal respiratory epithelium is preferable to the introduction of stratifying squamous epithelium.

Septal mucoperichondrial advancement flaps have been widely used to close small septal perforations. The flaps are advanced asymmetrically to provide nonopposed suture lines and a good mucoperichondrial blood supply to the remaining exposed cartilage. The length of the nose can be modified using composite septal flaps. A flap from the inferior turbinate-lateral nasal wall region may be used to close larger septal perforations. A two-stage technique is necessary. A long pedicled mucoperiosteal flap of the nasal floor can be used for thickness and strength, with a potential size of 2.5 × 4 cm in most cases. Middle turbinate flaps have been used to repair defects in the cribriform plate area and roof of the ethmoid bone.

A Z-plasty reconstruction often suffices to open the vestibule in cases of lateral vestibular stenosis. Composite lateral cartilage flaps also can be used in cases of vestibular stenosis after rhinoplasty. The buccal sulcus flap (Fig 4–12) is a regional flap providing good potential for multiple intranasal repairs. The long nasolabial fold flap and the island pedicle nasolabial flap (Fig 4–13) both have proved useful in anterior nasal reconstruction. A complex procedure for reconstructing a scarred nasal tip with stenosis is illustrated in Figure 4–14.

4–19 **Closure of Perforations of the Septum Including a Single-Session Method for Large Defects.** Rodolphe Meyer (Lausanne, Switzerland) and Alexander Berghaus (Berlin) believe that although the overall frequency of septal perforations has declined, the proportion of large nasal septal defects has increased. Trauma is the most common cause of septal perforations, but infections, metabolic disorders, and tumors also can cause these defects. Indications for closure depend on the presence of troublesome symptoms, particularly intense scab formation, recurrent bleeding, whistling noises, and deformity of the nose. Closure with obturators has been abandoned in favor of surgery when indicated. Surgical enlargement of the defect is, at best, a last resort in cases of a whistling defect. Total closure of the perforation is always sought.

Even large septal perforations are now closed by variations of the extramucosal approach. In closing small defects it is sufficient to mobilize a large area of mucoperichondrium and use adaptation sutures free of tension. Cartilage strips can be removed to reduce the size of the actual cartilage defect in the lamina quadrangularis. Alternatively, the mucoperichondrium and triangular cartilage on both sides can be rotated toward the front and down to close a lower, posterior perforation, and the upper lateral cartilage is shortened at its forward edge on both sides.

Defects up to 2 cm in diameter can be closed in a single session by the extramucosal technique, but larger defects are managed by a three-step method in which a spoon-shaped distant flap from the oral vestibule with cartilage attached is inserted into the perforation and then severed from its pedicle after the cartilage fragment, which is covered with mucosa on both sides, has grown into the septum. The flap is implanted 3 to 5 weeks after its preparation, and the final step is done after a further delay of 3 to 5 weeks.

(4–19) Head Neck Surg. 5:390–400, May–June 1983.

TRUNK AND EXTREMITIES

4-20 **Self-Consciousness of Disproportionate Breast Size: A Primary Psychologic Reaction to Abnormal Appearance.** Many psychiatrists and psychologists believe that self-consciousness of an esthetic abnormality, such as small-breasts, is due to an underlying personality disorder. D. L. Harris (Plymouth, England) proposes that such self-consciousness is for most subjects a primary psychologic reaction associated with normal personality structure. Symptoms result from an inherent need to feel confident that one's appearance is normal so that one can compete equally with others.

Individual susceptibility to self-consciousness depends on the circumstances and on such variables as sex and estheticality. Remarks by others may well lead to initial self-consciousness, which then is reinforced by critical attitudes of others. The subject comes to feel embarrassed and isolated from peers, and attempts may be made to conceal the characteristic in question. Defense mechanisms may lead to an artificial pattern of behavior. Eventually the subject may feel at a disadvantage as a socially competitive person, and a downgraded self-concept may result in difficulties in interpersonal relationships. Subjects with a problem that cannot be concealed, such as large breasts, may have more difficulties than others. Various circumstances can reawaken self-consciousness later in life.

Whether a given individual becomes self-conscious about an abnormal appearance depends on many factors, including age, site of the abnormality, teasing by others, and gender. Self-consciousness, once present, escalates and is reinforced by critical attitudes on the part of others. A compromised self-image leads to difficulties in relationships with other persons. The overall experience causes emotional distress and an impaired life-style and frequently leads a person to seek cosmetic surgery.

▶ [This paper tells us that women with disproportionate breast size are normal but self-conscious about their physical appearance as it relates to their breasts.— R.O.B.] ◀

4-21 **Use of Autologous Blood in Patients Undergoing Subcutaneous Mastectomy or Reduction Mammaplasty.** Some plastic operations such as breast reconstruction carry a risk of major blood loss, and autologous transfusions might reduce the risk of posttransfusion hepatitis in these cases. Forst E. Brown, Howard M. Rawnsley, and John E. Lawe (Dartmouth-Hitchcock Med. Center) evaluated autologous transfusion in patients scheduled for subcutaneous mastectomy or reduction mammaplasty over a 5-year period at a regional teaching hospital in a rural setting. Phlebotomy was scheduled for 10 to 14 days before operation, and patients used 250 mg of ferrous gluconate three times daily from a week before the scheduled phlebotomy. The hemoglobin concentration had to be 11 gm/dl or above, and the

(4-20) Br. J. Plast. Surg. 36:191–195, April 1983.
(4-21) Ann. Plast. Surg. 10:186–189, March 1983.

patient had to be in good general health. A single unit of blood was collected in citrate-phosphate-dextrose-adenine.

All but 16 of 88 patients who were offered autologous transfusion accepted. The mean reduction in hemoglobin concentration at admission for operation was 6.9%, an average of 10 days after phlebotomy. The average overall calculated blood loss was 959 ml. Twelve patients received no transfusions, 68 received one autologous transfusion, 4 received one homologous unit, and 4 received 2 units of blood. There were no transfusion reactions. The charge for an autologous blood transfusion was $20, compared with $63.50 for a homologous blood transfusion.

No complications resulted from the use of autologous transfusions in this series of patients undergoing breast reconstructions. Safer transfusions and a modest reduction in costs result from this policy. Blood is used more readily during operation. Patients given autologous transfusions have seemed to do better, and blood bank stocks are conserved. Autologous blood transfusion appears to be a valuable procedure and could be useful in many surgical specialties.

▶ [The authors have brought to our attention a procedure that our office has been using for a number of years.—R.O.B.] ◀

4–22 **Reduction Mammaplasty With Legal Implications.** Saul Hoffman and Anthony L. Schiavetti (New York) report a case of reduction mammaplasty in which the result was unsatisfactory because the nipples were too high. The patient instituted a lawsuit against the plastic surgeon, but lost the case. The patient was a 22-year-old woman who had had excessively large breasts since age 15 and had experienced back and shoulder pain as a result. She was pleased with the results of reduction mammaplasty postoperatively and expressed this in writing, but subsequently found that the nipples were too high and could be seen above her brassiere. Corrective surgery to lower the nipples left considerable scarring on the upper part of the breasts. Scar revisions on two occasions led to some improvement. The patient refused a settlement of $25,000, but eventually lost her malpractice action. The poor result probably was due to a technical error. Marking was carried out in the operating room rather than with the patient standing or sitting and fully cooperating.

Informed consent was not a factor in this case, since ordinarily scarring above the nipples is not expected. The results initially pleased the patient, even if they were not esthetically perfect. The case was tried less on the basis of its medical aspects than on the personalities of the parties involved. The physician was perceived as an understanding, attentive, responsible person with his patient's interests uppermost in his mind.

▶ [More and more suits are being filed by women dissatisfied with the results of surgery performed on their breasts.—R.O.B.] ◀

▶ ↓ The next two papers deal with the tuberous breast and the inverted nipple. The

(4–22) Ann. Plast. Surg. 9:506–507, December 1982.

author's technique for the snoopy breast certainly is appealing and I look forward to using it on the next patient that presents with this problem. The inverted nipple technique is not too dissimilar to what is being used today for nipple construction after a radical mastectomy.—R.O.B. ◄

4–23 **Surgical Correction of the Tuberous Breast** is described by Bahman Teimourian and Mehdi N. Adham (Georgetown Univ.). The tuberous breast, or domed nipple, is characterized by herniation of breast tissue into the nipple and areola, a deficient diameter of the base of the breast in each axis, and breast hypoplasia. All these deficiencies should be corrected. Previous techniques have failed to reduce the herniated tissue or, in the case of Vecchione's procedure, may compromise the blood and nerve supply to the nipple and areola.

TECHNIQUE.—A subpectoral augmentation is carried out through an inframammary skin incision, as shown in Figure 4–15. The skin between the two circles drawn on the areola is deepithelialized. The new areola is undermined to within about 1 cm of the base of the nipple. Four wedges of breast tissue are removed from beneath the new areola, and the four gaps are closed to

Fig 4–15.—Technique. *A,* appearance after subpectoral augmentation—"Snoopy nose" deformity. *B,* two circles are drawn on areola, outer at areola-skin junction. Skin between the two circles is deepithelialized to reduce diameter of areola to appropriate size. *C,* skin of new areola is undermined to within about 1 cm of base of nipple. *D* and *E,* four wedges of breast tissue are removed from four quadrants beneath new areola. *F* and *G,* gaps are closed with Vicryl sutures. *H,* new areola is stretched over deepithelialized area and closed to old areola-skin junction. *I,* result. (Courtesy of Teimourian, B., and Adham, M. N.: Ann. Plast. Surg. 10:190–193, March 1983.)

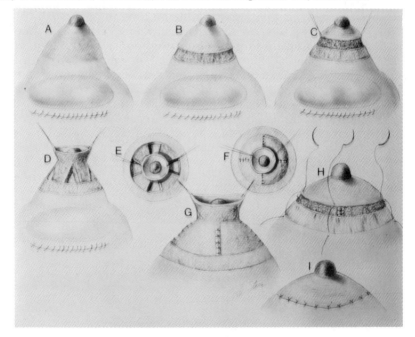

reduce the projection to an acceptable level. The new areola is then stretched over the deepithelialized area and closed to the old areola-skin junction with interrupted sutures. A small drain is left in place.

If the condition is unilateral, the other breast may require augmentation to achieve symmetry. This approach has been used in 6 patients, followed for 2 years, with satisfactory results. Closure of the gaps left by excising the four wedges of breast tissue from under the new areola results in reductions of both the herniated breast tissue and the areola.

4–24   **A Simple Method for Correction of the Inverted Nipple.** Nipple inversion usually is congenital in origin, although it can be caused by trauma or inflammation after pregnancy and lactation. This condition interferes with effective nursing and is an esthetic impairment. Corrective methods have been time-consuming, involving extensive skin incisions, or leading to undesirable scarring. Daniel J. Hauben and D. Mahler (Rotterdam, Netherlands) describe a short, simple procedure that produces desirable results in cases of nipple inversion.

TECHNIQUE.—The nipple is pulled out with a skin hook under infiltration

Fig 4–16.—Schematic design of radial (**top**) and vertical (**bottom**) undermining of areola to form new nipple. (Courtesy of Hauben, D. J., and Mahler, D.: Plast. Reconstr. Surg.: 71:556–559, April 1983.)

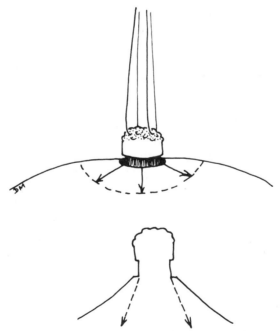

(4–24)   Plast. Reconstr. Surg. 71:556–559, April 1983.

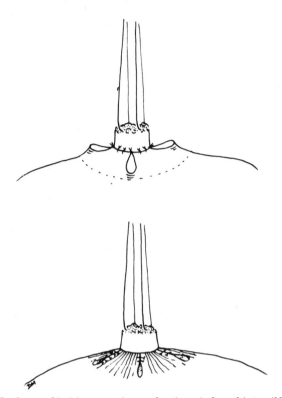

Fig 4–17.—In closure of incision, excessive areolar tissue is formed into mild "dog-ears" **(top)** to be absorbed spontaneously **(bottom).** (Courtesy of Hauben, D. J., and Mahler, D.: Plast. Reconstr. Surg. 71:556–559, April 1983.)

of local anesthesia. A circular incision is made around the nipple base, followed by wide circular undermining beneath the areola and backward toward the mammary gland (Fig 4–16). All tight bands of tissue around the nipple base are divided, creating a 1- to 2-cm pedicle below the original base. A 5-0 Dexon purse-string suture is tied around the pedicle base, which then is covered by the undermined areola, and the nipple-areola line is closed with four horizontal 5-0 nylon mattress sutures. "Dog-ears" of excess areolar tissue are pulled out and left to absorb spontaneously (Fig 4–17). A few more interrupted nylon sutures are passed between the areola and nipple. Lactiferous ducts are gently tightened within the pedicle by the purse-string suture.

This operation was performed 19 times on 11 patients. On follow-up for up to 18 months, 2 patients (3 operated nipples) had a recurrence of congenital inversion 2 months after operation. The recurrence was corrected by the same procedure in 1 patient by using a nonabsorbable purse-string suture.

No loss of lactiferous duct continuity occurs with this operation for nipple inversion, and the ability to nurse is not impaired. The nipple can erect without painful areolar tension. The operation is relatively simple and leaves minimal scarring and surgical deformity. It can be performed in the office under local anesthesia. No special dressing is necessary.

▶ ↓ The next two papers deal with placing the implant in the subpectoral position. Time will tell whether the subpectoral route gives a softer breast.—R.O.B. ◀

4–25 **Retropectoral Route for Breast Augmentation.** Dempsey and Latham proposed a "subpectoral" approach to insertion of a Silastic implant for breast augmentation. Dan Mahler, Jona Ben-Jakar, and Daniel J. Hauben (Beer-Sheva, Israel) have adopted this approach for both hypoplastic and ptotic-atrophied breasts. With local anesthesia, an inframammary incision is made beneath the hypoplastic breast, the pectoralis major is elevated from the serratus and ribs, the implant is inserted, and both the muscle and the dermis are closed in layers with 4-0 Dexon. The skin is closed with either 4-0 running nylon suture or Histoacryl glue. In the atrophied-ptotic breast, ptosis is corrected by the McKissock or superiorly based technique before the retropectoral area is prepared and the implant inserted through the lateral part of the incision. With the McKissock method, the vertical flap protects against further ptosis. Only after the muscle is closed is the excess medial skin trimmed away. All incisions are closed in layers. A drain is left in the cavity for 24 hours. A pleasing breast contour develops over 4 to 6 weeks after operation as swelling subsides.

The subpectoral approach has been used in 52 patients with hypoplastic or ptotic-atrophied breasts, with excellent results. The breasts remained soft in all patients but 1, who disregarded instructions regarding arm activity. Capsule formation was avoided. No lateral displacement was observed when the arms were elevated. This procedure is limited to implants of 210 ml or less in volume. The term "retropectoral" is suggested for this approach.

4–26 **Subpectoral-Transaxillary Method of Breast Augmentation in Orientals.** Many Oriental patients are quite flat-chested, and the scar from insertion of a breast prosthesis tends to be conspicuous. K. Watanabe, K. Tsurukiyi, and Y. Fugii (Tokyo) have used a combination of the subpectoral and the transaxillary approaches to breast augmentation in 47 patients operated on since 1979. General anesthesia is ideal. The 4- to 5-cm skin incision is similar to that used in the ordinary transaxillary approach. Dissection is done initially toward the lateral margin of the pectoralis major to avoid vascular structures in the deep part of the axilla. The interpectoral space is dissected, bluntly as far as is possible. The pectoralis major is usually cut at its inferior origin 2 to 3 cm beyond the inframammary fold dissection. The medial margin is not dissected sharply if feasible. Suction is continued for 48 hours after operation.

(4–25) Aesth. Plast. Surg. 6:237–242, 1982.
(4–26) Ibid., pp. 231–236.

This is a difficult operation, and hemostasis under direct vision is difficult, but the combined approach offers many advantages including an inconspicuous site of insertion of the prosthesis and a natural breast shape. Patients do not have discomfort from the prosthetic rim or fold. The rate of capsular contracture is low. This method appears to be especially suitable for use in Orientals, in whom the distance between the insertion site and the pocket is relatively short. Postoperative movement of the prosthesis can be avoided without completely severing the origin of the pectoralis major, and less hemorrhage occurs when this is possible.

4–27 **Anterior Periosteal Dermal Suspension With Suction Curettage for Lateral Thigh Lipectomy** is described by Bahman Teimourian and Mehdi N. Adham (Rockville, Md.). Some persons have excessive fat deposits in the area of the thighs and buttocks. The standard excisional approach to lipectomy now has been modified by the use of suction curettage, either as an adjunct or as a primary procedure. Curettage can be used to prepare and shape the flaps in patients with severe steatomeria or trochanteric obesity. Excision and periosteal dermal suspension sometimes are necessary to achieve adequate contour and lift. Suction curettage is carried out through a 2-cm incision made just posterior to the anterior superior iliac spine. Dermal fat suspension flaps then are developed as needed from the groin crease to the posterior superior iliac spine. From 2 to 3 cm are deepithelialized after adequate skin and fat resection; the flaps are rotated and suspended from the iliac periosteum and inguinal ligament with permanent monofilament nylon sutures. The upper flaps are sutured without tension in a vest-over-pants fashion using inverted interrupted 4-0 Vicryl sutures. Skin closure ideally is with intracuticular 3-0 monofilament sutures. Large drains are placed laterally and a pressure dressing is applied. The average hospital stay is 2–5 days.

Fourteen patients aged 28–60 years have had this procedure. Six had suction lipectomy and periosteal suspension in conjunction with other procedures. Two patients previously had standard excisional surgery. The only complication was a hematoma that was drained at the bedside. The scar is concealed well and undergoes less hypertrophy or widening than with other methods. The amount of lift can be individually adjusted with this approach. Suction contouring of the flaps above and below the incision, along with periosteal dermal suspension and use of buried dermal flaps, eliminates postoperative bulging. No significant ptosis occurred in any patient during follow-up for 3 years.

▶ [We are indebted to the authors for introducing to the medical community two anthropologic terms, steatomeria and steatopygia (localized fatness of thighs and buttocks, respectively). Suction lipectomy reduces incisions, scarring, operating time, and morbidity, and therefore can't be all bad.—F.J.M.] ◀

(4–27) Aesthetic Plast. Surg. 6:207–209, 1982.

5. Flaps, Grafts, and Transplants

CLINICAL

5–1 **Comparison of Synthetic Adhesive Moisture Vapor Permeable and Fine Mesh Gauze Dressings for Split-Thickness Skin Graft Donor Sites.** A new class of moisture vapor-permeable (SAM) dressings has been developed for use on skin graft donor sites. Andrew Barnett, R. Laurence Berkowitz, Robert Mills, and Lars M. Vistnes (Stanford Univ.) compared two of these products, Tegaderm and Op-Site, with fine mesh gauze in 60 consecutive skin graft donor sites. Grafts were taken at a depth of 0.012–0.015 inch at a variety of body sites, and epinephrine-soaked sponges were placed until the test dressings were applied. Daily activities were not altered to protect the dressings. The 24 patients in the study were aged 8 months to 81 years. Donor sites ranged from 80 to 800 sq cm in size; burn sizes ranged from 9% to 55% of total body surface. Both Tegaderm and Op-Site were used on 23 sites; fine mesh gauze was used on 14.

Clinical observations indicated that the SAM dressings were much superior to fine mesh gauze. Pain was nearly absent with the SAM dressings. Healing occurred much more rapidly than with fine mesh gauze. The SAM dressings were not occlusive. Four clinical infections due to *Pseudomonas aeruginosa* occurred; two under Tegaderm dressings and two under Op-Site dressings. Three of the four infections occurred in 1 colonized patient. The donor sites healed when the dressings were removed. No systemic infections occurred.

The SAM dressings are significantly superior to fine mesh gauze dressings for the healing of split-thickness skin graft donor sites. Healing occurs much more rapidly and with much less pain. Care is needed in using SAM dressings in patients colonized with *Pseudomonas*, although this is not an absolute contraindication. No clinically significant differences between Tegaderm and Op-Site were noted in the present study.

▶ [Synthetic adhesive moisture-permeable dressings, e.g., Op-Site and Tegaderm, have demonstrated effectiveness in donor site management. They cause little pain and prompt healing. A problem area is the large donor site, where adhesive attachment is difficult to maintain and there are increased opportunities for infection. When infection occurs, prompt drainage with dressing changes is mandated. Although G. D. Winter (Epidermal regeneration studied in the domestic pig, in Rovee D.T. and Marback J. (eds.): *Epidermal Wound Healing.* Chicago, Year Book Medical Publishers, 1972, pp. 71–112) demonstrated that epithelization is more rapid in a moist en-

---

(5–1) Am. J. Surg. 145:379–381, March 1983.

vironment, the exposed dry wound appears to be more resistant to infection.—
B.W.H.] ◄

5–2   **Gluteus Medius-Tensor Fasciae Latae Flap.** John W. Little, III, and James R. Lyons (Georgetown Univ.) describe an alternative method of repairing uncomplicated cutaneous defects of the trochanter, based on the proximal parts of the tensor fascia lata muscle and the neighboring gluteus medius. Closure is obtained through the rotation-advancement technique. The blood supply of the tensor fascia lata muscle and fascia is from a major branch of the lateral circumflex femoral artery of the profunda femoral system. The gluteus medius is served by the deep branch of the superior gluteal artery of the internal iliac system. Both structures are innervated by the superior gluteal nerve. The flap is outlined after ostectomy of the trochanter by inscribing a rotation arc, starting at the posterosuperior margin of the defect and rising to the height of the iliac crest; it ends near the site of the pedicle of the tensor fascia lata about 8 cm below. No muscles are divided beyond the anterior border of the tensor. After rotation of the flap the gluteus medius pad overlies the ostectomy site. Layered closure is carried out over multiple drains. The secondary defect is closed by direct advancement of the skin of the lower abdominal quadrant across the iliac crest. If the dense fascia over the crest has been lifted with the abdominal flap, it is advanced and secured to the fascia of the gluteus minimus.

Eight such flaps were prepared in paraplegic patients in a 2-year period. The defects ranged in size up to 8 × 12 cm. No skin grafts were necessary. All of the flaps survived completely without wound complications. Because the vascular pedicle is not disturbed, the entire traditional tensor fascia lata musculocutaneous flap remains available for later needs, as do virtually all useful axial flaps of the region that have been described. The flap has not been used in ambulatory patients. The tensor itself is expendable, but the gluteus medius is important for a normal gait, and total loss of this muscle probably would produce a Trendelenburg gait. The conventional tensor fascia lata flap therefore is preferable for use in ambulatory patients.

5–3   **Total Thigh and Rectus Abdominis Myocutaneous Flap for Closure of Extensive Hemipelvectomy Defects** was evaluated by Walley J. Temple, Walid Mnaymneh, and Alfred S. Ketcham (Univ. of Miami). Hemipelvectomy is important in the cure of selected patients with tumors in the upper thigh and hip. Consistent cure rates averaging 35% have been reported, with low surgical mortality and satisfactory rehabilitative potential; however, significant morbidity has resulted from inadequate closure or wound breakdown. Significant skin flap necrosis may occur in up to 50% of patients. Myocuta-

(5–2)   Plast. Reconstr. Surg. 71:366–371, March 1983.
(5–3)   Cancer 50:2524–2528, December 1982.

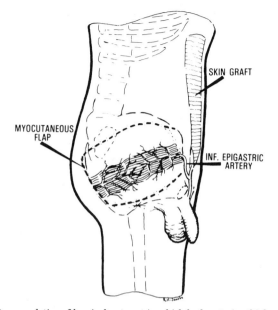

SKIN GRAFT

MYOCUTANEOUS
FLAP

INF. EPIGASTRIC
ARTERY

Fig 5–1.—After completion of hemipelvectomy, in which both anterior thigh and posterior buttock flaps were resected with the tumor, the myocutaneous flap was elevated off the posterior rectus sheath and transversalis fascia. The anterior rectus sheath was included in the inferior incision. The flap was then tunneled under a lateral skin bridge and sutured into place. The donor site was grafted with split-thickness skin. (Courtesy of Temple, W. J., et al.: Cancer 50:2524–2528, December 1982.)

neous flaps were used in 2 patients to close extensive hemipelvectomy defects. A rectus abdominis myocutaneous island flap was used to close a hemipelvectomy defect in a man aged 72 years with a femoral chondrosarcoma, as shown in Figure 5–1. A thigh myocutaneous flap was used to close a hemipelvectomy defect in a man aged 43 years with chondrosarcoma, as shown in Figure 5–2. Rehabilitation proceeded without complications in both cases.

The use of a myocutaneous flap for closure of an extensive hemipelvectomy defect contributes to the resectability of unusual pelvic and thigh tumors, and can minimize morbidity in these patients. The thigh flap is an excellent myocutaneous flap because of its large vascular pedicle. The full rectus muscle was used in the first patient described here. Because at least some of the flap was supported by random pattern vascularization, the procedure was staged to improve collateral flow. Angiographic delineation of the epigastric system may prove useful in predicting which patients will require a delay. This flap can be a useful adjunct in traumatic hemipelvectomies when both the thigh and buttock are sheared off or badly damaged.

With the availability of myocutaneous flaps, technical difficulty in closing hemipelvectomy wounds is no longer a reason for denying po-

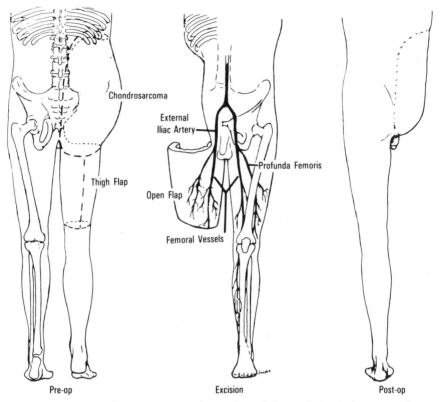

Pre-op   Excision   Post-op

Fig 5–2.—Drawing shows incision, vascular supply, and closure of a hemipelvectomy with anterior thigh flap pedicled on the iliac and femoral vessels. The incision on the thigh is carried down to the femur, and all soft tissues are elevated with the flap. Flap size can be modified as necessary to close the defect. (Courtesy of Temple, W. J., et al.: Cancer 50:2524–2528, December 1982.)

tentially curative surgery or for predicting the occurrence of unacceptable operative morbidity.

5–4 **The Exposed Knee Joint: Five Case Reports.** An injured, exposed knee always involves a threat to the extremity. After debridement, the knee should be covered with well-vascularized, mobile soft tissue to permit both early mobilization of the joint and immediate or delayed surgery on the underlying structures. Sirpa Asko-Seljavaara and Juhani Haajanen (Univ. of Helsinki) reviewed the emergency management of 3 patients with massive avulsion and 2 with deep, grossly infected wounds penetrating the knee cavity. The former patients incurred massive degloving injuries of the lower extremity in heavy vehicle accidents. After debridement of K wire suspension of the limb, when indicated, the exposed fascia and muscle were covered

(5–4) J. Trauma 22:1021–1025, December 1982.

with sheet or meshed split-skin grafts taken from the opposite limb or from avulsed skin flaps. The infected patients also had immediate excision of devitalized tissue and full soft tissue reconstruction at the same session. Gastrocnemius muscle or musculocutaneous flaps were used for closure in all 5 patients. The donor area was covered with a split-skin graft. No infectious complications resulted. Ligament reconstructions were carried out at the same time under the transposed muscle.

The exposed knee cavity in both accidental and contaminated wounds should be covered immediately, and the use of gastrocnemius muscle or musculocutaneous flaps appears feasible in these cases. The medial gastrocnemius musculocutaneous flap can be extended to cover the contralateral side of the joint. In smaller defects, a muscle flap covered with split-skin grafts provides a better cosmetic result. When adequate debridement is carried out, the well-vascularized gastrocnemius reconstruction permits full repair of knee structures at the same session. The gastrocnemius muscle mass later atrophies, forming elastic tissue over the joint and stabilizing its side movements. Secondary collateral ligament reconstructions are not always necessary.

5–5 **Combined Medial and Lateral Gastrocnemius Musculocutaneous V-Y Island Advancement Flap.** Reconstruction of soft tissue defects in the posterior ankle region remains a major challenge. Peter

Fig 5–3.—Drawing shows flap **A,** advanced and **B,** closed. Popliteal Z incision prevents flexion contracture and permits access to muscle origin and vessels. (Courtesy of Linton, P. C.: Plast. Reconstr. Surg. 70:490–493, October 1982.)

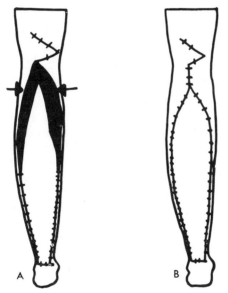

A   B

(5–5)   Plast. Reconstr. Surg. 70:490–493, October 1982.

C. Linton (Univ. of Vermont) advanced a functioning muscle-skin unit in simultaneous reconstruction of a distal skin defect and restoration of Achilles tendon integrity and function. A combined medial-lateral gastrocnemius musculocutaneous V-Y island advancement flap was used.

Man, 42, a sawmill operator, simultaneously amputated his right arm, cut through the anterior distal femur on the right, and sustained a compound fracture of the distal left tibia with avulsion of a large segment of soft tissue and Achilles tendon insertion. The ankle injury was initially managed by Hoffman fixation and skin grafting. The fixation was removed in 5 months. A defect 7 × 4.5 cm in size, consisting of healed skin graft on bone, remained. The graft procedure is illustrated in Figure 5–3. The medial and lateral gastrocnemius unit was advanced distally on the soleus bed. The V skin design permitted primary closure of the skin donor defect. The tendon was repaired with a Kessler suture of No. 1 Mersilene. The knee was splinted in 90 degrees of flexion and gradually extended over a period of months after secure tendon healing took place. Full knee extension was present at 1 year, when 20 degrees of active ankle plantar flexion from 90 degrees was possible.

Simultaneous reconstruction of Achilles tendon function and of a large defect of the Achilles insertion and soft tissue was achieved in this patient using the medial and lateral gastrocnemius musculocutaneous units, raised as a neurovascular island pedicle. The tissues can be advanced up to 4.5 cm distally, with primary V-Y closure of the popliteal defect.

▶ [This is an excellent adaptation of the possibilities of the gastrocnemius muscle-skin unit and the V-Y principle. It solves a difficult problem without doing violence to cosmetic considerations.—F.J.M.] ◀

5–6 **Free Flap Coverage of Deep Tissue Defects of the Foot.** Composite tissues are needed to reconstruct foot defects if periosteum or plantar skin is inadequate, or joints, tendons, or nerves are exposed. Free flaps are 1-stage procedures that reduce the total time required for anesthesia and surgery, as well as the time of immobilization and patient morbidity. James H. Roth, James R. Urbaniak, L. Andrew Koman, and J. Leonard Goldner performed seven cutaneous or myocutaneous free flap procedures to cover foot defects and followed up the patients for at least a year. The average age was 23 years, and the average size of the free flap was 8.6 × 13.1 cm. Four flaps covered heel defects, 2 covered forefoot defects, and 1 covered a tarsometatarsal amputation stump. Four cutaneous scapular flaps, 2 myocutaneous tensor fascia lata flaps, and 1 myocutaneous latissimus dorsi flap were transferred. The average length of anesthesia time was less than 8 hours. There were no failures, but 1 patient was reexplored and had revision of the venous anastomosis. Another responded to intraarterial thrombolysin administration for vascular insufficiency of the flap. The patients received low molecular weight dextran and Persantine postoperatively.

(5–6) Foot Ankle 3:150–157, Nov.–Dec. 1982.

Man, 23, sustained bilateral tibial and fibular fractures, as well as an open fracture dislocation of the left misfoot with loss of the entire heel pad. After fracture stabilization and wound debridement, the heel defect was covered with split-thickness skin, but weight-bearing caused a draining heel ulcer in the center of the grafted area. A cutaneous scapular free flap transfer was carried out as a 1-stage procedure, and the shoulder donor site was closed primarily. The circumflex scapular artery of the flap was joined to a branch of the posterior tibial artery of the left leg. The patient now walks without restriction. There was no flap ulceration.

No failures occurred in these patients, who were followed for an average of 19 months. The flaps provided good coverage and a good bed for further reconstructive surgery. The authors now prefer the cutaneous scapular free flap for covering foot defects. This surgery can be done in one stage with minimal immobilization and hospitalization. At present, innervated free flaps to the foot are not considered necessary. This surgery is contraindicated in feet with vascular insufficiency.

▶ [The authors briefly compare the advantages and disadvantages of free flaps and pedicled flaps. Not mentioned, however, is the often seen disadvantageous excessive bulk inherent (and uncontrollable) in many free flaps to the foot.—F.J.M.] ◀

5–7 **Experience With Ipsilateral Thigh Flap for Closure of Heel Defects in Children.** George B. Irons, Charles N. Verheyden, and Hamlet A. Peterson (Mayo Clinic and Found.) report results in 8 children in whom an ipsilateral thigh flap was used for soft tissue coverage of heel defects.

Boy, 6, incurred a lawn mower injury to his right heel. The wound extended from 7.6 cm below the popliteal crease to the plantar surface of the heel. A 10-cm segment of the posterior tibial neurovascular bundle was missing. The avulsed cartilaginous apophysis of the os calcis was reattached with 2 K wires, and the wound was debrided and skin grafted. The wound present 2½ weeks later was 10 cm in diameter, with the exposed os calcis at its base. A superiorly based flap 10 cm long and 8 cm wide was elevated from the posterior thigh, with its superior base just above the gluteal crease; the flap was sutured into place over the defect with the knee flexed. The lower limb was held in place with the Hoffmann apparatus. The donor site was closed primarily. The pedicle was divided 2 weeks later after fluorescein injection showed an adequate neovascular supply. The flap was inset on the heel 2 days later. The foot was completely healed within 14 months, and the patient walked without difficulty.

None of the flaps in this series was delayed, and all donor defects but 1 were closed primarily. The Hoffmann apparatus provides good immobilization, and the somewhat awkward position was accepted by the patients. The flaps were left attached for an average of 2 weeks. Knees regained mobility surprisingly quickly, without physical therapy being necessary. No flap loss occurred, although 2 patients required minor flap revisions. Use of the Hoffmann apparatus for immobilization precludes the need for a cumbersome cast. Also, the

(5–7) Plast. Reconstr. Surg. 70:561–567, November 1982.

surgeon has access to the flap, and the patient has reasonable mobility for turning in bed and moving about in a wheelchair or on crutches.

▶ [This is an excellent flap to use for children. I have also used it in young adults who had amputation of the opposite lower extremity and required heel coverage. It avoids the sometimes extensive deformities that occur in conspicuous areas when attempting coverage in a concealed area.—F.J.M.] ◀

5–8 **Direct Neurotization of Severely Damaged Muscles** is described by Giorgio Brunelli (Brescia, Italy). Several experimental studies found that denervated muscle accepts an implanted motor nerve and achieves functional innervation. The implanted nerve forms new motor end-plates. Studies in rabbits and rats showed the formation of new end-plates from the sprouts of a transposed motor nerve in an aneural zone of denervated muscle. When the distal end of the rat peroneal nerve was unraveled into fasciculi or group-subfascicular terminal units and these were implanted into muscle through small slits, newly formed motor end-plates were observed, particularly close to the nerve implant. Good contraction was obtained after 1 month on electrical stimulation of the peroneal nerve transplanted into the gastrocnemius muscle. Electron microscopy showed features of normal motor end-plates, including new synaptic contacts between the implanted nerve and muscle fibers, axonal branches rich in presynaptic vesicles in direct contact with the basal membrane of muscle fibers, and normal postsynaptic vesicles.

Nerve grafting was attempted in 13 patients to bridge large gaps between nerve and muscle after traumatic injury. Grafts split into several fasciculi were implanted into slits in the damaged muscle, and the proximal end was sutured to the original motor nerve of the denervated muscle. The graft was anchored by stitches joining the epineurium to the muscle fascia. The 11 evaluable patients had muscle ratings in the satisfactory range. Direct neurotization of damaged muscle appears to represent an option for treating patients with large nerve gaps resulting in significant muscle paralysis.

▶ [Brunelli's work, supported by both laboratory and clinical evidence, is highly exciting. Along with advances in microvascular techniques, it opens the door for early (immediate) reconstruction in avulsion-type injuries.—F.J.M.] ◀

5–9 **Experimental Study of Sleeve Technique in Microarterial Anastomoses.** Lance Sully, M. Gemma Nightingale, Bernard McC. O'Brien, and John V. Hurley (Melbourne) attempted to determine whether the results of anastomosing small arteries using a sleeve technique compare favorably with those of end-to-end anastomosis. Rabbit femoral arteries having a mean external diameter of 1 mm were transected and anastomosed just distal to the origin of the epigastric branch by routine end-to-end suture on one side and by sleeve anastomosis on the other. The technique of invaginating suture place-

(5–8)   J. Hand Surg. 7:572–579, November 1982.
(5–9)   Plast. Reconstr. Surg. 70:186–192, August 1982.

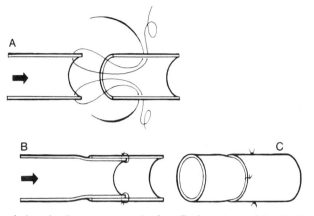

Fig 5–4.—**A,** invaginating sutures seen in place. **B,** sleeve is complete after invaginating sutures are tied and tacking sutures are inserted laterally. (Courtesy of Sully, L., et al.: Plast. Reconstr. Surg. 70:186–192, August 1982.)

ment in the sleeve technique is illustrated in Figure 5–4. The mean time required to complete sleeve anastomosis was 10.9 minutes, and for the conventional repair, 16.7 minutes, corresponding to the number of sutures used in the respective methods. The animals were explored 2 hours to 6 weeks after surgery.

The patency rate was 98% in the conventionally treated group and 84% in animals treated by sleeve anastomosis. Six of the 8 failures in the latter group showed poor flow on clamp removal and improved only after Xylocaine application. Less thrombotic deposit was present in the sleeve anastomoses, because of less suture material in the lumen and less disruption of the luminal surface. Reendothelialization occurred more rapidly after sleeve anastomosis, but narrowing was more marked than with conventional repair. The narrowing was a result of the combined effects of wall thickening and buildup of thrombus between the overlapping vessel ends.

A significantly lower patency rate was achieved by sleeve anastomosis of rabbit femoral arteries than by conventional end-to-end suture anastomosis in this study. This result is not outweighed by the shorter time required for sleeve repair or the supposed advantages of less luminal surface disruption and intraluminal suture exposure. This type of sleeve anastomosis may not be beneficial in clinical settings.

▶ [Another great idea that didn't work. It is well-executed and honestly reported by pioneers in the microvascular field. As Edison remarked at one point when asked if he wasn't discouraged by all of his failures in developing the incandescent light, "Not at all—I have now eliminated 300 ideas that won't work!"—F.J.M.] ◀

5–10 **Vascularized Autogenous Whole Joint Transfer in the Hand: Clinical Study.** Tsu-Min Tsai, Jesse B. Jupiter, Joseph E. Kutz, and

(5–10) J. Hand Surg. 7:335–342, July 1982.

Harold E. Kleinert (Univ. of Louisville) describe findings in 6 patients undergoing vascularized autogenous whole joint transfer to the hand; transfer of joints with an open epiphysis was done in 2. All 6 patients were males, aged 6–38 years, in whom severe trauma resulted in joint destruction. The proximal interphalangeal (PIP) joint was involved in 4 patients, the thumb metacarpophalangeal (MP) joint in 2, and the small finger MP joint in 1. The foot was the source of the autogenous joint in 5 patients, and 1 had an MP joint transferred from a digit that had sustained a more distal amputation. The dominant hand was involved in 5 patients. The technique is illustrated in Figure 5–5. Nine autogenous whole joint transfers were carried out. The mean follow-up was 2 years.

The transferred joints had a mean active range of motion of 22 degrees to 55 degrees, and a mean passive range of degrees to 64 degrees. All of the joints were painless, and all but one were stable. The transferred toe PIP joint tended to assume a flexed position, and a boutonniere deformity was present in 3 patients. Two expressed some dissatisfaction with the cosmetic outcome. Bony union occurred within 4 months in 5 of 6 patients. The articular space was maintained in all instances. Five patients required further surgery. All 4

Fig 5–5.—A, vascularized proximal interphalangeal (PIP) joint transfer is disarticulated through the distal interphalangeal joint with ligation of fibular-side articular branches. **B,** the PIP joint composite transfer includes an extensor mechanism as well as an island of overlying skin to function as a visible monitor of underlying circulation. (Courtesy of Tsai, T.-M., et al.: J. Hand Surg. 7:335–342, July 1982.)

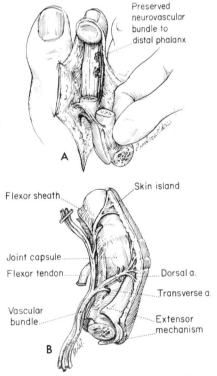

adults returned to their previous type of work, and all but 1 are satisfied with the overall surgical results.

These preliminary results indicate that the vascularized autogenous whole joint transfer is suitable for reconstructing severely injured or congenitally deficient joints in young patients. This approach could be used to manage the difficult congenital deformities associated with symphalangism, arthrogryposis multiplex congenita, brachydactyly, and congenitally fixed joint contractures. It also could be used to salvage a failed implant arthroplasty when there is significant loss of bone stock. The overlying soft tissue and neurovascular status must be intact, and the musculotendinous system of the joint capable of providing for function of the transferred joint.

5–11 **The Lymphatics of the Groin Flap** were studied by L. Clodius, P. J. Smith, J. Bruna, and D. Serafin. The concept of axial pattern flaps was developed when McGregor and Jackson described the groin flap in 1972. This flap was first used as a pedicle flap, but transfer of its vascular territory based on the axial vessels soon was undertaken to produce the so-called free flap. Edema did not occur after elevation of this flap and its transfer or transplantation to a new site. Suprailiac lymphography was performed in 10 patients to evaluate the lymphatics of the groin flap.

One to three major lymph collectors were seen in the filling phase, running parallel to the superficial circumflex iliac artery and the inguinal ligament. A beaded appearance indicated the presence of valves. In the storage phase of lymphography, the nodes lateral to the femoral vessels were filled. They lay within the confines of the groin flap. A pedicled groin flap was partially successful in a patient with lymphedema when a single-stage procedure was performed. Lympholymphatic anastomoses were not inhibited by excessive peripheral scar formation, but an insufficient number of new lymph vessels bypassed the area of obstruction. In a second patient, a vascularized groin flap failed because of insufficient lymphatic inflow, possibly resulting from a chemical lymphangitis secondary to lymphangiography.

Lympholymphatic anastomoses must become functional when flaps are transferred in order for adequate lymph drainage to be available. Scar tissue formation may have variable effects on this process. If possible, the deep lymphatic system should be drained. The groin flap appears to possess a self-contained lymphatic territory similar to its vascular system. It is possible with microsurgical methods to transplant lymph nodes with their vascular pedicle successfully.

5–12 **Successful Operation for Lymphedema Using Myocutaneous Flap as a "Wick."** Lymphatic bridge procedures are used less frequently because of the unsatisfactory results obtained. Sandor Med-

(5–11) Ann. Plast. Surg. 9:447–458, December 1982.
(5–12) Br. J. Plast. Surg. 36:64–66, January 1983.

gyesi (Copenhagen) reports the successful use of a new method of bypassing occluded lymphatic trunks in the axilla in a patient who had severe postmastectomy lymphedema for 2 years.

Woman, 73, underwent radical mastectomy 25 years previously with excision of axillary nodes for adenocarcinoma after preoperative irradiation. Marked lymphedema was present; the circumference of the left upper arm was 14 cm more than that of the right arm, and a 10-cm difference in the left forearm was present. No lymphatic trunks suitable for lymphangiography were found in the hand, but dye injection showed dermal backflow. An island flap 12 × 6 cm in size was raised on the border of the latissimus dorsi, and the muscle pedicle was drawn through a tunnel through the axilla into the arm. Fascia and some subcutaneous tissues were preserved on the muscle pedicle. The lymphedema was reduced significantly within a month of operation, and the arm appeared normal 3 years later. No compressive bandaging was necessary.

Undermining of the skin and transplantation of muscle tissue through the axilla may have reduced the risk of lymph drainage being compromised by additional scar tissue in this patient. There was no tension in the skin, and no scar tissue in the subcutaneous tissue. It also is possible that large lymph vessels were present in the island flap and its pedicle that formed anastomoses with lymph vessels in the arm during healing. The lymph vessels in the arm had not degenerated at the time of operation. A similar procedure in a patient with postmastectomy lymphedema for 3 months gave less satisfactory results, but the patient had far less tension in the arm postoperatively and the lymphedema has not increased in more than 1 year of follow-up.

▶ [If this "wick" operation stands the test of time (so many others have failed to do so), it will be a real contribution to the treatment of a long-standing and frustrating class of problems.—F.J.M.] ◀

5–13 **Autogenous Kinetic Dermis-Fat Orbital Implant: An Updated Technique** is described by Byron Smith, Stephen L. Bosniak, and Richard D. Lisman (New York). Extrusion and migration of spherical foreign bodies and integrated implants used to replace an enucleated globe have led to interest in the use of an autogenous orbital implant. The disinserted rectus muscles are isolated and sutured after standard enucleation (Fig 5–6). The upper outer quadrant of the buttock is preferred as a donor site. The diameter of the anterior lamella, the dermis, should be 18–25 mm, and the graft should be at least 25 mm deep. The implant is obtained after dermabrasion of the surface and placed within the extraocular muscle cone as shown in Figure 5–7. Interrupted 5–0 chromic sutures are used. Antibiotics are given for 2 weeks after surgery. A similar procedure is used when a spherical orbital implant has migrated or a nonautogenous orbital implant has extruded.

Forty-six operations have been done, and the patients were fol-

(5–13) Ophthalmology (Rochester) 89:1067–1071, September 1982.

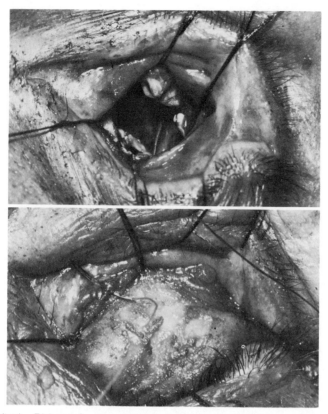

Fig 5–6 (top).—Disinserted rectus muscles are tagged with 5–0 Vicryl sutures that are attached to edge of graft at 12-, 3-, 6-, and 9-o'clock positions.
Fig 5–7 (bottom).—Two adjacent cardinal sutures are retracted so that edge of graft and conjunctiva may be sutured together more easily.
(Courtesy of Smith, B., et al.: Ophthalmology (Rochester) 89:1067–1071, September 1982.)

lowed up for as long as 4 years. Seven cases of contracted socket, 6 of implant migration, 9 of implant extrusion, and 11 of superior sulcus deformity were treated. Thirteen primary procedures were performed. The outcome in 1 case is shown in Figures 5–8 and 5–9. None of the 3 minor complications affected fitting of the prosthesis or detracted from the final outcome.

Placement of the autogenous kinetic dermis-fat orbital implant has been helpful in the management of difficult cases. In cases of multiple implant extrusions or injury where the fornices have contracted or conjunctiva is deficient, the procedure preserves existing conjunctiva and forms adequate fornices. In cases with deep superior sulci, the method permits the placement of a greater volume into the orbit without fear of extrusion. Excellent motility and little superior sulcus

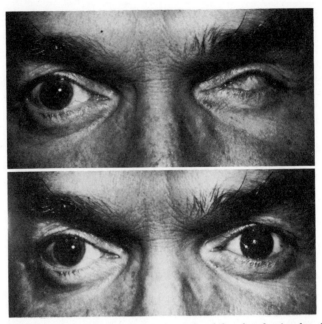

Fig 5–8 (top).—Patient 4 weeks after dermis-fat graft to left socket showing deep fornices and conjunctiva uniformly covering graft.

Fig 5–9 (bottom).—Patient wearing prosthesis 6 weeks after dermis-fat graft to left socket. (Courtesy of Smith, B., et al.: Ophthalmology (Rochester) 89:1067–1071, September 1982.)

deformity have resulted from dermis-fat grafting following enucleation.

▶ [The emphasis of the authors on using dermis to maintain a soft tissue socket is of concern to plastic surgeons dealing with anophthalmia. The donor site could, perhaps, be improved, but the principles are interesting.—L.A.W.] ◀

5–14   **Uses of Fascia in Ophthalmology and the Benefits of Autogenous Sources** are discussed by John S. Crawford and Timothy W. Doucet (Hosp. for Sick Children, Toronto). Indications for using fascia in ophthalmology have increased significantly in recent years. Autogenous fascia provides benefits not inherent in preserved fascia, particularly a lack of reabsorption. Congenital ptosis remains the most frequent indication for using fascia, when minimal or no levator function is present. Fascia also is used in cases of acquired ptosis, as in Marcus Gunn jaw-winking after levator disinsertion, congenital fibrosis syndrome, congenital third nerve palsy, myasthenia gravis, myopathies, and levator muscle injury from tumor surgery. Fascia also has been used to correct telecanthus. Strips of preserved fascia lata have been used in repair of certain types of retinal detachment in which the sclera is very thin or weak. Scleral wall defects can be

(5–14) J. Pediatr. Ophthalmol. Strabismus 19:21–25, July–Aug. 1982.

repaired with fascia. Other indications include implant extrusion or impending extrusion, lower lid ptosis, and upper lid retraction.

No failures occurred in using autogenous fascia in the repair of congenital ptosis. The use of stored fascia may result in failure from reabsorption or sterile abscess formation. Complications were infrequent with stored fascia, but they can be virtually eliminated with use of autogenous fascia. The morbidity and the extra operative time are warranted by the improved surgical results. The use of autogenous fascia is not recommended in children less than age 3½ years because of the small size of the leg. Occasionally, the excess fascia obtained from 1 patient was used in another.

▶ [The authors discuss procedures that have been known and used by plastic surgeons for decades.—L.A.W.] ◀

5–15 **Closure of Myelorachischisis Defects With Reverse Latissimus Dorsi Myocutaneous Flaps.** The surgical management of myelorachischisis defects is difficult and complicated. Dorothy H. Clark, John W. Walsh, and Edward A. Luce (Univ. of Kentucky) successfully rotated bilateral posteriorly based latissimus dorsi muscle flaps on 2 newborn infants with large thoracolumbar myelorachischisis. These "reverse" flaps were based on the paraspinal perforators. Coverage was uneventful in both instances. The procedure is illustrated in Figure 5–10. Follow-up at 2 years showed no compromise of upper limb function because of sacrifice of the latissimus dorsi. The children can

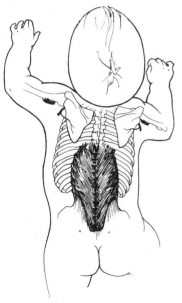

Fig 5–10.—Rotation of bilateral "reverse" latissimus dorsi muscle flaps following transection of humeral insertions and major vascular pedicles. Muscular closure is accomplished after closure of the dural defect. (Courtesy of Clark, D. H., et al.: Neurosurgery 11:423–425, September 1982.)

push up with their upper extremities and forcefully extend their shoulders.

Thoracolumbar myelorachischisis lesions are the most severe spina bifida defects and are associated with the poorest prognosis. The dura often is thin and friable, permitting only partial coverage of the neural tissue after it is in the spinal canal. The latissimus dorsi can be rotated nearly 360 degrees on the thoracodorsal artery. The posterior-based, or "reverse," latissimus dorsi flap has been used to cover posterior trunk defects. Blood loss can be significant, but was acceptable in the present infants. Few functional deficits have resulted from loss of the latissimus dorsi muscle. Children with thoracolumbar myelorachischisis are likely to be confined to a wheelchair, with transfer into and out of the chair being dependent on the latissimus dorsi, but the children described here appear to have compensated by recruiting efforts from other muscle groups.

▶ [It should be possible, perhaps in larger infants or smaller defects, to use only half of the latissimus dorsi muscle, leaving the humeral attachment intact and achieving partial preservation of its function.—F.J.M.] ◀

5–16   **Repair of the Thoracic and Pericardial Substance Loss Using a Net of Absorbable Material.** L. Toty and H. Bakdach describe a reparative technique used successfully in 30 cases to date after wide excision of the chest wall for primary tumor or bronchopulmonary carcinoma that involved the ribs. The resulting gap must be filled to prevent paradoxical respiration and its immediate functional consequences in the postoperative period.

Nonabsorbable materials are poorly tolerated in certain septic conditions, which suggested the use of a polyglactin 910 piece of netting, cut to size out of a 25 × 25-cm plaque and sutured between the ribs under tension. The slow absorption of this material (4–6 weeks) ensures thoracic stability and acts as support for readherence of the lung to the chest wall. The prosthesis resists coughing and is well-tolerated.

Major indication for its use are in cases of considerable costo-parietal resection associated with pulmonary excision in respiratory failure, or excision of a tumor-invaded pericardium with herniation of the heart.

▶ [This could be a valuable adjunct to chest reconstruction, particularly when cardiac support or widespan thoracic wall support is needed in conjunction with muscle or musculocutaneous flaps.—F.J.M.] ◀

5–17   **Reconstruction of Complex Thoracic Defects With Myocutaneous and Muscle Flaps: Applications of New Flap Refinements.** Gordon R. Tobin, Constantine Mavroudis, W. Robin Howe, and Laman A. Gray, Jr. (Univ. of Louisville) describe several modifications of latissimus dorsi and pectoralis major flap design that can be used in reconstructing complex thoracic defects. Both units can be

(5–16)   Nouv. Presse Med. 11:3265–3266, November 1982.
(5–17)   J. Thorac. Cardiovasc. Surg. 85:219–228, February 1983.

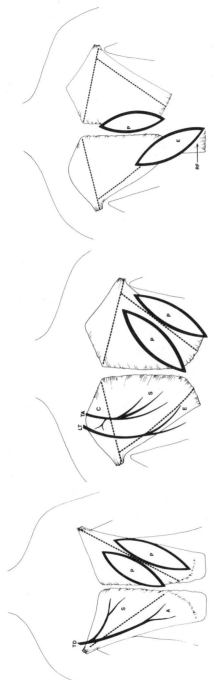

Fig 5–11 (left).—Anatomical basis for splitting latissimus dorsi flaps segmentally. On the left, thoracodorsal vessels *(TD)* bifurcate proximally to supply medial *(A)* and lateral *(S)* muscle segments, which can be split surgically *(dotted lines)*. On the right, either muscle segment can carry skin paddles *(P)* independently.

Fig 5–12 (center).—On the left (patient's right side), anatomical basis is shown for splitting pectoralis major flaps segmentally. Thoracoacromial vessel *(TA)* branches supply sternocostal *(S)* and clavicular *(C)* muscle segments. Lateral thoracic vessels *(LT)* supply external (abdominal) muscle

segment *(E)*. Muscle segments may be split surgically *(dotted lines)*. On the right side, each segment independently carries a myocutaneous flap *(P)*.

Fig 5–13 (right).—Anatomical basis is shown for extended pectoralis major fasciocutaneous flaps. On the left (patient's right side), the pectoralis muscle carries an abdominal skin paddle *(E)* on rectus abdominus fascia *(RF)*. On the right, a presternal skin paddle *(P)* also can be carried on the pectoralis major muscle.

(Courtesy of Tobin, G. R., et al.: J. Thorac. Cardiovasc. Surg. 85:219–228, February 1983.)

split into independent segments, each containing major intramuscular branches of the primary vascular pedicle. Segmental splitting of the latissimus dorsi flap is illustrated in Figure 5–11, and the pectoralis major flap in Figure 5–12. Muscle-carried skin paddles can be extended well beyond the distal muscle borders by preserving vascular connections that extend to adjacent myocutaneous territories on the muscle fascia and in the overlying subcutaneous tissue. In the thorax, either abdominal or presternal skin can be carried on a pectoralis major muscle pedicle (Fig 5–13). Flaps can be reversed and transferred on their caudal origins. Latissimus dorsi flaps can be reversed on posterior intercostal perforating vessels. Muscles can be converted to island vascular pedicle flaps that are transferred on a single vascular pedicle. This approach can be used for flap transfer through intercostal incisions to close intrathoracic defects and cavities when intact muscle pedicles restrict transfer because of excess bulk or insufficient length.

These refinements were used successfully to reconstruct complex thoracic and chest wall defects in 13 patients during a 4-year period. Three infected dehiscences of median sternotomy incisions were closed with split pectoralis major muscle advancement flaps developed from the sternocostal segment. Simultaneous thoracoplasty and closure of a bronchopleurocutaneous fistula were done with a split pectoralis major muscle advancement flap. Two massive chest wall defects from shotgun wounds were reconstructed with split latissimus dorsi and pectoralis major segmental flaps. A pectoralis major fasciocutaneous extended flap was used to reconstruct a precordial chest wall defect resulting from cancer resection. An exposed vein graft of the subclavian artery was covered with a split pectoralis major segmental muscle flap. Four wounds with exposed axillary nerves and vessels were covered with segmentally split myocutaneous flaps. An esophagopleurocutaneous fistula secondary to blunt trauma was closed by transfer of a rhomboid major muscle as an island vascular pedicle flap. These flaps can reliably protect vital structures and reconstruct massive defects. They provide a highly durable cover, permitting immediate or elective secondary restoration of architectural stability and elimination of large flail regions.

▶ [The feasibility of splitting pectoralis major and latissimus dorsi muscle flaps, and the use of cutaneous islands well beyond the muscle border, is beautifully demonstrated in this article. Caution: the reliability of these procedures in any but expert hands is not demonstrated.—F.J.M.] ◀

5–18 **Pectoralis Major Muscle Turnover Flaps for Closure of Infected Sternotomy Wound With Preservation of Form and Function.** Initially, mere coverage of a wound or control of infection was the goal in transposing muscles and muscle-skin units as flaps, but the original techniques now have been modified to preserve form

(5–18) Plast. Reconstr. Surg. 70:471–474, October 1982.

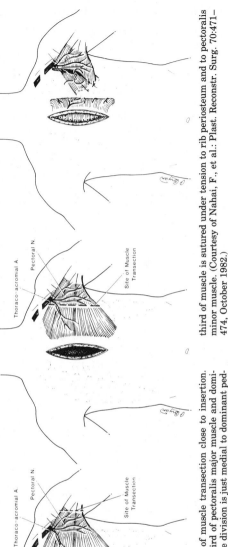

Fig 5–14.—Left, original site of muscle transection close to insertion. **Center,** preservation of lateral third of pectoralis major muscle and dominant neurovascular pedicle. Muscle division is just medial to dominant pedicle and nerves. **Right,** turnover flap of pectoralis major muscle. Lateral third of muscle is sutured under tension to rib periosteum and to pectoralis minor muscle. (Courtesy of Nahai, F., et al.: Plast. Reconstr. Surg. 70:471–474, October 1982.)

and function in the donor region. Foad Nahai, Louis Morales, Jr., David K. Bone, and John Bostwick, III (Emory Univ.) describe a modification in technique to preserve the anterior axillary fold after transposition of the pectoralis major muscle as a turnover flap to control an infected median sternotomy wound. After thorough debridement of the infected sternum, the muscle is divided as shown in Figure 5–14, the lateral third of the muscle is sutured under tension to the pectoralis minor and the rib periosteum. The skin is closed directly over the turnover flaps after placing suction drains in the mediastinum and in the donor areas.

Sixty patients with infected median sternotomy wounds underwent debridement and muscle flap closure in a 6-year period. Sixteen had the modified operation, with preservation of the anterior axillary fold and clinical evidence of muscle contraction resulting in all patients. Electromyography in 2 patients confirmed muscle innervation. Infection resolved completely in all 16 patients. Elevation of bilateral pectoralis major flaps was necessary in 15. A rectus abdominis muscle flap also was elevated in 12 patients and turned over as a flap into the lower mediastinum to cover the lower part of the defect. One patient had a hematoma in the donor area.

This modification preserves the anterior axillary fold in patients undergoing transposition of the pectoralis major muscle as a turnover flap in the mediastinum and sternal region. The resultant flaps controlled infection in the median sternotomy wound.

5–19 **Blood Pressure Drop as Result of Fluorescein Injection.** Fluorescein administered intravenously is widely used to assess flap viability, and the method is considered to be free of significant complications. Robert T. Buchanan and Norman S. Levine (Univ. of Oklahoma) used fluorescein for this purpose in 33 patients in a 2-year period. Adequate records were available for 29 patients having 39 procedures. Of these patients, 24% had a blood pressure drop of 20 mm Hg or more, and 33% (8% of the total group) had a fall in pressure of more than 60 mm Hg immediately after administration of fluorescein. The dose of fluorescein ranged from 6 to 25 mg/kg. Ephedrine was given to raise the blood pressure in 3 instances. In the other patients the pressure returned to baseline within 15–30 minutes with only increased fluid administration or other supportive measures.

Physicians using fluorescein in bolus form should be aware that a substantial fall in blood pressure can occur. Classic antigen-antibody reactions may develop with administration of iodinated contrast media, but there is no conclusive evidence. Deutsch points out that many patients experiencing reactions have received very large doses of fluorescein, and that the use of smaller doses might more safely permit determination of flap viability.   .

▶ [Caveat emptor!—R.J.H.] ◀

(5–19) Plast. Reconstr. Surg. 70:363–368, September 1982.

5–20 **The Fluorescence Camera: How to Use Fluorescein Dye in a Normally Illuminated Room.** Bert Myers, Myles Guber, and William Donovan (New Orleans) modified a Polaroid camera to produce instant pictures of fluorescence from fluorescein in normally illuminated rooms. The filter-modified camera was used to record fluorescence patterns in rats with caudally based flaps raised deep to the panniculus carnosus and replaced in their beds. Studies were done initially after the intraperitoneal injection of 0.5 ml of 25% fluorescein and were repeated a week later. The fluorescence camera also was used in 65 patients undergoing various flap procedures.

In the rat study, the mean dye level determined visually was close to the level determined in photograms and to actual survival (Fig 5–15). The mean values did not differ significantly. In the patient study, 1 or 2 gm of dye was used, the larger dose being given to very dark-skinned patients; 60 of the 65 flaps exhibited full fluorescence and survived completely. Five flaps had major nonfluorescent areas. Excess skin was present in 2 of these, and the remaining flap survived after unstained areas were removed. In 2 instances, unstained areas measuring more than 4 × 6 cm were left alone and the flaps necrosed, necessitating secondary operation. In 1 patient, an unstained area 3 × 5 cm in size was left alone and the flap survived.

Use of the modified fluorescence camera in illuminated rooms is as good as, but no better than, visual assessment in predicting skin flap

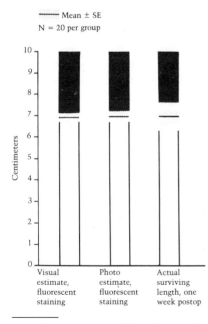

Fig 5–15.—Data from rat experiments using fluorescence camera. (Courtesy of Myers, B., et al.: Ann. Plast. Surg. 10:248–251, March 1983.)

(5–20) Ann. Plast. Surg. 10:248–251, March 1983.

viability. Use of this camera precludes the need for totally darkening the room and employing an ultraviolet lamp. Also, a permanent record is obtained for the chart.

5-21 **Comparison of Effect of Bacterial Inoculation in Musculocutaneous and Random-Pattern Flaps.** Muscle and musculocutaneous flaps are widely used in reconstructive surgery, but areas requiring coverage frequently are infected, thus the flap used should be able to contain and eliminate local infection. Ning Chang and Stephen J. Mathes (Univ. of California at San Francisco) injected live microorganisms into the undersides of random-pattern and musculocutaneous flaps in dogs. Cranial-based rectus abdominis musculocutaneous flaps 15 × 7 cm in size and random-pattern flaps of the same size and shape were used. A preparation of *Staphylococcus aureus* was injected intradermally and placed in wound cylinders.

No differences in susceptibility to bacterial challenge were observed in the different parts of musculocutaneous flaps and normal skin. More extensive necrosis occurred in the random-pattern flaps, in which the distal portions were significantly more vulnerable. The musculocutaneous flaps recovered rapidly from bacterial inoculation, but necrosis was seen in random-pattern flaps. Bacterial counts increased in the wound spaces surrounded by these flaps until full-thickness flap necrosis occurred. Bacterial counts decreased in wound spaces surrounded by musculocutaneous flaps, and there was evidence of healing around the wound cylinders.

Musculocutaneous and random-pattern flaps in the dog interact with pathogenic bacteria in reproducibly different ways. Musculocutaneous flaps exhibit a better ability to survive a bacterial challenge than do random-pattern flaps, both on their skin surfaces and at the interface of the muscle and wound.

5-22 **Anesthetic Management of Patients Undergoing Free Flap Transfer.** D. W. Robins (Bristol, England) reviewed experience with 31 patients having free flap transfer in a 4-year period, usually for correction of cutaneous, myocutaneous, or osteomyocutaneous defects of the lower limbs. Augmentation of tissue bulk in the face and scalp, fracture fixation, and nerve grafting also were performed. Most patients were young adults. Groin flap surgery was the most common procedure, and anesthesia often lasted for 9–10 hours.

Patients were premedicated with lorazepam and thymoxamine. Surgery was carried out under general anesthesia and ventilatory support. Alcuronium was used for tracheal intubation. Flucloxacillin usually was administered as prophylaxis. Humidified heated gases were used to prevent bronchial ciliary malfunction and drying of the respiratory mucosa. If the lower extremity was operated on, a lumbar extradural block with 0.5% bupivacaine was used in order to mini-

---

(5–21) Plast. Reconstr. Surg. 70:1–9, July 1982.
(5–22) Br. J. Plast. Surg. 36:231–234, April 1983.

mize vasoconstriction from sympathetic overactivity and increase blood flow to the lower limbs through dilatation of cutaneous vessels. With this approach, a lighter general anesthetic may be administered and better postoperative analgesia is possible. Thymoxamine was administered by infusion for up to 48 hours postoperatively to reduce the risk of skin flap necrosis; oral treatment was continued for up to 2 weeks. The central venous pressure was monitored as a guide to fluid and blood replacement.

The packed cell volume is not electively reduced, and high-molecular weight dextrans are not routinely administered. Heparin is used only if a free flap becomes ischemic and an attempt to avoid reexploring the graft is desired.

Arterial and central venous pressures are monitored overnight in intensive care after surgery. The patient is given 35% to 40% oxygen and is kept free of pain. Fluid and blood losses should be replaced accurately. No patient required intermittent positive-pressure ventilation postoperatively, and no deep vein thrombosis developed despite prolonged bed rest.

▶ [The view from beyond the ether screen.—R.J.H.] ◀

5–23 **Anesthesia For Patients Undergoing Prolonged Reconstructive and Microvascular Plastic Surgery.** The increase in the length of plastic surgery has raised new problems in anesthesiology. Markku Hynynen, Pirkko Eklund, and Per H. Rosenberg (Univ. of Helsinki) reviewed the anesthesia care given to 22 patients having reconstructive plastic or reimplantation procedures in 1977 to 1981. Seven had emergency replantation procedures, whereas 15 had elective operations. Three of the latter patients were in the American Society of Anesthesiologists' group II; the other patients were all in group I. Premedication was with pethidine and atropine; some patients also received diazepam. A "balanced" technique generally was performed with thiopentone, suxamethonium, alcuronium for maintenance of relaxation, fentanyl, and N_2O-oxygen. Enflurane was added in a few cases, and some patients received diazepam or droperidol as a supplement. Postoperative pain was relieved by intramuscular oxycodone. Care was taken to prevent heat loss during lengthy operations.

The patients were predominantly men and were relatively young. The mean duration of anesthesia was 8 hours, 45 minutes, in emergency cases and 8 hours in elective cases. Hemodilution during operations was achieved, with dextran in a majority of cases. Five electively operated-on patients and 1 in the replantation group required blood. Diuresis during surgery was adequate in all cases. Hemodynamics remained stable throughout the period of anesthesia. About 50% of the patients had nausea. Urinary tract symptoms also were frequent. Two electively operated-on patients had an unexpected fall

(5–23) Scand. J. Plast. Reconstr. Surg. 16:201–206, 1982.

in blood pressure at the time of extubation and awakening. One of them had received plasma protein solution immediately before the drop in pressure. No patient had evidence of deep venous thrombosis postoperatively. One emergency patient had laryngeal edema after extubation.

Few serious problems have occurred in patients who had a "balanced" anesthetic regimen for lengthy plastic surgical procedures. Regional anesthetic methods such as continuous axillary plexus block may be advantageous in some instances, such as in finger replantation.

▶ [Good communication and planning by the anesthesiologist and surgeon are necessary to minimize complications in these prolonged operations. All members of the surgical team should be familiar with the goals of the procedure and the potential complications.—S.H.M.] ◀

EXPERIMENTAL

5–24 **Axial-Pattern Flap Based on Arterialized Venous Network: Experimental Study in Rats.** Theodore Voukidis (Chepstow, Wales) examined the possibility of raising an axial-pattern flap in rats based on the blood supply from an arteriovenous fistula constructed 3 weeks previously. An arteriovenous fistula was made by end-to-side anastomosis of the superficial inferior epigastric vein and femoral artery. After 20–25 days, an abdominal flap 9 × 4 cm in size was raised with a line joining the xiphoid and the pubic symphysis as its medial border. The lateral thoracic vein was preserved as the venous outflow of the flap. A thin sheet of plastic foil was laid beneath the flap before suturing its back into place. The superficial inferior epigastric artery was ligated.

Five of 15 arteriovenous fistulas became thrombosed in the first 24 hours. All 10 arterialized flaps survived for a week after preparation, whereas all 5 control flaps sloughed. Groin swelling subsided within a week of construction of the arteriovenous fistula. No flap edema was observed. The thoracoepigastric and its branches were dilated for only a few hours after the flap was raised.

The goal of this approach was to reverse blood flow in the arteriovenous anatomoses to provide inflow to the nutrient arterioles from the venous network (Fig 5–16). Reversed venous flow becomes possible some 2–3 weeks after the fistula is made when the venous valves become incompetent. Clinically, this approach could be used to transform a random-pattern area of skin into an axial-pattern territory, permitting the use of unconventional donor areas in which "axial pattern" flaps can be raised without sacrificing the arterial system. The new flap would be bipolar, possibly with sensory innervation, and technically would be transferred relatively easily. The possibility exists of modifying the length of the vascular pedicle by performing the

(5–24) Br. J. Plast. Surg. 35:524–529, October 1982.

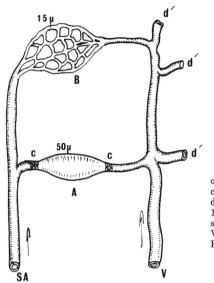

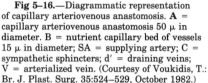

Fig 5–16.—Diagrammatic representation of capillary arteriovenous anastomosis. A = capillary arteriovenous anastomosis 50 μ in diameter. B = nutrient capillary bed of vessels 15 μ in diameter; SA = supplying artery; C = sympathetic sphincters; d' = draining veins; V = arterialized vein. (Courtesy of Voukidis, T.: Br. J. Plast. Surg. 35:524–529, October 1982.)

fistula at an appropriate level. More experimental work is needed before this technique is used in man.

▶ [An interesting innovation, one of many imaginative examples today in free flap physiologic research. The authors rightly emphasize the need for much more experimental work before clinical application of this principle.—R.J.H.] ◀

5–25 **Vascular Augmentation of Skin and Musculocutaneous Flaps.** With neovascularization by means of heterotopic vasculature, the construction of a cutaneous or musculocutaneous island flap by using a vascular pedicle is feasible. Yücel Erk, Franklin A. Rose, and Melvin Spira (Houston) attempted to develop a method of vascularly augmenting skin and musculocutaneous flaps by the surgical insertion of a vascular pedicle.

Vascular augmentation of a groin flap was attempted in the pig. Flaps were raised 4 weeks after ligating the superficial femoral vasculature with its surrounding areolar tissue at the level of the knee and bringing the vessels proximally for insertion under the groin skin. The flaps were elevated as island flaps, 10 × 15 cm, on the neopedicle only. A similar procedure was carried out in rats, in which a groin flap, 6 × 6 cm, was raised after a 2-month interval. Vascular augmentation of both skin and muscle was attempted in the dog by using the sartorius muscle and the adjacent femoral artery and vein. A groin flap, 10 × 12 cm, was raised 4 weeks later.

Marked fluorescence was present in the elevated groin flaps of the

(5–25) Ann. Plast. Surg. 10:341–348, May 1983.

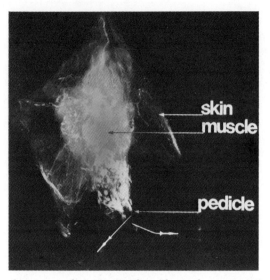

Fig 5–17.—Abundant neovascularization in a dog with vascular augmentation of both skin and muscle. (Courtesy of Erk, Y., et al.: Ann. Plast. Surg. 10:341–348, May 1983.)

4 pigs, and microangiography showed abundant transmural neovascularization from the neopedicle. In the 8 rats, abundant new capillaries arose from the upturned pedicle and supplied the groin flap. All flaps raised 8 weeks after implantation of the vascular pedicle survived totally. Marked neovascularization also was evident in the dog studies (Fig 5–17). In 1 of the 4 dogs the experiment failed because the vessels were excessively skeletonized before being sandwiched between the muscle and groin skin.

These studies show that it is possible to create a secondary island musculocutaneous flap at a site associated with minimal morbidity. The neopedicle of the secondary flap might provide a vascular pedicle on which to base clinical free flap transfer. The precise means by which neovascularization occurs in a delayed pedicle graft remains unclear. It is apparent, however, that transmural vascularization can follow simple complete immobilization, ligation, and transposition of a donor artery and vein without the need for an ischemic stimulus.

▶ [This novel and ingenious experimental work holds real promise for refined and improved survival both of pedicled flaps and free tissue transfers.—R.J.H.] ◀

▶ ↓ These articles are excellent and extensive studies on a difficult subject by ambitious and dedicated authors. The importance of the topic prompted a meeting of some members of the Plastic Surgery Research Council in July 1979 to standardize approaches to common problems in flap research. The critical discussions following these articles (Myers, B.: *Plast. Reconstr. Surg.* 71:408, March 1983; and Edstrom, L. E.: ibid., p. 409) refer to these difficulties in standardization, interpretation of data, and so on, and is highly recommended to the serious reader.—R.J.H. ◀

5–26   **A Study of the Pharmacologic Control of Blood Flow to Acute Skin Flaps Using Xenon Washout.** *Part I.*—The many methods used to increase the survival of skin flaps presumably share a capacity to increase capillary blood flow. Philip M. Hendel, David L. Lilien, and Harry J. Buncke (San Francisco) examined the mechanisms of the increase in blood flow by using the local xenon washout method to assess the effects of systemic vasoactive drugs in skin flaps and identical control areas. Differences in response were attributable to events within the flap that altered the local circulatory dynamics. Various surgical models of rats were used.

All types of vasodilators increased blood flow in skin flaps. No initial fall in flap circulation occurred with agents acting directly on vascular smooth muscle rather than on the adrenergic receptors. Decadron increased blood flow to flaps and control skin equally. Norepinephrine did not increase flap blood flow, but rather was associated with a steady decline in flap circulation. Methoxamine initially increased flow to both the flap and control skin; increasing doses reduced flow to the flap. Guanethidine and reserpine decreased flap perfusion initially, but flow then increased above baseline. Administration of systemic caffeine led to a drop in flap blood flow. α-Methyldopa increased and then decreased flap blood flow. All drug regimens studied, including dexamethasone, phenoxybenzamine, terbutaline, hydralazine, guanethidine, reserpine, and prazosin led to an increase in flap survival in the dose ranges predicted by the xenon studies.

These findings indicate that vasodilatation enhances both flap blood flow and flap survival, and that vasoconstriction reduces blood flow. Depletion of sympathetic nerve terminals enhances blood flow and flap survival. The vessels in an acutely elevated skin flap have greater vasospastic tone than is optimal for maximum nutrient blood flow. This may be a result of the release of catecholamines from sympathetic nerve terminals after flap elevation.

Part II.—Surgical delay is the chief method used in clinical work to increase skin flap survival. Hendel, Lilien, and Buncke examined the mechanism of blood flow changes resulting from the delay phenomenon by comparing the effects of vasoactive drugs on flow to acute and delayed flaps in the same rat. Blood flow was monitored by the xenon washout method. Ventral abdominal flaps were created. Xenon washout studies showed an increase in blood flow over time within flaps starting after 5 days in the proximal part of the flap and proceeding distally. A significant increase in flap survival beyond the midline occurred when the flap was surgically delayed.

Both norepinephrine and methoxamine decreased blood flow to acutely elevated flaps at lower doses than in delayed flaps. When the sympathetic nerve terminals were destroyed, flow to the delayed flap

(5–26)   Plast. Reconstr. Surg. 71:387–407, March 1983.

fell more rapidly than that to the acute flap. The catecholamine content of the distal part of the delayed flaps was much below that of acutely elevated flaps. Blood flow to an acutely elevated flap increased steadily with increasing doses of terbutaline. Flow to the delayed flap showed a relative decline.

These findings indicate that the delay phenomenon involves both passive vasodilation caused by loss of sympathetic nerve terminals in acutely elevated flaps, as well as active vasodilation that does not involve the loss of a second vasoconstrictor mechanism or sensitization of the β-adrenergic receptors. The characteristics of the latter component suggest that it acts directly at the smooth muscle or vascular-architecture level. Either an unidentified vasodilator or a structural change (e.g., vessel remodeling or denervation smooth-muscle atrophy) may be responsible.

5–27 **Altered Skin Flap Survival and Fluorescein Kinetics With Hemodilution.** There is evidence that isovolemic hemodilution can favorably alter blood flow in relatively ischemic tissues, on the basis of Poiseuille's law. Hemodilution reduces blood viscosity, and a reduction in either the blood cell concentration or the total serum protein concentration improves blood flow in skin flaps and their ultimate survival. John E. Gatti, Donato LaRossa, Samuel R. Neff, and David

Fig 5–18.—Skin flap survival in three hemodilution groups (Group A is control group). (Courtesy of Gatti, J. E., et al.: Surgery 92:200–205, August 1982.)

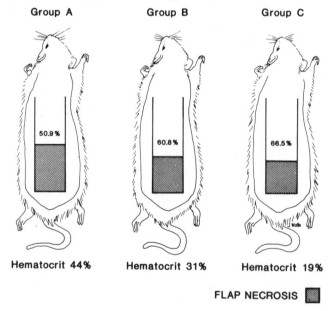

Group A   Group B   Group C

50.9%   60.8%   66.5%

Hematocrit 44%   Hematocrit 31%   Hematocrit 19%

FLAP NECROSIS ▨

(5–27) Surgery 92:200–205, August 1982.

G. Silverman (Philadelphia) examined blood flow and tissue survival in dorsal pedicle skin flaps in rats at varying hematocrit levels. Hemodilution was carried out by phlebotomy and crystalloid replacement to reduce the hematocrit from the control value of 44% to 31% and 19% in different groups of rats. The dye kinetics of intravenously injected fluorescein were examined by using the fiberoptic perfusion fluorometer.

Differences in skin flap survival among the groups are shown in Figure 5–18. Both study groups had significantly better flap survival than control rats. Fluorescein elimination was substantially accelerated in the hemodiluted groups, but no differences in uptake were noted. Reductions in concentration of total serum protein after flap elevation were not significantly different in the various groups. Hematocrit values increased slowly over 9 days of observations, but did not return to baseline values. Four of the most markedly hemodiluted animals died, presumably of hypothermia or infection.

These findings support the use of isovolemic hemodilution as a means of improving blood flow to ischemic tissues such as skin flaps. The reduction in red blood cell concentration appears to be more important than the change in concentration of total serum protein. Clinical application of the findings would seem to be empirically sound. Marginally ischemic tissues might benefit from a reduction in the hemoglobin of the patient before operation or from not replacing operative blood loss with more red cells. Microcirculatory stasis and thrombosis may be avoided, and the lower viscosity may help protect vascular anastomoses and improve the outcome of free flap transfer and replantation.

▶ [An imaginative and soundly controlled study which may find application in further enhancing the survival of flaps.—R.J.H.] ◀

5–28 **Vasospasm Control by Intra-Arterial Reserpine.** Vascular spasm caused by vascular trauma or embolism can complicate vascular surgery. It can impair flow across anastomoses and lead to thrombosis in microvascular surgery or replantation procedures. Reserpine has been used to treat vasospastic conditions of a chronic nature, and low-dose intra-arterial reserpine recently was administered to relieve acute vasospasm localized to an extremity. L. H. Hurst, H. B. Evans, and D. H. Brown (Univ. of Western Ontario, London) conducted a study in healthy persons in which a strong sympathetic vasoconstrictive response was produced by immersing both hands and forearms in water at 10 C for 2 minutes and either saline or reserpine in doses of 0.125 mg to 5 mg was injected. A response was consistently noted in the reserpine-injected arm, even with the lowest dose, and a classic dose-response curve was recorded. Differences in erythema, temperature, and pulse wave were noted. Systemic side effects occurred in all patients given more than 2 mg of reserpine.

(5–28) Plast. Reconstr. Surg. 70:595–599, November 1982.

Ten individuals in a clinical trial received 1.25 mg of reserpine via the brachial artery, with saline injected in the other arm. A marked temperature difference between the 2 arms occurred within 2 hours; the average difference was 8 C. The height of the pulse wave increased dramatically on reserpine injection in the setting of cold stimulation. No change in systemic or digital blood pressure was observed. The sympathectomy effects lasted for at least 48 hours, and in some persons they lasted for up to 2 weeks.

A single intra-arterial injection of 1.25 mg of reserpine produces prolonged chemical sympathectomy distal to the injection site, with minimal side effects. The mechanism of action of reserpine is not entirely clear, but it appears to exert a direct toxic effect on intraneuronal norepinephrine-containing vesicles. In addition, reserpine inhibits the storage of vasoactive amines in platelets, thereby reducing the vasospastic effect of extravasated blood.

5–29 **Monitoring Skin Flaps by Color Measurement.** Color change is the most frequently used gross clinical sign to detect circulatory compromise in flaps. Mechanical measurements of skin color might provide a more accurate indication of change than subjective estimates do. B. M. Jones, R. Sanders, and R. M. Greenhalgh used a technique based on reflection spectrophotometry to monitor cutaneous circulation in experimental skin flaps. Epigastric flaps were raised in CFY rats. Flaps were based on the femoral vessels, either as islands or as free flaps with microvascular anastomoses. The spectral reflectance curve was measured using a portable single-beam transmission spectrophotometer adapted for reflectance measurements. Measurements were made at 11 wavelengths in the range of 460–660 nm.

The method provided a rapid indication of both arterial and venous insufficiency in previously healthy flaps. Postoperative studies produced characteristic traces in cases of successful and unsuccessful free flap construction. The fate of a flap was clear within 16–24 hours postoperatively. An increasing value for the difference between baseline and current reflectance measurements always indicated a successful flap, whereas a marked decrease indicated venous failure; a constant value or a small decrease suggested arterial failure. Continuous monitoring of reflectance values postoperatively gave a clear indication of the eventual outcome of a free flap.

Because human and rat skin have similar reflectance properties, this method could be useful in the clinical monitoring of flaps, especially if a small, lightweight measuring head was developed that could be fixed to the flap skin. Reflectance spectrophotometry is an inexpensive method which responds rapidly to circulatory changes.

▶ [Color measurement for judging the viability of flaps is not a new idea (cholesterol crystals, fluorescein perfusion, clinical estimation of cyanosis). The attractive part of this study is that spectrophotometric monitoring of specific wavelengths were substi-

(5–29) Br. J. Plast. Surg. 36:88–94, January 1983.

tuted for evaluation of color by the human retina, which is known to vary genetically. With the further modifications suggested by the authors, this method should be of serious interest to all surgeons who transfer free or pedicled flaps.—R.J.H.] ◄

5–30   **Omnipotential Pig Buttock Flap.** Rollin K. Daniel and C. L. Kerrigan (McGill Univ., Montreal) designed an omnipotential buttock flap in the pig for use in skin flap research in an attempt to replicate clinical techniques. The flap, measuring 18 × 10 cm, is located with its cephalodorsal corner at the anterosuperior iliac spine. The neurovascular pedicle contains the deep circumflex iliac artery, paired venae comitantes, and the lateral femoral cutaneous nerve. White Poland-China pigs weighing about 20 kg are used. Either a proximally based random cutaneous flap or a distally based random flap is created and optionally delayed. A free flap can be created from an island flap by dividing the vessels and the flap replaced or transferred to a distant site.

In all, 152 buttock flaps of varying supply were created. Survival patterns are illustrated in Figure 5–19. The arterial buttock flap survived to a greater length than did the random cutaneous flap. The proximal cutaneous flap survived to a greater length than did the distally based random cutaneous flap. Innervated island flaps and denervated free flaps survived similarly, resembling arterial flaps in survival length. Survival of flaps delayed for 1–3 days was similar to that of standard arterial flaps.

Pig flap research, though costly, accurately replicates the cuta-

Fig 5–19.—Standard survival patterns of various pig buttock flaps. (Courtesy of Daniel, R. K., and Kerrigan, C. L.: Plast. Reconstr. Surg. 70:11–15, July 1982.)

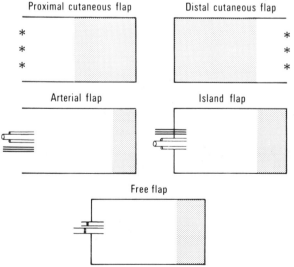

neous vascular supply in man and permits the creation of multiple flaps, including a control. Many flap configurations can be evaluated. The buttock flap technique provides consistent survival lengths and reliable anatomy. Postoperative observations are made readily at this site. Free flaps are technically easier to create than are flaps overlying thorax or abdomen, which moves with respiration.

5–31   **Tissue Glucose and Lactate Following Vascular Occlusion in Island Skin Flaps.** Venous occlusion may be more detrimental to island skin flaps than is arterial ligation. Chi-Tsung Su, Michael J. Im, and John E. Hoopes (Johns Hopkins Univ.) correlated tissue metabolite content with tissue viability in rat island flaps after vascular occlusions. Groin skin flaps measuring 3 × 6 cm were elevated as neurovascular island flaps. In some cases the deep and muscular branches of the femoral vein and the distal femoral vein were cauterized, leaving the femoral vein as the only venous drainage from the flap. In others, the same branches of the femoral artery were cauter-

Fig 5–20.—Tissue content of glucose and lactate and ratios of lactate to glucose in surviving and dying flaps measured in full-thickness skin at 24 hours after vascular clips were removed. (Courtesy of Su, C.-T., et al.: Plast. Reconstr. Surg. 70:202–205, August 1982.)

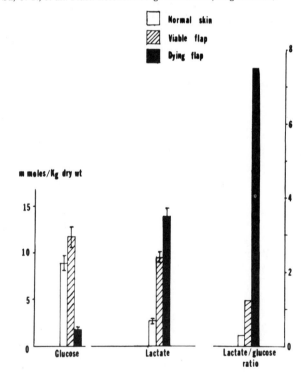

ized, leaving the femoral artery as the only arterial inflow, or the branches of both the femoral artery and vein were cauterized. The distal flap was biopsied after varying times of occlusion of the remaining vessels by microvascular clips and again 24 hours after removal of the clips.

Flap survival decreased progressively with increasing periods of venous occlusion. Flaps with venous occlusion for less than 2 hours exhibited no necrosis, whereas all of those subjected to 8 hours of venous occlusion were totally necrosed. Of flaps with arterial occlusion, 70% survived completely. Occlusion of both the artery and vein was followed by complete flap survival in about 30%. Glucose and lactate content in surviving flaps is shown in Figure 5–20. Viable flaps showed a 32% increase in glucose content and a 350% increase in lactate content, whereas dying flaps showed an 80% decrease in glucose content and a 50% increase in lactate content.

These findings indicate that venous occlusion is more harmful to the survival of neurovascular island skin flaps than is arterial occlusion. The ratio of tissue lactate content to glucose content may be a useful index of tissue viability.

▶ [These articles provide a good summation of the current clinical uses for selected free microvascular compound tissue flaps. A nice added touch is the anatomical demonstration of fascial "sleeves," which serve to protect the neurovascular supply to the flaps.—R.J.H.] ◀

5–32 **Irreplaceable Free Flaps in Reconstructive Surgery.**—*Part I.*—Robert M. Pearl (Kaiser-Permanente Med. Center, Santa Clara, Calif.) and Vincent R. Hentz (Stanford Univ.) point out that the microvascular free flap method is a reliable, safe means of managing difficult reconstructive problems. More versatile donor flaps now are available for use. The second generation of free compound tissue transfers is based on longer, larger vessels contained within fascial sleeves. Many problems previously associated with free-flap transfer have been overcome, and success rates exceeding 90% now are achieved commonly. In some situations a free flap is either the most reliable or the only available method of reconstruction.

The latissimus dorsi myocutaneous free flap can provide muscle alone or both skin and muscle. The flap is supplied by the thoracodorsal artery. The vascular hilum can be as long as 7 cm. The muscle can serve either for tissue coverage alone or as a functioning motor unit. Longitudinal orientation of the cutaneous portion permits the skin to extend to the posterior iliac crest. The transverse design results in a less conspicuous donor scar. The anterior part of the muscle is included unless excess bulk is a problem. If a functioning muscle is needed, the thoracodorsal nerve is included.

The tensor fascia lata myocutaneous flap can contain skin and muscle alone or, by incorporating the ascending division of the lateral

(5–32) Ann. Plast. Surg. 9:479–497, December 1982.

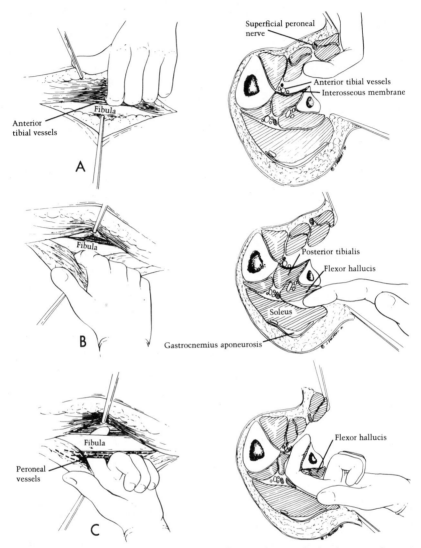

Fig 5–21.—Free fibula flap prepared using a sleeve technique. **A,** development of anterior sleeve. **B,** finger in posterior sleeve with plane of dissection between soleus and flexor hallucis longus muscles. **C,** connection between anterior and posterior sleeves. Peroneal artery is included with fibula, and nutrient artery as well as deep peroneal and posterior tibial nerves are excluded by means of prior dissection of anterior and posterior sleeves. (Courtesy of Pearl, R. M., and Hentz, V. R.: Ann. Plast. Surg. 9:479–497, December 1982.)

circumflex artery, bone as well. Two fascial sleeves are used to elevate this flap safely. The free flap can extend 12 cm posterior to a line drawn from the anterosuperior iliac spine to the lateral part of the patella and 75% of the way to the knee. The vascular supply is from the lateral circumflex artery. If bone is to be included, the ascending branch of the vessel must be preserved, although no sleeve exists for this part of the procedure. Disability from removal of the tensor fascia lata muscle is minimal, but enough muscle to preserve the ascending branch of the vascular axis should be resected, because injury to the gluteus muscles leads to a functional deficit.

Part II.—Pearl and Hentz describe several free flap procedures and the usefulness of such procedures generally in reconstructive surgery. The greater omentum is a very well-vascularized tissue and can be subdivided for refined reconstruction. An intra-abdominal approach is necessary, however, and there is a risk of adhesion formation. The free fibula flap is prepared using a sleeve technique to avoid damaging major neurovascular elements (Fig 5–21). The deep circumflex groin free flap is another possibility. A rapid dissection is carried out using the sleeve approach. The only added morbidity compared with standard nonvascularized iliac crest grafts is transection of one of the superficial sensory nerves of the thigh. Careful reconstruction is necessary to avoid herniation when skin is transferred in addition to bone and the flap contains portions of the abdominal wall muscles.

Free flaps are extremely useful for revascularizing ischemic tissues after extensive trauma or radiotherapy, for replacing muscle when there is no alternative, and for filling individual reconstructive needs. Microvascular free flaps can be used prophylactically when complications from radiotherapy are anticipated. Vascularized flaps of bone, or of skin and bone, can augment the blood supply, provide soft tissue coverage, and prevent or reverse bone healing problems when extensive trauma has occurred. Free flaps also can be used in hand rehabilitation after loss of flexor function. Little functional impairment generally results from free-flap procedures; donor site morbidity is not excessive compared with alternative reconstructive approaches. Most free-flap procedures require less than 6 hours.

Microvascular transfer of compound tissues permits the flexible tailoring of reconstructive procedures to specific patients. Revascularization of injured tissues is feasible using the free-flap transfer approach.

5–33   **The Irreplaceable Free Flap.**—*Part I. Skeletal reconstruction by microvascular free bone transfer.*—Vincent R. Hentz (Kaiser-Permanente Medical Center, Santa Clara, Calif.) and Robert M. Pearl (Stanford Univ.) point out that transplantation of autograft bone by conventional methods is much like free skin grafting, with healing viewed as a race between the impending death of transplanted tissues and their attempt to survive by reestablishment of vascularity. Even if the graft survives in part in a suboptimal milieu, union often is delayed or considerable reabsorption occurs. A means of transferring a bone graft with its nutrition intact now is available. Skeletal seg-

(5–33)   Ann. Plast. Surg. 10:36–54, January 1983.

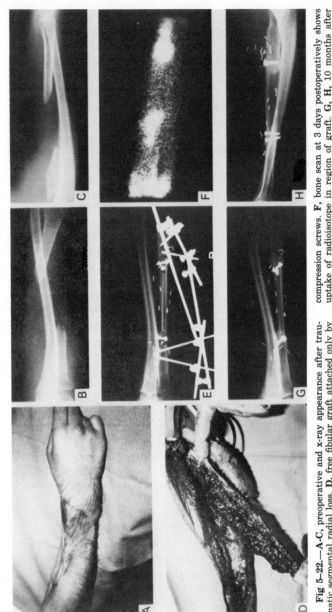

Fig 5-22.—A-C, preoperative and x-ray appearance after traumatic segmental radial loss. **D,** free fibular graft attached only by remaining peroneal vessels. **E,** immediate postoperative x-ray film shows stabilization of radial fragments by Roger-Anderson device. Lap joints between graft and radius stabilized with cortical compression screws. **F,** bone scan at 3 days postoperatively shows uptake of radioisotope in region of graft. **G, H,** 10 months after transplant, solid union with little callus is seen. (Courtesy of Hentz, V. R., and Pearl, R. M.: Ann. Plast. Surg. 10:36–54, January 1983.)

ments such as the rib and fibula have been transferred on their nutritional blood supply. Clavicle and iliac crest have been transferred on their periosteally derived nutrition as a component of composite regional osteocutaneous or osteomyocutaneous pedicle flaps. There remains a question of the level of nutrition provided by pedicled bone grafts, leading to development of the vascularized free bone transfer. The superiority of this approach was established in various experimental models. A graft that maintains vascularity can heal functionally, whereas no conventional bone graft can be expected to survive.

Uncontrolled clinical evidence supports laboratory findings of the feasibility of vascularized free bone transplantation. Recipient site irradiation or trauma is an indication for use of this method. If modern methods of osteosynthesis are used, the bone graft will heal by primary union rather than by creeping substitution, as in conventionally transferred autografts. Restructuring or remodeling begins im-

Fig 5–23.—**A,** lateral mandibular defect 1 year after resection for osteosarcoma. **B,** intraoperative photograph shows sagittal split of iliac crest. Probe in upper field is against hemorrhagic cancellous surface of graft attached only by its vascular pedicle, seen just inferior to graft. Iliac crest appears as transverse lighter colored line. **C,** bone scan 3 days postoperatively. **D,** 6 months after transfer, bony union is seen anteriorly and posteriorly. (Courtesy of Hentz, V. E., and Pearl, R. M.: Ann. Plast. Surg. 10:36–54, January 1983.)

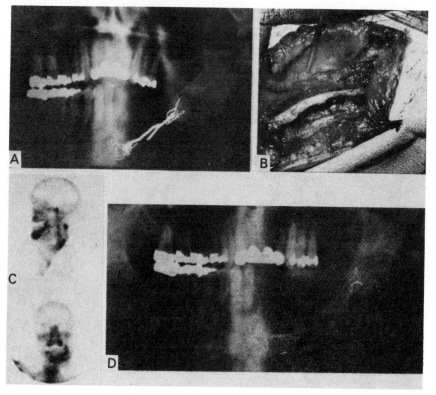

mediately in areas responsive to functional stimulation. Bone mass is better maintained after reconstructive augmentation of contour defects. Although a free vascularized graft probably cannot revascularize an ischemic area to the extent that a healthy muscle or a myocutaneous pedicle or free transfer can, it will not act as a parasite at the recipient site. The chief sources of bone at present are rib, fibula, and iliac bone. The use of newer vascularized grafts obviates some of the problems previously associated with free rib transfer.

Part II. Skeletal reconstruction by microvascular free bone transfer.—Hentz and Pearl describe alternatives to rib segments for use as free vascularized bone grafts. The rib does not lend itself readily to modern methods of osteosynthesis, and its dissection is tedious and not without hazard. The fibula may be used as a donor site to replace segmental defects in long bones when conventional grafts are likely to fail. A long length of strong cortical bone is provided. The method can be used in children if the remaining distal fibula is securely attached to the tibia. The proximal fibula can be transferred on the anterior tibial periosteal blood supply on the inferior lateral geniculate vessels through periosteal supply. An example is shown in Figure 5–22. The ilium also can be used as a source of a vascularized bone graft. This now is the preferred donor site for all except long segmental defects. The deep circumflex iliac artery is the best nutrient source. Donor site morbidity is minimized by sagitally splitting the ilium so as not to disturb muscle originating from the external cortex. An example of iliac grafting is shown in Figure 5–23.

Autogenous bone is the ideal material for use in skeletal reconstruction. Congenital pseudarthrosis of the tibia has been managed successfully by the microvascular free bone transfer technique. Functional whole-joint replacement by microvascular transfer from toe to digit holds promise. Rigid fixation by modern osteosynthesis methods enhances the success of this approach. External fixation devices have proved invaluable in stabilizing the bone fragments between which the vascularized bone graft is to be placed. Preliminary cadaver dissection is essential. Arteriography is necessary before the fibula can be harvested safely but it is not required if ilium is transferred. Two operative teams are desirable. Functional fixation is used whenever possible. No anticoagulant agents or antithrombotic drugs are used postoperatively.

5–34   **Experimental Free-Muscle Transplantation With Microneurovascular Anastomoses.** Manfred Frey, Helmut Gruber, Michael Havel, Erich Steiner, and Gerhard Freilinger (Univ. of Vienna) used the rabbit rectus femoris model to determine the best functional results to be expected after transplantation with microneurovascular anastomoses under optimal conditions. Direct vascular anastomoses and direct nerve suture were carried out with no tension. The artery

(5–34) Plast. Reconstr. Surg. 71:689–701, May 1983.

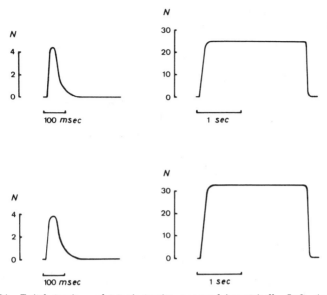

Fig 5–24.—Twitch tension and tetanic tension measured isometrically. **Left,** single twitch; **right,** tetanic contraction at a stimulation frequency of 100 Hz. **Upper row,** rectus femoris muscle 8 months after free transplantation with microneurovascular anastomoses. **Lower row,** normal, untreated rectus femoris muscle. (Courtesy of Frey, M., et al.: Plast. Reconstr. Surg. 71:689–701, May 1983.)

was anastomosed before the vein. The time of complete ischemia was about 30 minutes, and venous backflow was reestablished after an additional 20 minutes. Microvascular anastomoses were done with 11-0 sutures, and interfascicular suture of the bifascicular muscle nerve with 10-0 sutures. The animals were reassessed about 6 months postoperatively.

The muscles appeared healthy at follow-up. Optimal initial isometrically maximal tetanic and maximal twitch tensions were about 25% lower than in normal muscles (Fig 5–24). The proportion of atropic fibers correlated with impairment of function. On NADH staining, muscles with excellent force data exhibited clearly differentiated fiber types. With decreasing functional recovery the fiber types became more homogenous and lacked contrasts. Planimetry showed that the cumulative distribution deviated from normal for fiber area, but almost never for fiber perimeter. Enzyme content of the muscles could not be correlated with the degree of functional recovery, except for choline acetyltransferase, the content of which was greater in association with greater tetanic tension.

These findings demonstrate the value of muscle transplantation with microneurovascular anastomoses in restoring lost muscle function, even in extremities requiring strong forces. Survival of muscle fibers probably is greater than without microvascular anastomoses, and this technique may be considered indicated when force of contraction is the chief concern.

▶ [This is a particularly well-reasoned and elegantly executed experimental study. It illustrates the current concern that transplanted tissues should not just survive or the anastomoses remain patent, but that the tissues be chosen well in order to perform a missing function and that they replicate as nearly as possible that *quality* of function that was lost in the defect.—R.J.H.] ◀

5–35 **Use of Ultrasound Doppler Flowmeter in Reconstructive Microvascular Surgery.** An accurate test for anastomotic function that could be applied at the time of microvascular surgery would permit resection and revision of unsatisfactory anastomoses. B. M. Jones and R. M. Greenhalgh (London) used a directional ultrasound Doppler flowmeter in an attempt to predict the outcome of experimental free flaps at the time of surgery. Epigastric flaps were raised as either island or free flaps in CFY rats. A standard directional Doppler flowmeter with an 8-MHz probe was used. The arterial anastomosis was assessed alone or with the venous anastomosis.

The technique was 100% accurate when both the arterial and venous anastomoses were assessed individually. When only the arterial anastomosis was evaluated, the outcome was correctly predicted in 77% of instances. Spectral analysis of the Doppler signals provided information on the peripheral resistance within flaps.

A Doppler pulse tracing can be obtained from an artery 0.5 mm in diameter using a simple directional apparatus. The technique is of use both for evaluating microanastomoses and for predicting the outcome of free flaps. The arterial and venous anastomoses must be tested separately in free flaps. No flap failed in which an arterial pulse was heard 10 minutes after anastomosis and venous patency was provided. The accuracy of the Doppler method in predicting flap failures is not known. Data from spectrally analyzed true directional Doppler sonograms allow more detailed analysis than do those from conventional studies. The use of these methods may further improve the results of clinical microvascular reconstructive surgery. Postoperative monitoring is recommended.

5–36 **Skin-Flap Metabolism in Rats: Oxygen Consumption and Lactate Production.** Michael J. Im, Chi-Tsung Su, John E. Hoopes, and Robert M. Anthenelli (Johns Hopkins Univ.) examined the metabolism of pedicle skin flaps in female Sprague-Dawley rats by measuring rates of oxygen consumption and lactate production. Pedicle skin flaps 3 × 6 cm in size were based caudally on the lower right groin-abdominal area. The superficial epigastric neurovascular bundle was transected and the flap sutured back in place. Partial flap necrosis occurred in 22% of 23 animals. Biopsies were taken from the distal and proximal parts of the flap and from contralateral control sites 1, 3, and 7 days after flap elevation.

(5–35) Br. J. Plast. Surg. 36:245–253, April 1983.
(5–36) Plast. Reconstr. Surg. 71:685–688, May 1983.

Skin flaps had decreased glucose and glycogen levels and an increased lactate level in the first 3 days after flap elevation. Changes were greater in the distal than in the proximal halves of the flaps. The proximal halves had increased oxygen consumption rates at all postoperative intervals. The distal portions had lower rates of oxygen consumption than the proximal portions had on the first day, but no significant difference was noted thereafter. Lactate production was increased in flap tissues, especially in the distal portions, but the difference between the proximal and distal portions was not marked.

Increased oxygen consumption and lactate production are observed in pedicle skin flaps. The distal part of the flap is characterized by greater deposition of glucose than lactate in the first days after flap elevation. The contributions of glycolysis and of the oxidative paths to glucose metabolism in skin flaps approximate those in normal skin a week after flap elevation. The findings on determination of tissue glucose and lactate contents may be used as an index of microcirculation in skin flaps.

5–37 **Effect of Hypothermia and Tissue Perfusion on Extended Myocutaneous Flap Viability.** It is generally thought that cooling by perfusion extends the viability of organ homografts, but the role of perfusion in offsetting the endothelial injury and tissue edema that accompany prolonged ischemia remains unclear. Tsu-Min Tsai, Jesse B. Jupiter, Frank Serratoni, Toshiaki Seki, and Koichi Okubo examined the effects of hypothermia and tissue perfusion on the prolonged ischemic tolerance of the resting latissimus dorsi myocutaneous flap in adult dogs. Bilateral flaps about 7 × 7 cm in size were elevated and allowed to perfuse for 20 minutes before their pedicles were ligated and transected near their points of origin. After varying periods of hypothermic anoxia, a revascularization period of either 3 hours or 14 days was allowed. A single washout method employing iced Collins renal preservation solution was used. The flaps were transplanted into the groin by joining the thoracodorsal and femoral vessels. Some flaps were transplanted after 24 hours of ambient ischemia at 25–27 C.

In the acute flap study, nonperfused flaps gained more weight during hypothermic storage for up to 96 hours, but flaps maintained hypothermic for 120 hours followed a different pattern. Both perfused and nonperfused flaps in this group showed considerable interstitial hemorrhage, vascular congestion and thrombosis. In flaps maintained for a shorter time, morphological changes in muscle cells were greater in nonperfused flaps. In the extended flap study, perfusion before hypothermia was associated with much better survival than was observed for nonperfused flaps. No flaps transplanted after 48 hours of ambient ischemia survived. In flaps that survived after a long period of cool anoxia, much of the muscle tissue was replaced by proliferative fibrous connective tissue.

(5–37) Plast. Reconstr. Surg. 70:444–454, October 1982.

Both hypothermia and tissue perfusion extend the ischemic tolerance of canine latissimus dorsi myocutaneous flaps. Possible clinical applications include the hypothermic perfusion of major extremity amputations before replantation and temporary storage of free myocutaneous flaps.

5–38   **Genetic Control of Transplant Rejection** is discussed by Geoffrey W. Butcher and Jonathan C. Howard (Cambridge, England). Restriction of T cell specificity by the major histocompatibility complex (MHC) has important consequences for grafted tissues, even when MHC alloantigens themselves are the cause of rejection. Recent studies indicate that rejection of MHC-incompatible skin grafts can be under MHC-linked Ir gene control. The immune response gene Ir-RT1A appears to work at a regulatory rather than at an effector level of the immune response. Its properties are explicable only in terms of an antigen-specific, MHC-restricted regulatory function operating at some "administrative" level in the immune response to grafted tissues. It remains unclear whether host-processed alloantigen is responsible for the activation of T effector cells. Conventional cytotoxic T lymphocytes may have a specific determinative role in skin graft rejection. However, the case against these cells having a role in the destruction of some allografts is no better than the case against antibody.

Some findings in animal studies suggest that Ir genes could well exert significant effects on allograft survival in an outbred species such as man. The simplest means of starting a search for Ir genes in human organ transplantation would be to reexamine existing allograft data to sort for specific human leukocyte antigen (HLA) types in recipients with no reference to donor HLA type or to the precise incompatibility of the grafting. It then would be possible to learn whether any responder HLAs were present at a higher or lower frequency than that expected in graft-rejecting patients. Contact with transplantation antigens before organ grafting could have variable effects on the prognosis, depending on the patient's genotype. If Ir genes for organ transplantation prove to be important to graft survival, knowledge of their actions in certain donor-recipient combinations would improve the selection of grafts and treatments in individual patients.

▶ [This paper discusses the current views on the most significant of all persisting barriers to successful allogeneic organ transplantations—the genetic incompatibility between human donors and recipients via present-day concepts.—R.J.H.] ◀

5–39   **Cyclosporin A Prevents Appearance of Cell Surface "Activation" Antigens.** Cyclosporin A (CyA) inhibits the proliferation of human peripheral blood mononuclear cells cultured in vitro with stimulating alloantigens or mitogens. Stephen B. Leapman, Douglas M.

(5–38)   Transplantation 34:161–166, October 1982.
(5–39)   Ibid., pp. 94–96, August.

Strong, Ronald S. Filo, Edwin J. Smith, and Gail Lynn Brandt examined the mechanism by which CyA inhibits lymphocyte activation by studying cell surface markers on human peripheral mononuclear cells cultured in the presence and absence of CyA in a concentration of 1 μg/ml. Stimulator cells in allogeneic cultures were irradiated. Cells were incubated with monoclonal antibodies for 30 minutes.

Unstimulated cultured cells were unaffected by CyA except for an increase in background fluorescence. Cell surface Ia antigen was unaffected by CyA. The T cell subpopulations were similar in control and CyA-cultured cells, and the helper-suppressor T cell ratio was unchanged. Mixed lymphocyte reaction-stimulated cells in the presence of CyA had similar T cell subpopulation frequency when compared to cells cultured without CyA. A significant reduction in the frequencies of cells stained by monoclonal 7.2 and 5E9, markers of T cell activation, was observed in CyA-cultured cell populations.

The marked reduction in Ia-like antigen in cells treated with CyA indicates that CyA acts early in the activation process. The biochemical mechanism that prevents the appearance of this marker of activation by CyA remains to be determined. Inhibition of the 5E9 activation marker correlates with tritiated thymidine suppression. It may be that CyA prevents the expression of Ia cell surface markers.

▶ [This article provides some background information on the highly effective immunosuppressive agent CyA, which is responsible for the success of many of the recent organ allotransplants.—R.J.H.] ◀

5–40 **Cellular Target of Cyclosporin A Action in Humans.** Cyclosporin A (CyA) is a powerful immunosuppressive agent that may act by altering the balance of the regulatory T cell subpopulations that normally leads to transplant rejection. C. T. Van Buren, R. Kerman, G. Agostino, W. Payne, S. Flechner and B. D. Kahan (Univ. of Texas at Houston) determined the numbers and function of immunoregulatory helper and suppressor T cells in renal allograft recipients randomized to receive CyA or azathioprine after placement of a living related donor or cadaver donor kidney. Cyclosporin A was given orally in a dose of 14 mg/kg for 1 week, followed by 12 mg/kg for 2 weeks, 10 mg/kg for 1 month, and then 8 mg/kg. Doses were adjusted to maintain trough plasma levels below 200 ng/ml. Azathioprine was begun in a dose of 5 mg/kg and tapered to 2 mg/kg by 10 days postoperatively. Steroid therapy was the same for all patients.

The initial results suggest that graft survival may be better in CyA-treated patients than in those given azathioprine, in both the living related donor and cadaver donor recipients. Azathioprine-treated patients had a normal ratio of circulating helper-inducer to suppressor-cytotoxic cells in the peripheral blood, whereas CyA-treated patients had a reduced ratio owing to a decrease in number of helper T cells. Azathioprine-treated patients exhibited greater sup-

(5–40) Surgery 92:167–174, August 1982.

pressor cell activity than did normal persons or those given CyA. Helper T cell function was depressed in CyA-treated patients, but not in those given azathioprine, compared with findings in normal persons.

It appears that CyA therapy may improve graft survival in recipients of cadaveric or histoincompatible living related donor kidneys. Early graft rejection is less frequent in CyA recipients, and alloimmune reactions are attenuated and made more vulnerable to the effects of steroids. Allograft survival may be enhanced by CyA even in strong-responder recipients having relatively low suppressor cell activity.

5–41 **Vascularized Iliac Musculoperiosteal Free Flap Transfer: Case Report.** In order to obtain the full advantage of transferred periosteum, it should be properly vascularized or placed in a bed with good vascularity. Tetsuo Satoh, Masamitsu Tsuchiya, and Kiyonori Harii (Tokyo) report the use of a vascularized musculoperiosteal free flap transfer from the iliac bone in a patient with a severely comminuted tibial fracture.

Male, 17 years, sustained a comminuted fracture of the right lower leg with skin loss and underwent emergency wound excision and skeletal traction. The area of skin loss was 6×9 cm in size, with exposure of the fracture fragments. These were repositioned around an intramedullary nail 12 days after injury, and the anterior tibial vessels were exposed at the ankle. The deep circumflex iliac artery and vein were exposed in the left inguinal region; after dissection to the anterior superior iliac spine, a periosteal flap measuring 8×10 cm was removed with part of the iliacus muscle from the inner surface of the ilium (Fig 5–25). The flap was elevated as an island flap with a pedicle consisting of the deep circumflex vessels and immediately transferred to the recipient site, where microvascular revascularization was performed. The periosteal surface of the flap was spread out over the part of the

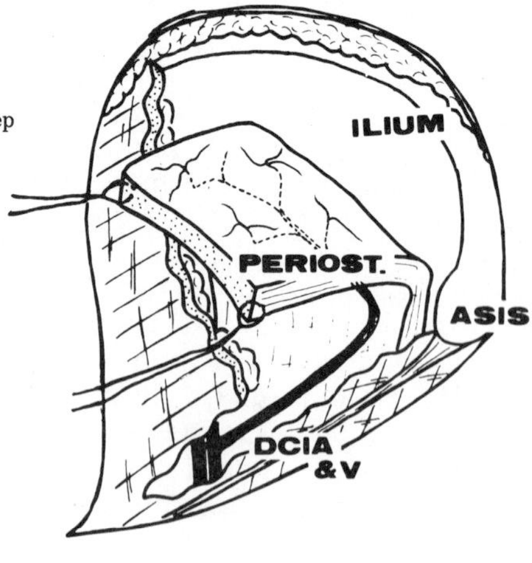

Fig 5–25.—Operation to harvest musculoperiosteal graft. DCIA and DCIV = deep circumflex iliac artery and vein; ASIS = anterior superior iliac spine; PERIOST = periosteum. (Courtesy of Satoh, T., et al.: Br. J. Plast. Surg. 36:109–112, January 1983.)

(5–41) Br. J. Plast. Surg. 36:109–112, January 1983.

injured tibia that had lost its periosteum, and the muscle surface was covered with split-thickness skin, which took completely. Linear callus formation was noted 6 weeks later. Complete bridging by newly formed bone and clinical bone union was confirmed 5 months after surgery. Full weight-bearing was allowed at 6 months.

The vascularized iliac musculoperiosteal free flap can provide well-vascularized soft tissue for covering exposed bone and enhance bony union beneath the surviving periosteum. It provides a possible means of treating tibial fractions associated with extensive soft tissue loss. Union is hastened by the addition of vascularized periosteum. An extensive skin and soft tissue defect can be covered in a single session. Donor site morbidity is minimal, because the iliac bone itself is left intact.

▶ [The theoretical advantages of periosteum over other vascularized soft tissue in bony union has not been universally demonstrated under clinical conditions. However, the choice of donor tissue in this case brilliantly combines a reliable vascular pattern, adequate coverage, and minimal donor site defect.—F.J.M.] ◀

5–42 **Revascularized Periosteum Transplantations.** Bridging a traumatic bone gap takes considerable time with the use of cancellous or cortical bone grafts, and several surgical procedures may be necessary. F. A. J. M. van den Wildenberg, R. J. A. Goris, and C. Boetes (Nijmegen, The Netherlands) examined the bone-forming capacity of 2 different revascularized periosteum grafts in midshaft tibial defects in African pygmy goats. Segments about 2 cm long were removed by osteotomy with the surrounding periosteum. Both nonvascularized and revascularized costal periosteum was transplanted around the defect. Revascularized rib transplants and revascularized tibial periosteal transplants also were evaluated.

Revascularized tibial periosteal grafts firmly bridged the defect within 8 weeks, whereas revascularized costal periosteum grafts did not. Complete consolidation was observed in several instances when revascularized tibial periosteal grafts were used. Bridging without complete consolidation usually occurred when revascularized rib transplants were used. No bridging of the defect was noted with the use of nonvascularized costal periosteum transplants.

Revascularized tibial periosteum can be used to bridge a segmental tibial defect in the African pygmy goat. Revascularized costal periosteum does not give comparable results in this model.

▶ [The surprising aspect of this study is not that bridging occurs but the speed with which it takes place.—F.J.M.] ◀

6. General Topics

6–1 **Influence of Hair Removal Methods on Wound Infections.** The practice of shaving operative sites was well established by the start of this century and has remained virtually inviolate until recently. J. Wesley Alexander, Josef E. Fischer, Michael Boyajian, Janet Palmquist, and Michael J. Morris (Univ. of Cincinnati) examined the influence of preoperative shaving and clipping on wound infection rates in a series of 1,013 patients having elective surgery at a single hospital. The patients were prospectively randomized to be either shaved or clipped the night before or on the morning of operation. All operative sites were scrubbed with an iodophor-containing detergent and painted with iodophor solution unless the patient was allergic to iodine.

The morning clipping method was associated with significantly fewer infections than the other regimens were, both at discharge and at 30-day follow-up. The effect was most marked in patients with clean wounds. The 1.8% infection rate for the morning clipping method at discharge was less than half that resulting from the other methods of hair removal. Stitch abscesses were more frequent in shaved than in clipped patients.

Clipping hair on the morning of operation was associated with fewer wound infections than was shaving or clipping on the night before surgery in this study. For every 1,000 patients treated, an estimated savings of about $275,000 could be realized if hair was clipped on the morning of surgery. Preoperative shaving is deleterious and should no longer be practiced. If at least half of all surgical patients have hair removed, more than $3 billion could be saved each year in the United States if preoperative shaving were replaced by clipping or by use of a depilatory on the morning of operation.

▶ [With the advent of osteomyocutaneous free flaps and other reconstructive procedures in which every last detail is of critical importance to tissue survival, this authoritative article should give pause for thought.—R.J.H.] ◀

6–2 **Operating Room Practices for the Control of Infection in U.S. Hospitals, October 1976 to July 1977.** Julia S. Garner, T. Grace Emori, and Robert W. Haley (Centers for Disease Control (CDC), Atlanta) report the findings of a survey of operating room supervisors in 433 U.S. hospitals regarding infection control practices in use during the period October 1976 to July 1977 and compared selected prac-

(6–1) Arch. Surg. 118:347–352, March 1983.
(6–2) Surg. Gynecol. Obstet. 155:873–880, December 1982.

tices with published statements and recommendations from the Medical Research Council of Great Britain, the U.S. Public Health Service Centers for Disease Control, the American Hospital Association, and the American College of Surgeons.

Preoperative shave was performed the night before the operation in 58% of the hospitals, no sooner than 5 hours before operation in 8%, 1 to 4 hours before operation in 17%, and within 1 hour before operation in 14%. The timing of the preoperative shave was determined by hospital policy in 64% of the hospitals. Almost all (97%) of the hospitals used iodophor compounds for preoperative preparation of the incision site and 57.5% used it exclusively. Iodophors were available for surgeon's hand scrub in 91% of the hospitals and a hexachlorophene emulsion was available in 58%. Surgeons and other operating room personnel were allowed to wear beards in the operating room in 94% of the hospitals and 87% of the hospitals routinely provided high-efficiency disposable masks. Nurses generally wore trouser-style scrub suits in the operating room in 54% of the hospitals. In 92% of the hospitals, operating room personnel who did not wear cover gowns when leaving the operating room were required to change scrub suits before reentering the operating room. Shoe coverings were required by only 53% of the operating rooms. Most hospitals (84%) reported using different housekeeping procedures for clean and dirty cases. Special mats, such as tacky or disinfectant mats, were used at the entrance to the operating room by 44% of the hospitals; most of these hospitals reported changing these mats at least once a day. Only 15% reported having a laminar, unidirectional, air flow unit in at least one operating room and only 4% used ultraviolet lights. Seventy-seven percent of the hospitals reported taking cultures of walls, floors, and table tops to monitor bacterial contamination in the operating room and 43% performed cultures of air samples obtained in the operating room. Nose or throat cultures were obtained routinely in 16% of the hospitals to monitor operating room personnel. Almost all (97%) operating room supervisors reported that some kinds of data were collected regarding the occurrence of postoperative wound infections.

Guidelines from the Centers for Disease Control for operating room antiseptic practices are shown in the table. The survey results confirm that practices that have not received scientific or budgetary scrutiny have become part of the perioperative routine in many hospitals. Almost 50% of the hospitals used nonrecommended tacky or disinfectant mats at operating room entrances and more than 75% were performing nonrecommended environmental cultures in the operating room at an estimated cost of $2,000 to $20,000 per year. When routine nose and throat cultures were taken of operating room personnel, an obvious pecking order was used, rather than a scientific rationale for culturing. Wide variations in practices also were observed. This nonuniformity may reflect such factors as a lack of a convincing sci-

RECOMMENDATIONS FOR SELECTED OPERATING ROOM PRACTICES FROM CENTERS FOR DISEASE CONTROL GUIDELINES FOR PREVENTING SURGICAL WOUND INFECTIONS, 1982

Practice	Recommendation*
Timing of preoperative shave	Unless hair near the operative site is so thick that it will interfere with the surgical procedure, it should not be removed. If hair removal is necessary, it should be done as near the time of operation as possible, preferably immediately before. Category II
Antiseptics for preparation of skin around incision sites	Tincture of chlorhexidine, iodophors and tincture of iodine are the recommended antiseptic products for preparing the operative site. Plain soap, alcohol or hexachlorophene are not recommended as single agents for operative site preparation, unless a patient's skin is sensitive to the recommended antiseptic products. Aqueous quaternary ammonium compounds should not be used. Category I
Surgeon's handscrubbing agent	Chlorhexidine, iodophors and hexachlorophene are the recommended active antimicrobial ingredients for the surgical handscrub. Aqueous quaternary ammonium compounds should not be used. Category I
Routine environmental culturing	Routine culturing of the operating room environment should not be done. Category I
Routine personnel culturing	Routine culturing of personnel using the operating room should not be done. Category I

*Strength of recommendations. Category I: strongly recommended. Measures in category I should be supported strongly by well-designed and controlled clinical studies that show effectiveness in reducing the risk of nosocomial infections or be viewed as useful by an overwhelming consensus of reasonable and informed experts in the field. Category-I recommendations should be applicable to most hospitals regardless of size, patient population, or endemic nosocomial infection rates and should be practical to implement. Category II: moderately recommended. These measures are supported by highly suggestive clinical studies or by definitive studies in institutions that might not be representative of other hospitals. Measures that have not been studied adequately but have a logical or strong theoretical rationale indicating that they might be quite effective are included in this category. Category-II recommendations should be practical to implement but should not be considered standard practice for every hospital.

(Courtesy of Garner, J. S., et al.: Surg. Gynecol. Obstet. 155:873–880, December 1982.)

entific basis for evaluating the relative efficacy of alternative practices, the strong influence of industry marketing, the individual preferences of surgeons and operating room supervisors, and the lack of completeness and agreement of statements from various scientific and professional organizations.

▶ [A practical and valuable article for those who are interested in cost-containment in our operating rooms, which should be all of us.—B.W.H.] ◀

6–3 **Acute Bupivacaine Toxicity as a Result of Venous Leakage Under Tourniquet Cuff During Bier Block.** Several cardiovascular complications may result from rapid absorption or unintentional intravascular injection of the newer local anesthetics. Per H. Rosenberg, Eija A. Kalso, Marjatta K. Tuominen, and Hans B. Lindén (Helsinki Univ.) observed a patient in whom bupivacaine intoxication developed soon after injection of the anesthetic; the tourniquet cuff appeared to be intact. Tourniquet phlebography of the arm was carried out in this patient and in 6 others to determine whether local anesthetic was entering the general circulation.

Man, 71, taking digoxin and pindolol for atrial fibrillation, was scheduled for excision of a Dupuytren's contracture. Diazepam and meperidine were given preoperatively. The arm was exsanguinated and the proximal cuff was inflated to 300 mm Hg before regional anesthesia was induced by injecting 80 ml of 0.25% bupivacaine into a wrist vein for about 30 seconds. Bradycardia and cyanosis developed after about 2 minutes and the patient lost consciousness; seizures occurred and arterial blood pressure was absent. Ventilation was controlled, thiopental and succinylcholine given and tracheal intubation carried out. Epinephrine, $CaCl_2$, and atropine were administered, as well as 270 mEq of sodium bicarbonate. The circulation was maintained with dopamine and nitroprusside infusions. Consciousness returned after 30 minutes, and the cardiovascular status returned to baseline. The arterial bupivacaine level 10 minutes after the toxic symptoms appeared was 1.8 µg/ml. The tourniquet was deflated after 55 minutes, and the bupivacaine level in the ipsilateral subclavian venous blood 1 minute later was 1.05 µg/ml.

When phlebography of the upper extremity was performed 2 days later, leakage of Urografin under the inflated cuff was observed in the first roentgenograms. In 2 of 3 other patients with measurable bupivacaine in the venous blood while a tourniquet cuff was inflated, contrast fluid was seen proximal to the cuff within 15 seconds of injection. Contrast leakage also occurred in 2 of 3 volunteers at a cuff pressure of 250 mm Hg.

Even a tourniquet cuff pressure that is 110 mm Hg above the preanesthetic systolic arterial pressure may not prevent venous leakage of anesthetic under the cuff. The risk may be greater in large patients, in whom venous compression by the cuff may be inadequate. Toxic reactions may be prevented by slow injection of anesthetic from a distal vein, restriction of the volume used, and close patient observation.

(6–3) Anesthesiology 58:95–98, January 1983.

6–4 **Study of Carcinogenic Effects of In Vitro Argon Laser Exposure of Fibroblasts. David B. Apfelberg, Benny Chadi, Morton R. Maser, and Harvey Lash** (Palo Alto, Calif.) present the first laboratory validation of the safety of the argon laser. Mouse fibroblasts were grown in tissue culture and exposed to varying energy levels of the argon laser for nine generations to determine their potential for malignant transformation. The cells were irradiated with both x-rays and the argon laser at up to 4 W × 40 seconds. The exposure of mouse fibroblasts of the BALB/3T3 strain to argon laser energy did not result in a significant transformation frequency compared with frequencies in x-irradiation or untreated controls.

Findings from this first study of argon laser energy in the induction of malignant change supports the lack of unusual malignant potential observed in long-term follow-up studies of large series of patients who had argon laser therapy. In addition, long-range histologic studies have suggested that laser wounds are permanent and stable, without the occurrence of ongoing changes likely to result in malignancy.

▶ [This is an important area of investigation which must be pursued vigorously. The malignant potential of therapeutic and diagnostic x-ray was not recognized for many years. Does the lack of malignant transformation in this experimental study prove that it won't occur in vivo in a different species or in a different cell type (i.e., epithelial)? Careful, long-term follow-up of patients treated with this modality must continue and be reported as data accumulate.—S.H.M.] ◀

6–5 **Medicinal Leech and Its Use in Plastic Surgery: A Possible Cause for Infection** is discussed by M. R. Whitlock, P. M. O'Hare, R. Sanders, and N. C. Morrow. The medicinal leech (Fig 6–1) feeds by sucking the blood of mammals and is remarkably adept at removing a considerable amount of blood from the host. Interest in the leech has increased recently; it has been used to treat periorbital hematoma, and in microsurgery to treat venous congestion. Studies were done on 9 medicinal leeches that had been fed on human blood 4 months previously. Heavy growth of a "pseudomonad" was observed

Fig 6–1.—Medicinal leech, characterized by anterior suckers and more powerful posterior suckers. (Courtesy of Whitlock, M. R., et al.: Br. J. Plast. Surg. 36:240–244, April 1983.)

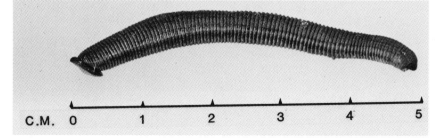

C.M. 0 1 2 3 4 5

(6–4) Plast. Reconstr. Surg. 71:92–97, January 1983.
(6–5) Br. J. Plast. Surg. 36:240–244, April 1983.

after 24 hours in all instances. The "pseudomonad" was cultured from both the anterior and posterior suckers of the leeches, and also from the gut. The organism was identified as *Aeromonas hydrophila*. It was resistant to penicillin, ampicillin, and streptomycin, but sensitive to tetracycline, erythromycin, and tobramycin.

Use of the live medicinal leech may carry a significant risk of infection by *A. hydrophila,* which is pathogenic in man. Pharmaceutical preparations are available that can achieve the same effect as use of the medicinal leech. For example, Hirudoid cream contains an organo-heparinoid of animal origin that is claimed to inhibit proteolysis and the spread of hyaluronidase, promoting edema absorption. Poor blood flow in a thumb replant improved markedly within 3 hours of application of the cream. Also, the cream appeared to have some local anesthetic effect. Topical glyceryl trinitrate has been suggested for use in patients with Raynaud's disease, and it may well improve circulation after microvascular procedures.

▶ [This is an article for those who wondered what became of the once ubiquitous leech or for those who might still entertain its clinical use.—R.J.H.] ◀

6-6 **Erectile Dysfunction: Progress in Evaluation and Treatment** is reviewed by Lee W. Vliet and Jon K. Meyer. Erectile failure occurring as often as once in every four attempts calls for investigation and treatment. Organic causes may be primary in as many as half the cases of sexual dysfunction. The most common medical cause is diabetes mellitus. In addition, drugs can affect any phase of the human sexual response cycle. Many psychological, social, cultural, environmental, and experiential factors have been implicated in the development of erectile dysfunction. Diagnostic evaluation may include, besides a biopsychosocial history and physical and mental status examinations, nocturnal penile tumescence monitoring, Doppler study of penile blood flow dynamics, and measurements of bulbocavernosus activity and reflex response latency time. Internal pudendal arteriography may be indicated rarely. Nocturnal monitoring is carried out in the course of 3 nights of polysomnographic study.

Patients with medical disorders are managed by appropriate treatment of these disorders. The efficacy of testosterone is not established, except possibly in patients undergoing renal dialysis and in those in whom the serum testosterone level is low. Patients with chiefly physiologic causes of erectile failure may benefit from brief supportive counseling. Several researchers consider men whose erectile dysfunction is organically based but not amenable to less conservative measures to be candidates for implantation of a penile prosthesis. A relatively rigid, fixed silicone rod prosthesis and an inflatable prosthesis are available. Success rates generally are in the 85%–95% range regardless of the type of prosthesis used.

Psychotherapy is indicated when erectile dysfunction is mainly due

(6–6) Johns Hopkins Med. J. 151:246–258, November 1982.

to psychosocial factors and when organic dysfunction is associated with significant psychological distress. The available approaches include behaviorally oriented sex therapy for couples, Kaplan's psychodynamically oriented sex therapy for couples, psychoanalysis and analytically oriented individual therapies, brief individual psychotherapy, behavior therapy, and biofeedback training.

▶ [We, as plastic surgeons, need to be aware of this problem and suggested treatment. The article should probably be read in its entirety.—R.O.B.] ◀

Subject Index

A

Abdominal flap (*see* Flap, abdominal)
Adhesive
  in dressing for skin graft donor site,
    219
  fibrin adhesive system and bone
    healing rate, 186
  fibrinogen tissue, in nerve
    anastomosis, 181
  tape, zinc, in keloids and hypertrophic
    scar, 170
Adrenal
  response to repeated hemorrhage, 170
Aged
  head and neck cancer of, 86
Alveolar
  cleft, bone graft in, 15
  process reconstruction, plate
    augmentation in, 119
Amniotic membranes
  in burn wound care, 141
Amputation
  of penis, reconstruction after, in
    children, 136
Anastomosis
  arteriovenous, in absent venous
    drainage in replantation, 125
  microarterial, sleeve technique in, 226
  microneurovascular, in muscle
    transplant, 256
  nerve, by fibrinogen tissue adhesive,
    181
Anergy
  after burns, 152
  in high-risk surgical patients, 165
Anesthesia, 240 ff.
  for flap transfer, 240
  for osteotomy, craniofacial, 53
  for plastic surgery, reconstructive and
    microvascular, 241
Angiodema
  vibratory, with carpal tunnel
    syndrome, 120
Angiogenesis
  study of, 181
Angioma
  of face and scalp, electrothrombosis in,
    59

Anomalies
  boutonniere, traumatic, repair, 124
  capillary-venous, fibrosing agent in,
    62
  craniofacial (*see* Craniofacial
    anomalies)
  dentofacial, mobilization of maxilla
    and mandible in, 43, 51
  "hook-nail," "antenna" procedure in,
    129
  stiff swan-neck, palmar arthroplasty
    in, 126
  thumb-in-palm, flexor policis longus
    abductor-plasty in, 122
Anophthalmic orbit
  temporalis muscle transposition into,
    70
Anoplasty
  in anal stricture, 95
"Antenna" procedure
  for "hook-nail" deformity, 129
Antibiotics
  prophylactic, in burns, 143
Antibody(ies)
  monoclonal, after burns, 153
Antidiuretic hormone syndrome
  inappropriate, in craniofacial surgery,
    44
Antigen(s)
  cell surface "activation," and
    cyclosporin A, 260
Antiserum
  to *Escherichia coli,* in bacteremia and
    shock, 154
Anus
  stricture, anoplasty in, 95
Apnea
  sleep, in mandibular hypoplasia, 20
Argon laser
  exposure of fibroblasts, carcinogenic
    effects, 269
Arterialized venous network
  in axial-pattern flap (in rat), 242
Arteriovenous anastomosis
  in absent venous drainage in
    replantation, 125
Arthritis
  rheumatoid, wrist arthroplasty in,
    97

273

Index to Authors